FOOD AND BEVERAGE CONSUMPTION AND HEALTH

PEANUTS

PRODUCTION, NUTRITIONAL CONTENT AND HEALTH IMPLICATIONS

FOOD AND BEVERAGE CONSUMPTION AND HEALTH

Additional books in this series can be found on Nova's website under the Series tab.

Additional e-books in this series can be found on Nova's website under the e-book tab.

FOOD AND BEVERAGE CONSUMPTION AND HEALTH

PEANUTS

PRODUCTION, NUTRITIONAL CONTENT AND HEALTH IMPLICATIONS

RICHARD W. COOK
EDITOR

nova publishers
New York

For permission to use material from this book please contact us:
Telephone 631-231-7269; Fax 631-231-8175
Web Site: http://www.novapublishers.com

Library of Congress Cataloging-in-Publication Data

ISBN: 978-1-63321-013-4

Library of Congress Control Number: 2014939496

Published by Nova Science Publishers, Inc. † New York

CONTENTS

PREFACE

Peanuts are among the most popular oilseeds in the world. When their price is considered, they present a competitive advantage in comparison to other nuts such as macadamia, walnuts, hazelnuts, Brazil nuts and cashew nuts. Peanuts are a good source of protein, and, depending on the cultivar, may render amounts of up to 80% unsaturated fatty acids. Tocopherol, also known as vitamin E, is found in high concentration in peanuts. Furthermore, peanuts are recognized by their high polyphenol contents. Phenolic compounds from several classes, namely, phenolic acids, flavonoids, and stilbenes have been identified in peanuts. Polyphenols have antimicrobial, anti-inflammatory, anticarcinogenic, and antioxidant properties. As such, peanuts may be beneficial to consumers through the prevention of chronic diseases. This book discusses information regarding the nutritional and possible nutraceutical potential of peanuts and peanut products, as well as the anticipated impacts of production of new cultivars and processing on their content. The value of peanuts as a source of nutrients and nutraceuticals, and its production is also highlighted and discussed.

Chapter 1 – Due to their health benefits, availability and affordability, peanuts (*Arachis hypogaea)* and peanut products are routinely found within the daily diet. Dietary inclusion of peanuts and peanut products has increased the number of sensitized consumers. In fact, for unknown health reasons, peanut allergy has doubled within the last decade. It has been hypothesized that a dramatic rise in sensitization to food allergens is consequential to reduced breastfeeding and intensive modern environmental sterilization practices that prevent early colonization of commensal microorganisms within the gut. It has been proposed that commensal microorganisms enhance mucosal immunity and reduce the likelihood of allergic reactions to food proteins. Allergenic food proteins are stable to digestion, are absorbed across the intestinal lumen and subsequently elicit an immunological response. Thus, the authors aimed to determine the digestibility of peanut proteins to digestive proteases found within the mammalian gut using an *in vitro* digestibility model with acid denaturation, pepsin and pancreatin. Their second research aim was to determine and identify protease stable peanut proteins and determine their immunoreactivity using reducing gel electrophoresis and immunoblotting analysis.

The authors determined that peanut proteins ≤ 14 kDa were pepsin stable and immunoreactive for up to 80 minutes with *in vitro* digestion, while peanut proteins of 50 kDa, 30 kDa, and 21 kDa pancreatin stable and immunoreactive for up to 80 minutes. The findings indicate that some peanut proteins and their fragments are pepsin- and pancreatin-stable, and immunoreactive for up to at least 1 hour. Thus a digestion model utilizing pepsin and pancreatin stability may provide more accurate safety assessment of allergenic versus non-allergic food proteins.

Lastly, the authors aimed to determine whether early probiotic administration may attenuate hypersensitivity reactions to peanut proteins using a validated murine model to parallel pediatric peanut allergy. Probiotic administration has been shown to attenuate Th2-biased cellular immunity and predisposition to food allergies. To test this hypothesis the authors provided *ad libitum* a probiotic-supplemented or control diet to lactating dams with suckling pups and weaned pups until 10 weeks of age. Weaned mice were sensitized/challenged with peanut extract, saline or adjuvant at 6, 8 and 10 weeks of age. At 3, 6, 8 and 10 weeks, fecal samples were collected for microbial analysis, while blood samples were analyzed for total plasma IgE levels. At termination, splenic T lymphocyte population subtypes were determined using FACS analysis and Th1/Th2/Th17 gene expression by PCR array. Mice given the probiotic supplemented diet had significantly enhanced *Lactobacillus acidophilus* fecal counts compared to controls at 3, 6, 8 and 10 weeks. Moreover, mice fed the probiotic supplemented diet had enhanced splenic naturally occurring T regulatory cell populations, and reduced splenic gene expression of allergic mediator IL-13 compared to controls. These results provide evidence that early probiotic supplementation may provide host protection to hypersensitivity reactions to food allergens by attenuating food allergen inflammatory responses.

Chapter 2 – Peanut skins are low cost feedstock generated by the industrial peanut blanching process. However, its high antioxidant phytochemical constituents still lack effective industrial application of their extractable compounds. For efficient recovery of these target compounds, the present work combined antioxidant assays and statistical tools to achieve its goals. Response surface methodology (RSM) was used to fit predictive mathematical models. By matching all predicted responses a global standardized response was generated, which found a high positive correlation between observed and predicted responses (r = 0.9921, $p < 0.01$). Thus, Tukey's multiple test ($p < 0.05$) was carried out to define the best extraction conditions (2.5% peanut skin extracted with 50.0% ethanol over 20 min). Under optimized conditions, total phenolic content (TPC) and ferric reducing antioxidant power (FRAP) were 91.87 mg GAE/g and 135.07 mmol Fe^{2+}/g of peanut skins, respectively. Trolox equivalent antioxidant capacity (TEAC) values for DPPH, ABTS, and ORAC assays were 585.61, 2093.64 and 1206.87 μmol/g of peanut skins, respectively. It was possible to reduce the time of extraction and the solvent concentration as compared to the literature. Through RSM and further statistical analysis it was possible set extraction conditions at which the antioxidant extracts overlapped the reaction mechanism of FRAP, DPPH, ABTS, and ORAC assays.

Chapter 3 – In-shell peanuts were submitted to gamma irradiation (2.5, 5.0, 7.5 and 10.0 kGy) and evaluated on their microbiological safety. Yeasts and molds were detected in non-irradiated samples but not in irradiated ones. 5.0 kGy was suitable in reducing the total coliform count by two log cycles, thus 5.0 kGy was chosen to be the highest dose for further analyses. Peroxide value and hexanal content significantly increased at 5.0 and 2.5 kGy, respectively. Taste was the only sensory attribute statistically different and this was noticed only at 5.0 kGy. However, there was no rejection in this sample. The purchase intent was not affected by any gamma irradiation dose. 2.5 kGy can be used to improve microbiological safety but better results are reached with 5.0 kGy. To the best of the authors' knowledge there is no other publication that addresses the microbiological safety, oxidation status and their relation on sensory results of in-shell gamma irradiated peanuts. Also, it is not common to achieve sensory acceptance of nuts with doses as high as 5.0 kGy, therefore this report will be helpful for the peanut industry.

Chapter 4 – Peanuts are among the most popular oilseeds in the world. When their price is considered, they present a competitive advantage in comparison to other nuts such as macadamia, walnuts, hazelnuts, Brazil nuts and cashew nuts. Peanuts are a good source of protein, and, depending on the cultivar, may render amounts of up to 80% unsaturated fatty acids. Tocopherol, also known as vitamin E, is found in high concentration in peanuts. Furthermore, peanuts are recognized by their high polyphenol contents. Phenolic compounds from several classes, namely, phenolic acids, flavonoids, and stilbenes have been identified in peanuts. Polyphenols have antimicrobial, anti-inflammatory, anticarcinogenic, and antioxidant properties. As such, peanuts may be beneficial to consumers through the prevention of chronic diseases. This review summarizes information regarding the nutritional and possible nutraceutical potential of peanuts and peanut products, as well as the anticipated impacts of production of new cultivars and processing on their content. The value of peanuts as a source of nutrients and nutraceuticals is also highlighted and discussed.

Chapter 5 – Peanuts, as a groundnut, are in constant contact with soil population of aflatoxigenic fungi from section *Flavi*, thus they may be infected by *A. flavus* before harvesting. Aflatoxins are recognized as carcinogens produced mostly by *A. flavus* and *A. parasiticus*. As such, their concentrations in peanuts and peanut products are limited to 20 μg/kg in Brazil or less in other countries. In the present study, a commercial product containing a non-toxigenic strain of *A. flavus* was evaluated as a biological control to avoid production of aflatoxin B1 (AFB1). The competitive effect of *A. flavus* NRRL 21882 (Afla-guard®) for the reduction of AFB1 contamination was evaluated under field conditions in peanuts of Valencia type (cv. IAC Tatu ST) at a low rainfall condition. Planting and crop management for aerial pest and disease control followed Brazilian recommended practices. The field was irrigated to induce germination and plant growth until 72 days after planting; after which, irrigation was suppressed to impose drought stress until harvesting for 34 days. The product containing *A. flavus* NRRL 21882 was applied 60 days after planting (22.4 kg/ha). Peanuts from four large plots (two treated and two devoid of the product) were evaluated for AFB1 contamination. A total of 20 samples per plot was evaluated. Pod samples were mechanically shelled and two subsamples were taken: subsample A (8 – 10 kg) denominated field kernel sample (FK), whose kernels were not segregated; subsample B (2 kg) denominated edible grade kernel (EK), comprising hand-picked kernels, free of damages and commercially graded. Peanuts grown in soil devoid of the product containing *A. flavus* NRRL 21882 were contaminated by AFB1 in concentrations of 1444 and 41 μg/kg in FK and EK, respectively. On the other hand, peanuts grown in soil treated with the product contained AFB1 in concentrations of 248 and 5.6 μg/kg in FK and EK, respectively. In both FK and EK, a highly significant ($p < 0.0001$) reduction of AFB1 concentration (84 and 83%, respectively) was observed for peanuts grown in soil with the product containing non-toxigenic strains of *A. flavus*.

Chapter 6 – Seed crops with high oleate content proved to have better keeping quality. High oleate diet helps to lower the harmful low density lipoprotein cholesterol level. Other health benefits of high oleate peanut include, increased sensitivity to insulin, amelioration in some inflammatory diseases, and preventive effects on tumorigenesis. In addition, high oleate peanut genotypes are considered more suitable for biodiesel production than their normal oleate counterparts. Significant progress in the genetic improvement of the cultivated peanut for high oleate has been made since the identification of the natural mutant F435 in University of Florida. The present chapter reviews recent technical advances in peanut fatty acid determination, genetics of oleate content, molecular basis of the high oleate phenotype, factors affecting oleate content, and peanut germplasm enhancement in high oleate content.

In: Peanuts
Editor: Richard W. Cook

ISBN: 978-1-63321-013-4

Chapter 1

DETERMINATION OF PEANUT DIGESTIBILITY AND ALLERGENICITY USING *IN VITRO* AND *IN VIVO* EXPERIMENTAL MODELS

Ondulla T. Toomer*[*], *Martine Ferguson, Andrew Do, Marion Pereira and Kristina Williams
U.S. Food and Drug Administration, Laurel, Maryland, US

ABSTRACT

Due to their health benefits, availability and affordability, peanuts (*Arachis hypogaea)* and peanut products are routinely found within the daily diet. Dietary inclusion of peanuts and peanut products has increased the number of sensitized consumers. In fact, for unknown health reasons, peanut allergy has doubled within the last decade. It has been hypothesized that a dramatic rise in sensitization to food allergens is consequential to reduced breastfeeding and intensive modern environmental sterilization practices that prevent early colonization of commensal microorganisms within the gut. It has been proposed that

* Please address correspondence to: Ondulla Toomer, PhD, Immunobiology Branch, Division of Virulence Assessment, Office of Applied Research and Safety Assessment, Center for Food Safety and Applied, United States Department of Food and Drug Administration, 8301 Muirkirk Road, MOD-1, Room 2007, Laurel, MD 20708. Office 402.240-3430; Fax 301.210.4769. Email address: Ondulla.Toomer@fda.hhs.gov.

commensal microorganisms enhance mucosal immunity and reduce the likelihood of allergic reactions to food proteins. Allergenic food proteins are stable to digestion, are absorbed across the intestinal lumen and subsequently elicit an immunological response. Thus, we aimed to determine the digestibility of peanut proteins to digestive proteases found within the mammalian gut using an *in vitro* digestibility model with acid denaturation, pepsin and pancreatin. Our second research aim was to determine and identify protease stable peanut proteins and determine their immunoreactivity using reducing gel electrophoresis and immunoblotting analysis. We determined that peanut proteins ≤ 14 kDa were pepsin stable and immunoreactive for up to 80 minutes with *in vitro* digestion, while peanut proteins of 50 kDa, 30 kDa, and 21 kDa pancreatin stable and immunoreactive for up to 80 minutes. The findings indicate that some peanut proteins and their fragments are pepsin- and pancreatin-stable, and immunoreactive for up to at least 1 hour. Thus a digestion model utilizing pepsin and pancreatin stability may provide more accurate safety assessment of allergenic versus non-allergic food proteins.

Lastly, we aimed to determine whether early probiotic administration may attenuate hypersensitivity reactions to peanut proteins using a validated murine model to parallel pediatric peanut allergy. Probiotic administration has been shown to attenuate Th2-biased cellular immunity and predisposition to food allergies. To test this hypothesis we provided *ad libitum* a probiotic-supplemented or control diet to lactating dams with suckling pups and weaned pups until 10 weeks of age. Weaned mice were sensitized/challenged with peanut extract, saline or adjuvant at 6, 8 and 10 weeks of age. At 3, 6, 8 and 10 weeks, fecal samples were collected for microbial analysis, while blood samples were analyzed for total plasma IgE levels. At termination, splenic T lymphocyte population subtypes were determined using FACS analysis and Th1/Th2/Th17 gene expression by PCR array. Mice given the probiotic supplemented diet had significantly enhanced *Lactobacillus acidophilus* fecal counts compared to controls at 3, 6, 8 and 10 weeks. Moreover, mice fed the probiotic supplemented diet had enhanced splenic naturally occurring T regulatory cell populations, and reduced splenic gene expression of allergic mediator IL-13 compared to controls. These results provide evidence that early probiotic supplementation may provide host protection to hypersensitivity reactions to food allergens by attenuating food allergen inflammatory responses.

INTRODUCTION

Peanuts (*Arachis hypogaea*), also known as ground nuts are technically legumes, more closely related to chickpeas and soybeans than to almonds, walnuts or other tree nuts. Because peanuts are legumes, they are more protein rich and their protein content is more nutritionally complete than other tree nuts (Ros, 2010). Peanuts and tree nuts are a great vegetarian source of protein, fiber and healthy fats, and dietary inclusion has been linked to reduced heart disease (Jones et al., 2014), certain types of cancers (Gonzalez and Salas-Salvadó, 2006) and improved weight management (Moreno et al., 2013). Peanuts are rich in the antioxidant resveratrol, having heart-protective and cancer preventive qualities (Sales and Resurreccion, 2014); with boiled peanuts having 10-fold greater resveratrol content in comparison to roasted peanuts or peanut butter (Rudolf, 2003). Peanuts are also rich in phytoesterols, known to promote healthy cholesterol levels, important to heart disease prevention (Bouchenak and Lamri-Senhadji, 2013). Consequently, due to the many health benefits of peanuts, wide availability and affordability, peanuts and peanut products are widely consumed and found with the daily diet worldwide.

For reasons not specifically known, peanut allergy has increased during recent decades and now affects 1% to 2% of young children (Boyce et al., 2010). However, the scientific community hypothesizes that the increased incidence of pediatric peanut allergy may be associated with increased sterilization and reduced breastfeeding within industrialized countries leading to reduced childhood immunity and increased risk for the development of hypersensitivity reactions to food proteins. A large fraction of all food-induced anaphylactic reactions and lethal food-allergic responses are caused by peanuts (Sampson, 2004), with the a typical peanut dose causing allergic reactions in the range of 100-1000mg, and in some sensitive patients with very low doses of approximately 100ug of peanut protein eliciting adverse reactions (Wensing et al., 2002). Unlike other food allergies, peanut allergy is rarely outgrown after childhood and often has lifelong persistence (Carr, 2005) and with no treatment options and/or cure, dietary avoidance is the only option for the peanut-sensitive population, an approach that is complicated by the wide-spread use of peanut products as a food ingredient, and the cross contamination of peanut products in a wide variety of processed and packaged foods.

Studies have shown that establishment of food allergy occurs early in life and in genetically predisposed individuals food allergen sensitization occurs with exposure to food allergens in the gut, causing IgE-mediated food allergic responses (Eigenmann et al., 1998). Immunological responses of the gut to food proteins have been shown to be greatly influenced by gut microbiota, with children who develop food allergies within the first two years of life having fewer *Bifodobacteria* and *Enterococci* within the gut and more *Staphylococcus aureus* and *Clostridium*, in comparison to non-allergic infants and toddlers (Bjorksten et al., 2001). Studies have shown that prenatal oral *Lactobacillus* GG supplementation reduced allergy in infants/toddlers (birth to two years of age) born to mothers genetically predisposed to allergy (Kalliomaki et al., 2001), suggesting that probiotic microorganisms may play a role in early development of oral tolerance to food antigens and balance type 1 T helper cell (Th1)/type 2 T helper cell function during postnatal development.

Thus our aim was to identify the immunological mechanisms of sensitization to peanut proteins and how early administration of probiotic microorganisms may attenuate hypersensitivity immunological responses to peanut proteins using a validated murine model for food allergy to parallel pediatric peanut food allergy. To test this hypothesis we provided *ad libitum* a probiotic-supplemented or control diet to lactating dams and/or mouse pups for 10 weeks and orally sensitized/challenged weaned mice with peanut protein extracts.

The major peanut allergens Ara h 1, Ara h 2, and Ara h 3 have been well characterized, cloned, and sequenced with their IgE-binding and T-cell epitopes identified (Burks et al., 1998; Schmidt et al., 2010). Ara h 1, a ~64 kDa glycoprotein, is recognized by more than 95% of peanut allergic patients, with Ara h 1 being initially identified by IgE immunoblot analysis with pooled serum from peanut allergic patients (Burks et al., 1998). Ara h 1 occurs naturally in trimeric form of approximately 185 kDa via non-covalent interactions (Koppelman et al., 2010). Ara h 2 migrates as a doublet at approximately 20 kDa, consisting of two isoforms (de Jong et al., 1998). Ara h 3 is a post-translationally proteolytically processed protein consisting of 42-45 kDa and 25 kDa subunits, with less prominent bands at 12-18 kDa (de Jong et al., 1998).

Current *in vitro* and *in vivo* studies have demonstrated that purified Ara h 2 triggers the release of histamine from basophils containing peanut specific IgE, and reactivity in skin prick test with peanut allergic individuals was far more pronounced for Ara h 2 compared to Ara h 1 (Koppelman et al., 2010). Ara h 6 (15 kDa) IgE binding and histamine release from basophils has been found to be very similar to Ara h 2 activity (Koppelman et al., 2005). The percentage of patients recognizing Ara h 3 is much lower than that of patients recognizing Ara h 1 and Ara h 2, and the ability of Ara h 3 to trigger histamine release is much lower than Ara h 2 and Ara h6, but in the range of Ara h 1 (Koppelman et al., 2004). These differences in allergenicity and immunoreactivity have been attributed to the random differences in human subjects and study populations (Koppelman et al., 2004, 2005, 2010).

While peanut allergens Ara h 1, 2, 3, 4, 5, 6, 7, 8, 9, and Ara h 10 have been well identified and characterized, a paucity of studies have closely examined the stability of the Ara h proteins to the digestive enzymes of the mammalian gut and subsequently, the immunoreactivity of these allergens. Peanut allergen Ara h 2, recognized by more than 90% of peanut-allergic patients, is resistant to pepsin, trypsin, and chymotrypsin cleavage due to the protection provided by the secondary and tertiary protein structure (Sen et al., 2002). Current models of digestibility utilize pepsin stability for safety assessment of allergenic food proteins. However, dietary protein digestion *in vivo* requires acid denaturation and protease cleavage by pepsin, trypsin, and/or chymotrypsin. Therefore, the ability of this approach to identify food protein stability in the mammalian gut may be limited. We aimed to determine the temporal stability and immunoreactivity of peanut proteins using simulated physiologic gastric and intestinal digestive conditions *in vitro* to more accurately identify potential allergenic peanut proteins that are stable to *in vivo* digestion within the gut.

MATERIALS AND METHODS

Materials-*In Vitro* Digestibility

Pre-packaged peanuts were purchased from local grocery stores. Peanuts were ground with a mortar and pestle and 100 g of the ground mixture nut was dissolved in hexane and filtered using Whatman paper. This process was repeated three times and the sample filtrate was collected and allowed to air dry overnight. Several different 100g samples were dissolved in hexane and filtered once using a glass funnel lined with Whatman paper, positioned over a glass beaker. The collected filtrate from each different 100g sample was pooled and stored at -20°C.

Total proteins were extracted from defatted flour (flour to buffer ratio 1:10 w/v) in 20 mM Tris-HCL pH 8.1 buffer supplemented with 1% HALT protease inhibitor (Thermo Scientific, Rockford, IL, USA). Samples were vortexed and centrifuged for 10 min at 4ºC and the supernatants were used for analysis. Total soluble protein was determined using a BCA Protein Assay Kit purchased from Thermo Scientific. Protein extracts were aliquoted and stored at -20ºC.

Pepsin, (2546 U/mg activity) and pancreatin (26296 U/mg activity) were purchased from Sigma Chemical Company (St. Louis, MO, USA) in the highest available purity. The gels and running buffer for sodium dodecyl sulfate-polyacrylamide gel electrophoresis (SDS-PAGE) Mini-PROTEAN TGX were purchased from Bio-Rad (Hercules, CA, USA) and reducing sample buffer was purchased from Thermo Scientific. Western blots were performed using the Trans-Blot Turbo Mini System and Nitrocellulose Transfer Packs purchased from Bio-Rad. Immunoreactive proteins were detected using rabbit anti-peanut primary antibodies raised in-house, donkey anti-rabbit IgG- horseradish peroxidase (HRP) secondary antibodies from Santa Cruz Biotechnology (Santa Cruz, CA, USA), and chromogenic substrates chloronaphthol and diaminobenzidine (CN/DAB) from ThermoScientific. Allergenic proteins were detected using peanut-specific primary antibodies collected from allergic and non-allergic human donors purchased commercially from Plasma Lab International (Everett, WA, USA), goat anti-human IgE- HRP secondary antibodies from KPL (Gaithersburg, MD, USA), and CN/DAB from ThermoScientific.

Simulated Gastric Fluid Digestion Assay

The protocols of Astwood et al. (1996) were followed with some modifications. Simulated gastric fluid (SGF) was prepared as described in the United States Pharmacopeia (2006): 1 mg/mL solution comprised 2.546 U pepsin/μL in 0.03 mol/L NaCL (pH 1.2). SGF was aliquoted (500 μL) to a 5.0-mL glass tube for each time interval (0, 0.5, 5, 15, 30, 60, 80 and minutes) and incubated in a 37°C water bath for 10 min. Test protein (1600 μg) was added to each tube to begin the temporal SGF digestion assay, and 75 μL of 1 N NaOH was added to each vial to stop the reaction. SGF digestive products were subsequently stored at -20°C until analyzed.

Simulated Intestinal Fluid Digestion Assay

Simulated intestinal fluid (SIF) was prepared as described in the United States Pharmacopeia (2006): 10 mg/mL pancreatin (chymotrypsin, trypsin, amylase, and lipase) in 0.05 mol/L KH2PO4, (pH 7.5) containing 26,296 U pancreatin/mL12. SIF was aliquoted (500 μL) to a 5.0-mL glass tube for each time interval (0, 0.5, 5, 15, 30, 60, and 80 minutes) and incubated in a 37°C water bath for 10 min. Test protein (1600 μg) was added to each tube to begin the temporal SIF digestion assay at an 8:1 ratio. The reaction was immediately stopped by placing each tube in a boiling water bath for 10 min. All digestive products were subsequently stored at -20°C until analyzed.

Production of Allergen-specific Rabbit Antibodies

Rabbit antibodies were prepared by subcutaneous inoculation of adult New Zealand White rabbits (>2.0 kg). Prepared antigens were peanut proteins extracted from defatted peanut flour using phosphate-buffered saline, pH 8. Antigens were dialyzed overnight against normal saline, and suspended to a final concentration of 1.0 mg/ml. One hundred micrograms of antigen was injected into multiple sites on the shaved back of the rabbit. The initial injection was antigen suspended 1:1 in normal saline: Complete Freund's adjuvant. Rabbits were inoculated 2-3 weeks later with antigen suspended 1:1 in normal saline: Incomplete Freund's adjuvant. Two bsequent injections consisted of 100 ug protein suspended in normal saline. For blood collection, animals were anesthetized with an intramuscular injection of ketamine/xylazine/acepromazine. Rabbits were euthanized using intravenous injection of potassium chloride. All procedures were approved by the Institutional Animal Care and Use Committee (IACUC) and rabbits were housed in an AAALAC (Association for Assessment and Accreditation of Laboratory Animal Care) accredited facility.

SDS-PAGE Analysis and Immunoblotting

Digested or undigested test proteins (40 μg for immunoblots with rabbit primary antibodies or 80 μg for immunoblots with human primary antibodies) were loaded per lane on either a 4-20% or 10% polyacrylamide Tris-glycine gel and electrophoretically separated under constant voltage with Tris/Glycine/SDS buffer according to the manufacturer's instructions. Proteins were visualized by Coomassie Brilliant Blue staining and digitally imaged. To detect allergen specific IgE-binding peptides, immunoblot analysis was performed using allergen-specific antibodies generated in rabbits in-house. SDS-PAGE resolved proteins were transferred to nitrocellulose membranes electrophoretically according to the manufacturer's instructions. The membranes were then washed three times in Tris-buffered saline with 0.1%

Tween (TBST) and subsequently blocked in 5% non-fat dry milk (NFDM) in TBST for 2 h at room temperature. The membranes were incubated at 4ºC overnight in 1:1000 dilution of rabbit allergen-specific antibody in 5% NFDM in TBST or 1:2 dilution of human plasma from allergic donors in 5% NFDM in TBST. The membranes were washed three times in TBST and incubated in secondary antibodies (donkey anti-rabbit IgG-HRP dilution 1:1000 in 5% NFDM in TBST or goat anti-human IgE-HRP 1:10 dilution in 5% NFDM in TBST) at room temperature for 1 h. Bio-detection was determined utilizing chromogenic peroxidase substrate CN/DAB-based detection of HRP activity.

Materials-*In Vivo* Mouse Model

Mice and Reagents

We hypothesize that maternal (nursing dams) and postnatal (3 to 10 weeks of postnatal age) dietary probiotic supplementation will attenuate Th2-biased phenotype, thereby providing a balanced Th1/Th2 cytokine profile and provide host protection against food allergy development. To test this hypothesis, two day old C3H/HeJ mice pups and lactating dams were purchased from Jackson Laboratory (Bar Harbor, ME) and housed in an AAALAC-accredited facility at the Center for Food Safety and Applied Nutrition, Module-1 in Laurel, Maryland. Lactating dams and suckling pups were provided bi-weekly sterile water and fed either Purina Mouse Lab Diet 5015(Control diet) or Purina Mouse Lab Diet 5015 supplemented with Primalac 454 Feed Grade Microbials (Star-Labs/Forage Research) at 0.1% inclusion (Probiotic diet) *ad libitum* from week 1 to week 6 prior to peanut sensitization. Primalac 454 Feed Grade Microbials (Star-Labs/Forage Research) freeze-dried probiotic, was supplemented within the Purina Certified Mouse Diet 5015 prior to the pelleting at an inclusion of 0.05714 grams of Primalac 454 feed grade microbials per gram of Certified Mouse Diet 5015. The probiotic supplemented diet was formulated such that each mouse received 2.0 X 10^9 *Lactobacillus acidophilus* microorganisms per week based upon the average daily intake for rodents (National Research Council, Nutrient Requirements for the Mouse, 1995). This level of supplementation was based upon previous reports demonstrating immuno-enhancing effects of weekly *Lactobacillus acidophilus* supplementation with 1.0 X 10^9 microorganisms using a murine model (Chen et al., 2005, Foye et al., 2012). Primalac 454 Feed Grade Microbials utilized contained a proprietary blend of *Lactobacillus acidophilus, Lactobacillus casei, Bifido bacterium bifidium*, and *Enterococcus faecium*, (primarily *Lactobacillus acidophilus* and *Lactobacillus casei*). Peanut extract was purchased from Greer Source Materials (Lenoir, North Carolina). Cholera toxin B (CT) utilized as an adjuvant was purchased from List Biological Laboratories (Campbell, California).

In Vivo-Experimental Design

Mouse pups were housed with approximately 5 to 10 suckling pups per lactating dam from 2 to 21 days of postnatal age. Three independent *in vivo* experiments were conducted in which 2 day old suckling pups were divided into 5 treatment groups (Experimental Design), with each treatment group containing 10 to 15 suckling pups each: Control Diet-PBS challenge, Probiotic Diet-PBS challenge, Control Diet-Peanut + CT challenge, Probiotic Diet-Peanut+ CT challenge, Control Diet-CT challenge. Lactating dams with suckling pups were fed experimental diets from postnatal day 2 of age until weaning. Mouse pups were weaned at 3 weeks of age and individually caged and fed aforementioned experimental diets. At 6 weeks of age, mice in treatment groups Control Diet-Peanut + CT and Probiotic Diet-Peanut + CT were orally sensitized with 1 mg of Peanut extract + 10μg CT in 0.2mL of sterile phosphate buffered saline (PBS). Alternatively, mice of treatment groups Control Diet-PBS and Probiotic Diet-PBS were orally administered 0.2mL of sterile PBS, while mice of treatment group Control Diet-CT were orally administered 10μg of CT in 0.2 mL of sterile PBS.

At 8 weeks of age, mice were orally challenged with 2 mg of peanut extract + 10μg of CT in 0.2mL of sterile PBS. Negative and positive controls were orally administered 0.2mL of sterile PBS (treatment group Control Diet-PBS) or 0.2mL of sterile PBS consisting 10μg of CT (treatment group Control Diet-CT), respectively. After allergen, PBS or CT challenge, mice were observed twice daily for allergic symptoms. At 10 weeks of age, mice were orally challenged with 2 mg of peanut extract + 10μg of CT in 0.2mL of sterile PBS, 0.2mL of sterile PBS (treatment group Control Diet-PBS) or 0.2mL of sterile PBS containing 10μg of CT (treatment group Control Diet-CT). Four hours after oral challenge, mice were sacrificed and tissues collected for immunological analysis. All animal experiments were approved by the Institutional Animal Care and Use Committee.

Experimental Design

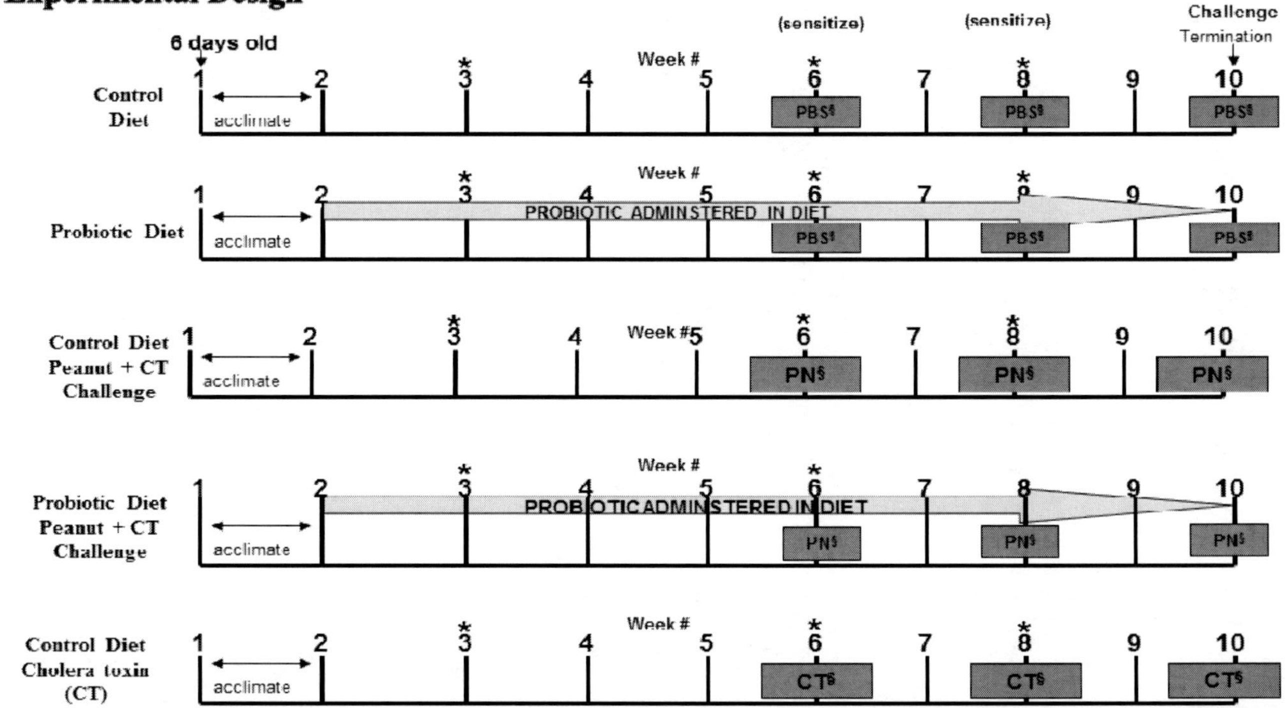

Experimental Design. *submandibular blood samples taken; PN–Peanut extract, PBS–phosphate buffered saline, CT–cholera toxin B. Mice were sensitized at 6 and 8 weeks of age with PBS alone, Peanut extract + CT, or CT alone. At 10 weeks of age, mice were orally challenged with PBS alone, Peanut extract +CT, or CT alone and euthanized 4 hours post oral challenge. CT was utilized as an adjuvant in PN challenge.

Fluorescence Activated Cell Sorter (FACS) Analysis

Surface Staining Procedures

Splenocytes were harvested by pressing through a nylon mesh at 10 weeks of age. Red blood cells were lysed using Red Blood Cell Lysis Buffer (Promega, Madison, Wisconsin). Lymphocyte populations were identified using PE Rat Anti-mouse CD8a, FITC Rat Anti-mouse CD4, PE Hamster Anti-mouse CD3e, APC Rat Anti-mouse CD25 and PE Rat anti-mouse FoxP3 antibodies (BD Pharmingen) and respective PE, FITC, and APC labeled isotype controls. The stained samples were analyzed on a BD Biosciences FACScan with Cell Quest software. Dead cells and debris were excluded from analysis by gates set on forward and side angle light scatter.

Intracellular Staining Procedures

Cell suspensions were activated for 3 hours with Leukocyte Activation Cocktail with BD Golgi Plug (BD Pharmingen). BD Pharmingen Stain Buffer (FBS) was used to wash cells, followed by Mouse BD Fc Block purified anti-mouse CD16/CD32 mAb to block cells from binding to non-specific antigens. Lymphocyte populations were identified using APC Rat anti-mouse $CD4^+$ and PE-Cy7 Rat anti-mouse $CD25^+$ labeled antibodies. PE Rat anti-mouse $FoxP3^+$ labeled antibody was used for intracellular staining. (BD Pharmingen, Franklin Lakes, New Jersey). Fixation and permeabilization procedures were followed as recommended by BD Pharmingen Mouse FoxP3 Fixation/ Permeabilization Buffer Set. Approximately 60,000 events were collected. A sample containing unstained cells and single stained cell samples for PE CD4, APC $CD4^+$ and PE-Cy7 $CD25^+$ respectively, were used to establish the compensation for the analysis. Dead cells and debris were excluded from analysis by gates set on forward and side angle light scatter. Results from events within the $CD4^+$ subpopulation gate were expressed as percentages of $CD25^+FoxP3^+$ from $CD4^+$ parent events and analyzed using BD FACSDiva software.

Th1/Th2/Th17 Gene Expression Array

Total RNA was isolated from fresh spleen sections using manufacturer's instructions described for RNeasy Mini Kit (Qiagen). A column containing DNase I digest was utilized to digest and remove contaminating genomic DNA before elution of total RNA. The concentration and A260/A280 ratio of total RNA were determined using NanoDrop 2000 (Thermo Scientific) and subsequently stored at −80°C. First strand cDNA was generated per manufacturer's instructions using RT² First Strand Kit (Qiagen) using 1.0μg of total RNA. Th1 and Th2 Pathway-Focused Gene Expression profiling was conducted using a 96 well format per manufacturer's instructions and analysis for RT² Profiler™ PCR Array Mouse Th1 & Th2 Responses with diluted first strand cDNA (SA Biosciences/Qiagen).

Statistical Analysis

All results were expressed as the mean ± standard error of the mean and each animal served as an experimental unit for statistical analysis by ANOVA in SAS (version 9.4, 2013). Treatment variables that were significantly different were assigned differing subscripts at the $p<0.05$ significance level. PCR Array statistical analysis was conducted using manufacturer's software available at: http://pcrdataanalysis.sabiosciences.com/pcr/arrayanalysis.php. Fold regulation was calculated using the ΔΔCt method: fold change = $2^{(-\Delta\Delta Ct),}$ where ΔΔCt = [(ΔCt) experimental group] [(ΔCt) control group]. The ΔCt for each tissue-treatment combination was calculated using: ΔCt = (average Ct gene of interest − average Ct endogenous housekeeping gene). Average Ct values represent the mean Ct values of data pooled for three independent *in vivo* experiments. The p values were calculated based on a Student's t-test of the replicate $2^{(-\text{Delta Ct})}$ values for each gene in the control group and treatment groups, at $p \leq 0.05$ significance level.

Results

In Vitro Peanut Digestibility and Immunoreactivity

Upon reducing SDS-PAGE analysis (4-20% SDS-PAGE), the control non-digested peanut proteins resolved as protein bands of molecular weights of 75, 65, 39, 35, 30, 23, 14, and 12 kDa. Protein bands at 65, 35, and 23 kDa are prominent (Figure 1A), which parallels findings by Koppelman et al.' (2010). Protein bands of 23, 30, and 65 kDa were pepsin-stable for 0 to 30 min of digestion, and absent in the 60- and 80-min pepsin-digested samples, with decreasing visibility of the banding pattern indicative of temporal pepsin digestion (Figure 1A). Of the pepsin-digested peanut preparations (0 to 80 minutes), protein bands of 35-37 kDa (braced area) are resolved and may also correlate with the known molecular weight of porcine pepsin (Sigma Chemical Company) of approximately 34-36 kDa (Figure 1A). Peanut protein bands of 14 and 12 kDa were pepsin stable up to 0.5 minutes of *in vitro* digestion, while resolved protein bands less than 12 kDa appear in the 5 to 60 minute pepsin digested samples suggesting that these are peptide fragments products of pepsin digestion (Figure 1A).

With immunoblotting procedures, protein bands 75, 65, 54, 35, 17, and 14 kDa of the control non-digested peanut proteins were reactive to rabbit anti-peanut IgG (Figure 1B). Protein band of 75 kDa was pepsin stable and immunoreactive with rabbit anti-peanut IgG from 0 to 15 minutes of *in vitro* digestion, while protein bands ≤ 14 kDa (bracketed area) were pepsin stable and immunoreactive with rabbit anti-peanut IgG for up to 80 minutes of *in vitro* digestion (Figure 1B).

Vieths et al., (1999) demonstrated that substantial proteolytic digestion with pepsin did not alter the IgE-binding properties of many peanut allergens[36]. In our study, peanut protein bands in the control non-digested sample predominately between 75 to 50 kDa were immunoreactive to antibodies in the plasma of a peanut allergic donor patient (Figure 1C) and no reactivity after 0, 30, and 80 minutes of *in vitro* pepsin digestion (Figure 1C).

Electrophoretically-separated (10% SDS-PAGE) pancreatin-digested peanut proteins bands of 70-118 kDa (bracket), 50 kDa (black circle), and 23-27 kDa (brace) were stable from 0 to 80 min of digestion *in vitro* under simulated physiologic conditions (Figure 2A). While porcine pancreatin amylase (51-54 kDa), trypsin (≈24 kDa) and carboxypeptidase (≈34 kDa) are present within the pancreatin-digested peanut samples resolved with electrophoresis (0 to 80 minutes), only digestive stable peanut proteins of 50 kDa, 30 kDa, and 21 kDa (asterick) were immunoreactive to rabbit peanut IgG (Figure 2B). Peanut protein bands in the control non-digested sample between 75to 50 kDa were immunoreactive to antibodies in the plasma of peanut allergic donor patient (Figures 1C and 2C), with immunoreactive protein bands of 75 kDa and 43 kDa present in the 0 minute, 30 minute, and 80 minute pancreatin digested samples (Figure 2C), suggesting that these proteins are pancreatin-stable and potentially allergenic. Also, as a negative control immunoblot, control non-digested and digested (pepsin, pancreatin) peanut proteins were non-reactive to IgE antibodies in the plasma of a non-allergic (peanut and tree nut) donor patient or conjugated secondary antibodies, with immunoblot analysis of the (data not shown).

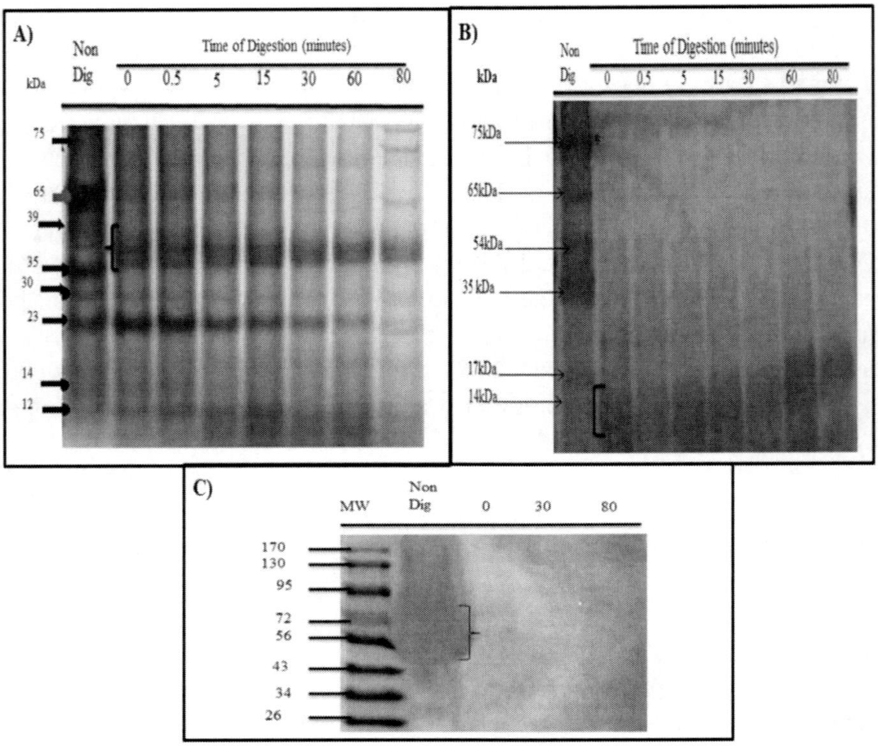

Figure 1. Temporal Pepsin Stability and Immunoreactivity of Extracted Peanut Proteins.

A.) Control non-digested or pepsin digested peanut proteins (40 μg) were separated by SDS-PAGE (4-20%) under reducing conditions and stained with Coomassie Brilliant Blue. Lanes: MW=molecular weight marker; Non-Dig=control non-digested peanut proteins; and 0, 0.5, 5, 15, 30, 60, 80 = time (minutes) of *in vitro* pepsin digestion under physiologic conditions. B.) Electrophoretically (4-20% SDS-PAGE)-separated digested and control non-digested peanut proteins were transferred to a nitrocellulose membrane and immunoblotted with using rabbit anti-peanut antibodies (1:1000) to determine the immunoreactivity of peanut digested proteins. Lanes: MW=molecular weight marker; Non-Dig=control non-digested peanut proteins; and 0, 0.5, 5, 15, 30, 60, 80 = time (minutes) of *in vitro* pepsin digestion. C.) Electrophoretically separated peanut proteins were transferred to a nitrocellulose membrane and immunoblotted with antibodies from peanut allergic patient (1:2) to determine immunoreactivity. Lanes: Non-Dig=control non-digested peanut proteins; and 0, 30, and 80 = time (minutes) of digestion. MW=Molecular weight marker.

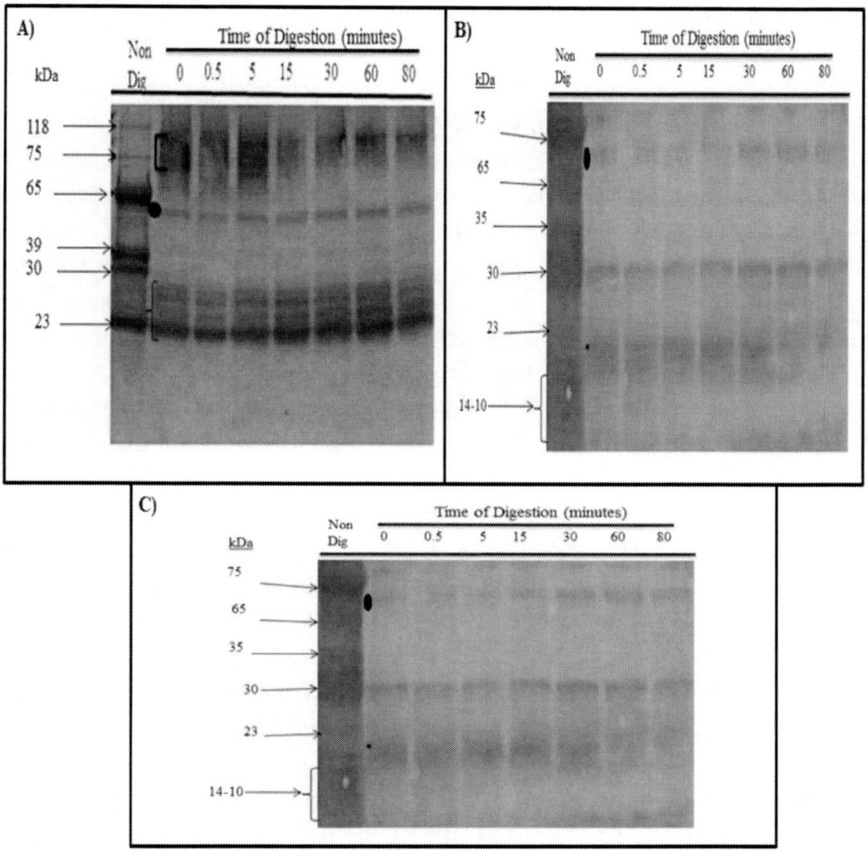

Figure 2. Temporal Pancreatin Stability and Immunoreactivity of Extracted Peanut Proteins.

A.) Control non-digested or pepsin digested peanut proteins (40 μg) were separated by SDS-PAGE (4-20%) under reducing conditions and stained with Coomassie Brilliant Blue. Lanes: MW=molecular weight marker; Non-Dig=control non-digested peanut proteins; and 0, 0.5, 5, 15, 30, 60, 80 and 120 = time (minutes) of *in vitro* pancreatin digestion under physiologic conditions. B.) Electrophoretically (10% SDS-PAGE)-separated digested and non-digested peanut proteins were transferred to a nitrocellulose membrane and immunoblotted with using rabbit anti-peanut antibodies (1:1000) to determine the immunoreactivity of peanut digested proteins. Lanes: MW=molecular weight marker; Non-Dig=control non-digested peanut proteins; and 0, 0.5, 5, 15, 30, 60, 80 and 120 = time (minutes) of *in vitro* pancreatin digestion. C.) Electrophoretically separated peanut proteins were transferred to a nitrocellulose membrane and immunoblotted with antibodies from peanut allergic patient (1:2) to determine immunoreactivity. Lanes: Non-Dig=control non-digested peanut proteins; and 0, 30, and 80 = time (minutes) of digestion. MW=Molecular weight marker.

Results-Murine Model of Peanut Allergy

Elevation of total plasma IgE levels are often used as an indicator of clinical allergy, therefore in this study we aimed to use this as an indices to hypersensitivity responses to allergenic peanut proteins. Total plasma IgE levels were determined over the course of 10 weeks (3, 6, 8 and 10 weeks of age). Total plasma IgE levels were significantly enhanced in peanut extract + CT challenged mice fed the probiotic-supplemented in comparison to mice fed the control diet and peanut extract + CT challenged at 3 weeks of age ($p=0.0101$, Figure 3A). Also, mice fed the probiotic diet and PBS challenged had significantly greater total plasma IgE levels than all other treatment groups with the exception of control diet-PBS challenged treatment group at 3 weeks of age ($p<0.05$, Figure 3A). However, there were no significant differences in total plasma IgE levels between treatment groups at any of the remaining time points measured (6 weeks of age, Figure 3B; 8 weeks of age, Figure 3C; 10 weeks of age, Figure 3D) at $p<0.05$ or $p<0.10$ significance levels.

The effect of probiotic supplementation and sensitization to peanut proteins on splenic lymphocyte populations was determined using surface and intracellular cell staining procedures and fluorescence activated cell sorter analysis (FACS). We utilized surface staining of $CD3^+$ glycoprotein to identify the total T cell population of treatment groups. Mice fed the probiotic-supplemented diet and orally challenged with peanut allergen + CT had a significantly larger splenic total T cell population in comparison to all other treatment groups (Table 1, $p=0.0140$). T helper cells are key players of adaptive immunity and critical to almost all adaptive immunological responses. Hence, we used $CD3^+CD4^+$ surface staining procedures and FACS analysis to identify this activated sub-population of T helper cells. Mice fed the probiotic-supplemented diet (Probiotic Diet-PBS and Probiotic Diet-PN + CT) had significantly more splenic $CD3^+CD4^+$ lymphocyte populations in comparison to mice of control groups (Control Diet-PBS, Control Diet-PN + CT, and Control Diet-CT; Table1, $p\leq 0.02$). $CD8^+$ glycoprotein cell surface staining procedures were utilized to identify and quantify splenic cytotoxic T cells and/or natural killer cells. Mice fed the probiotic diet and challenged with PBS, had a significantly greater splenic lymphocyte $CD3^+CD8^+$ population in comparison to mice of all other treatment groups, while mice fed the control diet and challenged with CT had a significantly smaller $CD3^+CD8^+$ splenic lymphocyte population compared to all other treatment groups ($p<0.0001$, Table1).

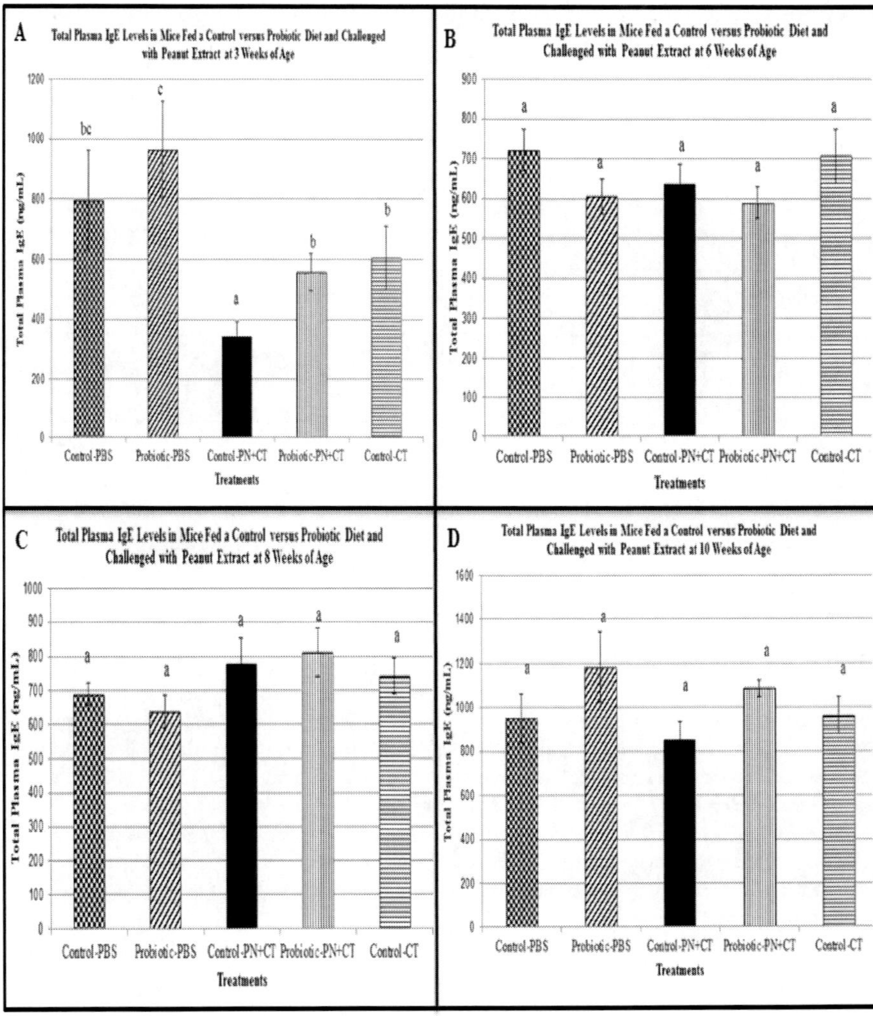

Figure 3. Maternal and Postnatal Dietary Probiotic Supplementation Enhances Early Total IgE Plasma Levels in Peanut Sensitized Mice. All data represent the mean value ± standard error of data pooled for 3 independent experiments and treatment effects were evaluated by age A) 3 weeks of age, B) 6 weeks of age, C) 8 weeks of age and D) 10 weeks of age). [a,b,c,d] Statistical differences were determined using a nested ANOVA model in SAS (version 9.4, 2013). Nested ANOVA tests were significant at $p<0.05$, and subsequently treatments were separated by least squares means (t-test) for comparisons between each treatment group. Bar graphs with differing superscripts were significantly different at $p<0.05$ level.

Table 1. Maternal and Postnatal Dietary Probiotic Supplementation Enhances Splenic T Cell Propulations in Peanut Sensitized Mice[1]

	Dietary Treatments[2]				
	Control Diet-PBS	**Probiotic Diet-PBS**	**Control Diet-PN + CT**	**Probiotic Diet-PN + CT**	**Control Diet-CT**
Lymphocytes	**% Marker-positive of parent population**				
$CD3^+$	59.02± 2.13[a]	62.51±1.2[a]	61.11±5.37[a]	76.28±2.92[b]	57.62±5.93[a]
$CD3^+CD4^+$	28.29±0.84[a]	51.59±2.4[c]	27.80±2.93[a]	35.58±1.67[b]	24.25±1.90[a]
$CD3^+CD8^+$	14.91±0.34[b]	17.2±0.71[c]	12.19±1.13[b]	13.98±0.78[b]	8.27±1.52[a]
$CD4+CD25^+$	1.83±0.15[a]	3.81±0.34[b]	3.90±0.46[b]	5.31±0.28[c]	5.03±0.53[c]

Table 1) Splenic T cell lymphocyte populations were determined using surface cell staining procedures and fluorescence activate cell sorter analysis. [1]All data represent the mean value ± standard error of data pooled for 3 independent experiments of 45-60 animals per treatment. [2]Dietary Treatments= Lactating dams and weaned pups were fed a control mouse chow or probiotic-supplemented mouse chow diet for 10 weeks (2days of age to 10 weeks of age), and sensitized (6 weeks of age) with 0.2mL of sterile PBS, or 10µg of cholera toxin (CT) in 0.2mL of PBS, or 1 mg of peanut extract (PN) + 10µg CT in 0.2mL of PBS. At 8 and 10 weeks of age, mice were orally challenged with 0.2mL of sterile PBS, or 10µg CT in 0.2mL of PBS, or 2 mg of PN + 10µg of CT in 0.2mL of PBS. [a,b,c,d,e]Statistical differences were determined using a nested ANOVA model in SAS (version 9.4, 2013). Nested ANOVA tests were significant at $p<0.05$, and subsequently treatments were separated by least squares means (t-test) for comparisons between each treatment group.

We utilized $CD4^+CD25^+$ surface staining to identify and quantitate this subtype of T cells, which serves as a biomarker for regulatory or suppressor cells (Lan et al., 2012). Interestingly, mice fed the probiotic-supplemented diet and orally sensitized and challenged with peanut allergen (Probiotic Diet-PN + CT) had a significantly enhanced $CD4^+CD25^+$ splenic lymphocyte population in comparison to the respective control groups, Control Diet-PBS and Control Diet-PN + CT ($p<0.01$, Table1). However, because CD25+ is an activation marker for lymphocytes the utility of CD25 surface expression as cell population biomarker for T regulatory cells is limited since it does not discriminate between activated T effector cells and regulatory T cells. Hence, in our final in *vivo* mouse experiment we aimed to more specifically identify naturally occurring and adaptive T regulatory cell populations, using intracellular $FoxP3^+$ and $CD4^+CD25^+$ and $CD4^+CD25^-$ surface staining procedures, respectively (Lan et al., 2012; Su et al., 2012; Fontenot et al., 2003).

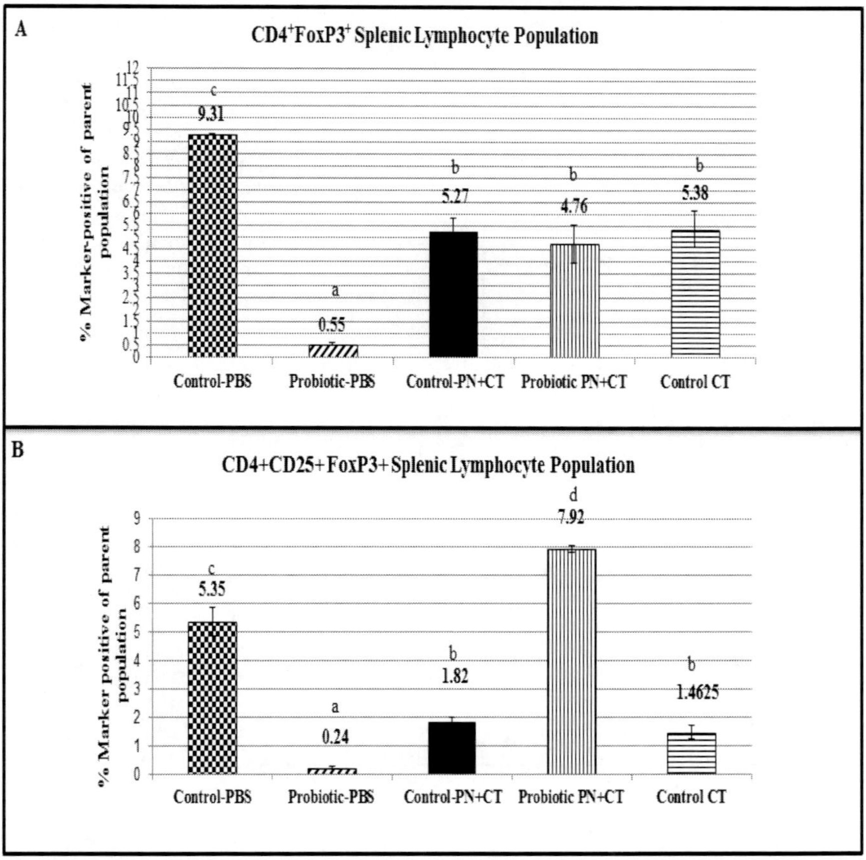

Figure 4. Maternal and Postnatal Dietary Probiotic Supplementation and Peanut Challenge Enhances Naturally-Occurring Splenic T Regulatory Cell Populations in Treated Mice.

Splenic T cell lymphocyte populations were determined using surface and intracellular cell staining procedures and fluorescence activate cell sorter analysis. All data represent the mean value ± standard error. [a,b,c,d] Statistical differences were determined using a nested ANOVA model in SAS (version 9.4, 2013). Nested ANOVA tests were significant at $P<0.05$, and subsequently treatments were separated by least squares means (t-test) for comparisons between each treatment group. Bar graphs with differing superscripts are significantly different ($P<0.01$).

Table 2. Peanut Sensitization and Probiotic Administration Alters Th1/Th2/Th17-Associated Splenic Gene Expression[1]

Gene	Probiotic Diet-PBS	Control Diet-Peanut+CT	Probiotic Diet-Peanut+CT	Control Diet-CT
	Fold Regulation Comparing to Control Diet-PBS (p-value)			
TGFβ	↓1.174 (0.941)	↓1.674 (0.161)	↓1.700 (0.037)	↓1.344 (0.298)
IL-4	↓1.234 (0.111)	↓1.412 (0.890)	↓1.185 (0.681)	↓1.739 (0.620)
IL-17	↓2.237 (0.010)	↓3.547 (0.001)	↓3.475 (0.0003)	↓3.283 (0.922)
IFNγ	↓1.181 (0.431)	↓2.618 (0.178)	↓2.122 (0.186)	↓2.404 (0.384)
TNFα	↓2.704 (0.007)	↓3.252 (0.008)	↓4.949 (0.001)	↓2.780 (0.440)
IL-27	↓1.236 (0.667)	↓1.791 (0.230)	↓1.435 (0.200)	↓1.095 (0.603)
CCL11	↓1.383 (0.819)	↓3.270 (0.031)	↓4.406 (0.001)	↓3.176 (0.026)
CCL7	↓6.451 (0.016)	↓10.300 (0.005)	↓21.965 (<0.001)	↓14.952 (0.008)
IL-13	↓2.705 (0.018)	↓5.451 (0.004)	↓6.886 (<0.001)	↓8.283 (0.014)
IL-6	↓4.634 (0.008)	↓9.011 (0.001)	↓18.668 (<0.001)	↓13.349 (0.006)
IL-7	↓2.237 (0.010)	↓3.547 (0.001)	↓3.475 (<0.001)	↓3.283 (0.922)
IL-7R	↓3.494 (0.010)	↓3.858 (0.005)	↓5.830 (<0.001)	↓6.815 (0.009)
IL-9	↓2.793 (0.010)	↓5.986 (0.005)	↓10.546 (<0.001)	↓11.266 (0.010)

Table 2) Splenic gene expression was determined using total RNA isolated from fresh spleen sections. First strand cDNA was generated and Th1/Th2/Th17 pathway-focused gene expression profiling was conducted using RT² Profiler™ PCR Array. [1] All data represent pooled data for 3 independent *in vivo* experiments. [2] Fold regulation was calculated using the ΔΔCt method: fold change = $2^{(-\Delta\Delta Ct)}$, where ΔΔCt = [(ΔCt)experimental group] − [(ΔCt)control group] The ΔCt for each tissue-treatment combination was calculated using : ΔCt = (average Ct gene of interest – average Ct endogenous housekeeping gene. Average Ct values represent the mean Ct values of data pooled for 3 independent experiments. P-values < 0.05 were significant.

There were no significant differences in the induced splenic T regulatory cell population ($CD4^+FoxP3^+$ positive) between mice orally challenged with peanut + CT fed the control diet or probiotic-supplemented diet (Figure 4A). However, mice fed the probiotic-supplemented diet and orally challenged with peanut + CT had a significantly enhanced (~4-fold) naturally occurring T regulatory cell population ($CD4^+CD25^+FoxP3^+$ positive) in comparison to the corresponding control group and all other treatment groups (Figure 4B, $p<0.01$).

Our final objective was to determine the effect of maternal and postnatal dietary probiotic supplementation on splenic expression of Th1, Th2 and Th17 associated gene expression utilizing the Mouse Th1 & Th2 RT² Profiler PCR

Array profiling the expression of 84 genes involved in T helper cell immune responses using real-time PCR. Splenic gene expression of chemokine CCL11 and cytokine IL-13 (mediators of allergic inflammatory responses) were down-regulated by approximately 4- and 7-fold, respectively in mice fed the probiotic-supplemented diet and orally challenged with peanut allergen + CT relative to gene expression in mice fed the control diet and PBS challenged (Table 2, $p \leq 0.001$).

There was a significant reduction in splenic gene expression of Th2-associated cytokines IL-6 and IL-9 in mice of the following treatment groups: Probiotic Diet-PBS, Control Diet-Peanut + CT, Probiotic Diet-Peanut+ CT and Control Diet-CT relative to control mice (Control Diet-PBS). Mice fed the probiotic-supplemented diet and challenged with peanut + CT ha d 19-fold reduction in IL-6 splenic gene expression relative to the controls ($p<0.05$, Table 2). Among the Th1-assoaciated cytokines analyzed (IFN-γ, IL-27 and TNF-α) only TNF-α splenic expression levels were significantly reduced in mice of treatments: Probiotic Diet-PBS, Control Diet-Peanut + CT, and Probiotic-Diet-Peanut + CT relative to mice of the control group ($p<0.05$, Table 2). Most interestingly, this effect was more pronounced in mice fed the probiotic-supplemented diet and orally challenged with peanut + CT with a 5-fold reduction in TNF-α splenic gene expression relative to mice of the control group (Control Diet-PBS).

Splenic gene expression of cytokine IL-17 (pro-inflammatory cytokine secreted by associated with the Th17 subpopulation of T helper cells) and IL-7 were significantly down-regulated in mice of treatment groups Probiotic Diet-PBS, Control Diet-Peanut+ CT, and Probiotic Diet-Peanut + CT relative to mice of the control group, Control Diet-PBS ($p<0.05$, Table 2). While there was significant reduction in splenic gene expression of CCL7 in mice of treatments Probiotic Diet-PBS, Control Diet-Peanut + CT, and Probiotic Diet-Peanut+ CT, mice fed the probiotic-supplemented diet and orally challenged with peanut + CT had a 22-fold reduction in splenic gene expression of chemokine CCL7 relative to control mice, Control Diet-PBS ($p<0.05$, Table 2).

DISCUSSION AND CONCLUSION

Many food allergen proteins have strong intramolecular disulfide bonds, which makes them resistant to acid denaturation and contribute to their allergenicity[37]. Allergenicity of peanut allergen Ara h 2 is diminished after reduction of the intramolecular disulfide bonds, allowing rapid digestion with pepsin, chymotrypsin, or trypsin[6]. Maleki et al. reported that Ara h 1 is very resistant to protease digestion and denaturation due to structural protection as a stable trimeric complex, allowing passage of Ara h 1 with several intact IgE binding epitopes across the small intestine. Conversely, Astwood et al. (1996) found that Ara h 1 loses immunoreactivity within 15 seconds of *in vitro* pepsin digestion based on a digestibility model and immunoblotting analysis[11]. While this study demonstrates the stability and immunoreactivity of peanut protein bands of 75 kDa and ≤ 14 kDa, these bands cannot be positively identified as any of the Ara h allergenic peanut proteins without protein sequencing. Additionally, variations in allergenicity and potency of peanut allergens between study subjects and human study populations makes interpretation and identification of immunoblotting results more complex. Nevertheless, studies that parallel *in vivo* digestion of orally consumed allergenic containing-foods are necessary for the identification of non-allergenic and allergenic food proteins, their epitope-binding and IgE reactivity.

We elected to use total peanut proteins and not purified allergenic proteins in each of the temporal digestion assays to more closely parallel *in vivo* conditions, in which peanuts are orally consumed in the diet. This approach proves to be more challenging in the complexity of the data, since we are using a pool of various allergenic and non-allergenic proteins and digested protein fragments rather than a single purified allergenic protein. Nevertheless, the use of total peanut protein more closely parallels the pool of digested dietary proteins found in the mammalian gut and available for nutrient absorption following consumption of peanut-containing foods. In summary, the findings of the present study indicate that some peanut proteins and their fragments are pepsin-stable, pancreatin-stable, and immunoreactive for up to at least 1 hour, while these models are representative of human digestion (gastric and intestinal), they do not predict protein half-life or protein stability *in vivo*. However, understanding the stability and allergenicity of these digestive-stable proteins may be helpful in identifying *in vivo* mechanisms of food allergen sensitization.

Peanut allergy affects approximately 1.1% of the population of the United States, similarly for the adult and pediatric populations for unknown scientific reasons (Sicherer et al., 1999).

Peanut allergies persist beyond childhood (Carr, 2005) and with no or cure and/or effective treatment options, we aimed to determine how oral probiotic supplementation may attenuate peanut allergens hypersensitivity immunological responses using a validated murine model to parallel human infantile and childhood peanut allergy. Studies using C3H/HeJ mice have reported numerous benefits of therapeutic probiotic treatment to prevent food allergy to the shellfish allergen tropomyosin, (Schiavi et al., 2011), egg allergen ovalbumin (Kim et al., 2005; 2008) and milk allergen β-Lactoglobulin (Thang et al., 2013). However, most of these studies have explored the immunological effects of acute probiotic administration (bi-weekly oral gavage) on allergen sensitization using weaned animals.

Studies with probiotic supplementation of the maternal diet have demonstrated that maternally derived commensal microorganisms, which colonize the intestine of vaginally delivered and breast-fed infants and persist up to 2 years of age (Tannock et al., 1990) may have protective effects against allergy development (Kim et al., 2010; Abrahamsson et al., 2007; Kalliomäki et al., 2001; Wickens et al., 2008). In this study we demonstrate that at weaning, pups suckled by dams fed the probiotic-supplemented diet had enhanced fecal counts of *Lactobacillus acidophilus* (predominate probiotic strain) relative to treatment controls, suggesting the maternal transfer of the probiotic microorganisms to suckling pups during early development. However, in our study, we could not ascertain maternal transfer of commensals with certainty due to the limitations of sampling imposed by suckling pups co-housed with lactating dams, which prevent microbiological analysis of maternal milk and excreta. Nonetheless, after weaning, enhanced *Lactobacillus acidophilus* fecal counts were maintained in these offspring up to 10 weeks of age in the probiotic-supplemented treatment groups (Probiotic Diet-PBS, Probiotic Diet-Peanut+ CT) relative to treatment controls.

T regulatory cells are a component of the immune system that suppresses immune responses critically needed for immunological tolerance of innocuous antigens and preventing autoimmunity (Lan et al., 2012). "Naturally-occurring" T regulatory cells arise within the thymus and have intracellular molecule, transcription factor forkhead box protein 3 ($FoxP3^+$) and surface glycoproteins $CD4^+CD25^+$ (Su et al., 2012; Lan et al., 2012). Induced T regulatory cells develop outside the thymus after antigen presentation and activation under a variety of conditions (non-inflammatory, inflammatory, infections) distinguishable as $CD4^+CD25^-FoxP3^+$ (Su et al., 2012; Lan et al., 2012). In this study we demonstrate that maternal and post-weaning probiotic dietary supplementation provide immunological enhancement by enhancing T helper cell, cytotoxic T cell and/or natural killer cell and naturally-occurring T regulatory cell populations which may attenuate hypersensitivity responses to food allergens. Our results are supported by previous reports demonstrating that acute probiotic supplementation enhances activated Th17 helper (Donkor et al., 2012) and T regulatory cell populations (Lavasani et al., 2010, Schiavi et al., 2011) and secretion and/or expression of regulatory cytokine TGFβ (Chen et al., 2005, Schiavi et al., 2011, Foye et al., 2012). Induced regulatory T cells have been shown to inhibit macrophage function *in vitro* and to attenuate established macrophage-driven skin contact hypersensitivity after *in vivo* transfer via TGF-β mediated mechanisms (Su et al., 2012).

In summary, this study demonstrates that probiotic dietary supplementation may attenuate peanut allergen hypersensitivity reactions by the reduction of pro-inflammatory cytokines (TNF-α, IL-17) and immunological mediators of allergy (IL-13 and CCL11). Previous reports have demonstrated enhanced secretion and expression of regulatory cytokines TGFβ and/or IL-10 in response to therapeutic probiotic administration (Donkor et al., 2012; Kobayashi et al., 2012). As a consequence, in future probiotic feeding studies we aim to determine the effect of probiotic dietary supplementation and food allergens on splenic secretion and expression of Th1- and Th2-associated cytokines.

In contrast to other probiotic feeding studies demonstrating a reduction in total plasma IgE levels in allergen sensitized subjects, in this study we demonstrate that probiotic dietary supplementation does not reduce total plasma IgE levels in peanut challenged mice. Kim et al., (2010) reported that prenatal and postnatal supplementation with a mixture of probiotic strains reduced the incidence of offspring atopic eczema during the first year, while there were no differences in serum total IgE and food allergen specific IgE between probiotic supplemented and placebo groups in infants at high risk for allergy development. While total plasma IgE levels are often utilized as a potential predictor of allergic sensitization in animal (Thang et al., 2013) and human studies (Satwani et al., 2009) measurement of total plasma IgE levels have been shown to be of little diagnostic value, due to the potential of numerous mitogenic factors (virus, bacteria, parasites, environmental adjuvants), which may enhance the production of total plasma IgE levels not associated with allergen-specific IgE sensitization. Therefore, it is our aim in all future probiotic feeding studies to analyze peanut-specific plasma IgE levels in addition to total plasma IgE levels, dependent upon the availability of plasma from treated mice.

The overall objective of this study was to determine the effect of maternal and postnatal probiotic dietary supplementation (2 days of age to10 weeks of age) on gut *Lactobacillus acidophilus* colonization, total plasma IgE levels, the dynamics of the T helper cell splenic population, and splenic expression profile of Th1/Th2/Th17 associated genes using a validated mouse model to parallel hypersensitivity reactions to peanut in humans. In summary, our data demonstrate that probiotic dietary supplementation enhances gut colonization of the predominate commensal microbe, *Lactobacillus acidophilus*, and enhancement of regulatory T helper and cytotoxic/natural killer T cell populations in mice challenged with peanut allergens.

Our data parallel the findings of other reports utilizing oral probiotic supplementation protocols, suggesting that prolonged probiotic supplementation (2 days of age to 10 weeks of age) in the diet may provide additive immunological benefits by preventing host development of hypersensitivity reactions to food allergens. While the majority of probiotic microorganisms have not been shown to cause illness, additional research is needed to determine the safety, dose responses and efficacy of probiotic supplementation especially in high risk populations, such as infants and young children. Nevertheless, numerous studies imply that probiotic supplementation may serve as an effective therapeutic strategy in the prevention and treatment of food allergies. In conclusion, these results suggest that the probiotic strains present in the feed grade microbials utilized in this study may be good candidates for clinical research in peanut allergy.

References

Abrahamsson, T.R., Jakobsson, T., Böttcher, M.F., Fredrikson, M., Jenmalm, M.C., Björkstén, B., & Oldaeus, G. (2007). Probiotics in prevention of IgE-associated eczema: a double-blind, randomized, placebo-controlled trial. *J. Allergy Clin. Immunol., 119(5),* 1174-1180.

Astwood, J., Leach, J., & Fuchs, R. (1996). Stability of food allergens to digestion in vitro. *Nat. Biotechnol., 14,* 1269-1273.

Björkstén, B., Sepp, E., Julge, K., Voor, T., & Mikelsaar, M. (2001). Allergy development and the intestinal microflora during the first year of life. *J. Allergy Clin. Immunol., 108(4),* 516-520.

Bouchenak, M. & Lamri-Senhadji, M. (2013). Nutritional quality of legumes, and their role in cardiometabolic risk prevention: a review. *J Med Food, 16(3),* 185-198.

Boyce, J.A., Assa'ad, A., Burks, A.W., Jones, S.M., Sampson, H.A., Wood, R.A., Plaut, M., Cooper, S.F., Fenton, M.J., Arshad, S.H., Bahna, S.L., Beck, L.A., Byrd-Bredbenner, C., Camargo, C.A. Jr, Eichenfield, L., Furuta, G.T., Hanifin, J.M., Jones, C., Kraft, M., Levy, B.D., Lieberman, P., Luccioli, S., McCall, K.M., Schneider, L.C., Simon, R.A., Simons,

F.E., Teach, S.J., Yawn, B.P., & Schwaninger, J.M. (2006). Guidelines for the diagnosis and management of food allergy in the United States: summary of the NIAID-sponsored expert panel report. *J. Allergy Clin. Immunol., 126,* 1105-1118.

Burks, W., Sampson, H.A., & Bannon, G.A. (1998). Peanut allergens. *Allergy, 53,* 725-730.

Carr, W.W. (2005). Clinical pearls and pitfalls: peanut allergy. *Allergy Asthma Proc.. 26(2),* 145-7.

Chen, C.C., Louie, S., Shi, H.N., & Walker, W.A. (2005). Preinoculation with the probiotic Lactobacillus acidophilus early in life effectively inhibits murine Citrobacter rodentium colitis. *Pediatric Research, 58,* 1185-1191.

De Jong E.C., Van Zijverden M., Spanhaak S., Koppelman SJ., Pellegrom H., & Penninks A.H. (1998). Identification and partial characterization of multiple major allergens in peanut proteins. *Clin Exp Allergy, 28(6),* 743-51.

Donkor, O.N., Ravikumar, M., Proudfoot, O., Day, S.L., Apostolopoulos, V., Paukovics, G., Vasiljevic, T., Nutt, S.L., & Gill, H. (2012). Cytokine profile and induction of T helper type 17 and regulatory T cells by human peripheral mononuclear cells after microbial exposure. *Clin. Exp. Immunol, 167(2),* 282-295.

Eigenmann, P.A., Sicherer, S.H., Borkowski, T.A., Cohen, B.A., & Sampson, H.A. (1998). Prevalence of IgE-mediated food allergy among children with atopic dermatitis. *Pediatrics, 101(3),* E8-14.

Foye, O.T., Huang, I.F., Chiou, C.C., Walker, W.A., & Shi, H.N. (2012). Early administration of probiotic Lactobacillus acidophilus and/or prebiotic inulin attenuates pathogen-mediated intestinal inflammation and Smad 7 cell signaling. *FEMS Immunol. Med. Microbiol., 65(3),* 467-480.

Gonzalez, C.A., & Salas-Salvadó, J. (2006). The potential of nuts in the prevention of cancer. *Br. J. Nutr., 96*, S87-S94.

Jones, J.B., Provost, M., Keaver, L., Breen, C., Ludy. M.J., & Mattes, R.D. (2014). A randomized trial on the effects of flavorings on the health benefits of daily peanut consumption. *Am J Clin Nutr., 99(3),* 490-496

Kalliomäki, M., Salminen, S., Arvilommi, H., Kero, P., Koskinen, P., & Isolauri, E. (2001). Probiotics in primary prevention of atopic disease: a randomised placebo-controlled trial. *Lancet. 357(9262),* 1076-1079.

Kim, H., Kwack, K., Kim, D.Y., & Ji, G.E. (2005). Oral probiotic bacterial administration suppressed allergic responses in an ovalbumin-induced allergy mouse model. *FEMS Immunol. Med. Microbiol., 45(2),* 259-267.

Kim, J.Y., Choi, Y.O., & Ji, G.E. (2008). Effect of oral probiotics (*Bifidobacterium lactis* AD011 and *Lactobacillus acidophilus* AD031) administration on ovalbumin-induced food allergy mouse model. *J. Microbiol. Biotechnol., 18(8),* 1393-1400.

Kim, J.Y., Kwon, J.H., Ahn, S.H., Lee, S.I., Han, Y.S., Choi, Y.O., Lee, S.Y., Ahn, K.M., & Ji, G.E. (2010). Effect of probiotic mix (Bifidobacterium bifidum, Bifidobacterium lactis, *Lactobacillus acidophilus*) in the primary prevention of eczema: a double-blind, randomized, placebo-controlled trial. *Pediatr. Allergy Immunol. 21*, 386–393

Kobayashi, T., Suzuki, T., Kaji, R., Serata, M., Nagata, T., Ando, M., Iizuka, R., Tsujibe, S., Murakami, J., Kiyoshima-Shibata, J., Kato, I., Nanno, M., & Shida, K. (2012). Probiotic upregulation of peripheral IL-17 responses does not exacerbate neurological symptoms in experimental autoimmune encephalomyelitis mouse models. *Immunopharmacol. Immunotoxicol., 34(3),* 423-433.

Koppelman, S.J., Hefle, S.L., Taylor, S.L., & de Jong, G.A. (2010). Digestion of peanut allergens Ara h 1, Ara h 2, Ara h 3, and Ara h 6: a comparative in vitro study and partial characterization of digestion-resistant peptides. *Mol Nutr Food Res., 54,* 1711-1721.

Koppelman, S.J., de Jong, G.A., Laaper-Ertmann, M., Peeters, K.A., Knulst, A.C., Hefle, S.L., & Knol, E.F. (2005). Purification and immunoglobulin E-binding properties of peanut allergen Ara h 6: evidence for cross-reactivity with Ara h 2. *Clin Exp Allergy., 35,* 490-497.

Koppelman, S.J., Wensing, M., Ertmann, M., Knulst, A.C., & Knol, E.F. (2004). Relevance of Ara h1, Ara h2 and Ara h3 in peanut-allergic patients, as determined by immunoglobulin E Western blotting, basophil-histamine release and intracutaneous testing: Ara h2 is the most important peanut allergen. *Clin Exp Allergy., 34,* 583-590.

Lan, Q., Fan, H., Quesniaux, V., Ryffel, B., Liu, Z., & Zheng, S.G. (2012). Induced FoxP3(+) regulatory T cells: a potential new weapon to treat autoimmune and inflammatory diseases? *J Mol Cell Biol. 4(1),* 22-28.

Lavasani, S., Dzhambazov, B., Nouri, M., Fåk, F., Buske, S., Molin, G., Thorlacius, H., Alenfall, J., Jeppsson, B., & Weström, B. (2010). A novel probiotic mixture exerts a therapeutic effect on experimental autoimmune encephalomyelitis mediated by IL-10 producing regulatory T cells. *PLoS One. 5(2),* e9009.

Lehrer, S.B., Horner, W.E., & Reese, G. (1996). Why are some proteins allergenic? Implications for biotechnology. *Crit. Rev. Food Sci. Nutr., 36,* 553-564.

Maleki, S.J., Kopper, R.A., Shin, D.S., Park, C.W., Compadre, C.M., Sampson, H., Burks, A.W., & Bannon, G.A. (2000). Structure of the major peanut allergen Ara h 1 may protect IgE-binding epitopes from degradation. *J. Immunol., 164*, 5844-5849.

Moreno, J.P., Johnston, C.A., El-Mubasher, A.A., Papaioannou, M.A., Tyler C., Gee, M., & Foreyt, J.P. (2013). Peanut consumption in adolescents is associated with improved weight status. *Nutr Res., 33(7),* 552-556.

Ros E. (2010). Health benefits of nut consumption. *Nutrients, 2(7),* 652-682.

Rudolf, J. L. (2003). Development of an HPLC Method for Resveratrol and OptimizationofPost-HarvestStresstoInduceProductioninPeanuts. *Master's thesis*, University of Georgia, Athens, GA.

Sales, J,M., & Resurreccion, A.V. (2014). Resveratrol in peanuts. *Crit Rev Food Sci Nutr., 54(6)*, 734-770.

Sampson, H.A. (2004). Update on food allergy. *J Allergy Clin Immunol., 113(5),* 805-819.

Satwani, H., Rehman, A., Ashraf, S., & Hassan, A. (2009). Is serum total IgE levels a good predictor of allergies in children? *J. Pak. Med. Assoc., 59(10),* 698-702.

Schiavi, E, Barletta, B., Butteroni, C., Corinti, S., Boirivant, M., & Di Felice, G. (2011). Oral therapeutic administration of a probiotic mixture suppresses established Th2 responses and systemic anaphylaxis in a murine model of food allergy. *Allergy, 66(4),* 499-508.

Schmidt, H., Krause, S., Gelhaus, C., Petersen, A., Janssen, O., & Becker, W.M. (2010). Detection and structural characterization of natural Ara h 7, the third peanut allergen of the 2S albumin family. *J. Proteome Res., 9,* 3701-3709.

Sen, M., Kopper, R., Pons, L., Abraham, E.C., Burks, A.W., & Bannon, G.A. (2002). Protein structure plays a critical role in peanut allergen stability and may determine immunodominant IgE-binding epitopes. *J. Immunol., 169,* 882-887.

Su, W., Fan, H., Chen, M., Wang, J., Brand, D., He, X., Quesniaux, V., Ryffel, B., Zhu, L., Liang, D., & Zheng, S.G. (2012). Induced CD4+ forkhead box protein-positive T cells inhibit mast cell function and established contact hypersensitivity through TGF-β1. *J. Allergy Clin. Immunol., 130(2),* 444-452.

Tannock, G.W., Fuller, R., Smith, S.L., & Hall, M.A. (1990). Plasmid profiling of members of the family Enterobacteriaceae, lactobacilli, and bifidobacteria to study the transmission of bacteria from mother to infant. *J. Clin. Microbiol., 28(6),* 1225-1228.

Thang, C.L., Boye, J.I., & Zhao, X. (2013). Low doses of allergen and probiotic supplementation separately or in combination alleviate allergic reactions to cow β-lactoglobulin in mice. *J. Nutr., 143(2),*136-141.

United States Pharmacopeia 23. (1996). Simulated Gastric Fluid and Simulated Intestinal Fluid, The National Formulary 18 (3171). Rockville, MD: The United States Pharmacopeial Convention Inc.

Wickens, K., Black, P.N., Stanley, T.V., Mitchell, E., Fitzharris, P., Tannock, G.W., Purdie, G., & Crane, J. (2008). A differential effect of 2 probiotics in the prevention of eczema and atopy: a double-blind, randomized, placebo-controlled trial. *J. Allergy Clin. Immunol., 122(4),* 788-794.

Wensing, M., Penninks A.H., Hefle, S.L., Koppelman, S.J., Bruijnzeel-Koomen, C.A., & Knulst, A.C. (2002). The distribution of individual threshold doses eliciting allergic reactions in a population with peanut allergy. *J Allergy Clin Immunol., 110(6),* 915-920.

In: Peanuts
Editor: Richard W. Cook
ISBN: 978-1-63321-013-4

Chapter 2

Lower Solvent Concentration and Time for Extraction of Peanut Skin Antioxidants at Optimized Conditions

Adriano Costa de Camargo*[*]*,
Thais Maria Ferreira de Souza Vieira,
Gabriela Boscariol Rasera,
Solange Guidolin Canniatti-Brazaca,
Severino Matias de Alencar
and Marisa Aparecida Bismara Regitano-d'Arce
Department of Agri-Food Industry, Food & Nutrition,
"Luiz de Queiroz" College of Agriculture, (ESALQ/USP),
University of São Paulo, Brazil

Abstract

Peanut skins are low cost feedstock generated by the industrial peanut blanching process. However, its high antioxidant phytochemical constituents still lack effective industrial application of their extractable compounds. For efficient recovery of these target compounds, the present work combined antioxidant assays and statistical tools to achieve its goals. Response surface methodology (RSM) was used to fit predictive

---

[*] Corresponding author: E-Mail: adrianoesalq@gmail.com.

mathematical models. By matching all predicted responses a global standardized response was generated, which found a high positive correlation between observed and predicted responses (r = 0.9921, $p < 0.01$). Thus, Tukey's multiple test ($p < 0.05$) was carried out to define the best extraction conditions (2.5% peanut skin extracted with 50.0% ethanol over 20 min). Under optimized conditions, total phenolic content (TPC) and ferric reducing antioxidant power (FRAP) were 91.87 mg GAE/g and 135.07 mmol Fe^{2+}/g of peanut skins, respectively. Trolox equivalent antioxidant capacity (TEAC) values for DPPH, ABTS, and ORAC assays were 585.61, 2093.64 and 1206.87 μmol/g of peanut skins, respectively. It was possible to reduce the time of extraction and the solvent concentration as compared to the literature. Through RSM and further statistical analysis it was possible set extraction conditions at which the antioxidant extracts overlapped the reaction mechanism of FRAP, DPPH, ABTS, and ORAC assays.

Keywords: by-product, response surface methodology, polyphenols, FRAP, DPPH, ABTS, ORAC

1. INTRODUCTION

The antioxidant properties of phenolic compounds have been reported. Antioxidants are able to neutralize free radicals. Studies on vegetables [1], fruits [2], cereals [3], spices [4], tea [5], nuts [6] and other foods have highlighted the potential use of polyphenols. By-products such as grape seed [7] and peanut skins [8] are also source of antioxidants. Polyphenols were reported as having positive *in vivo* effect in reducing visceral fat obesity [9], and potential anti-inflammatory [10], anticarcinogenic [11], and management of pre-diabetes and/or diabetes [12].

Peanut skin, which is generated in the blanching process of peanuts has already been studied by our research group [13]. It showed a high phenolic content, condensed tannins, and antioxidant capacity against DPPH and ABTS radicals and, most importantly, the effective antioxidant property of peanut skin extracts in soybean oil model system. Furthermore, it was demonstrated that peanut skin antioxidants from IAC-Runner 886 cultivar were more efficient at delaying oxidative damage than butylated hydroxytoluene (BHT) by using Oil Stability Index Rancimat method, which applies temperatures as high as 110 ºC. The literature also provides data supporting the hypothesis of peanut skins as having higher antioxidant properties than green tea [14], trolox and vitamin C [15].

Peanut skins and its extracts have been studied by several research groups. The presence of proanthocyanidins was reported in several publications [16-19]. The effect of the process used for removal of peanut skin (e.g., direct peeling, blanching, and roasting) on the concentration of procyanidins was also studied [15]. The isolation of flavonoids was reported by Lou et al. [20]. Resveratrol was identified by Ballard et al. [21,22], and the presence of phenolic acids, flavonoids and stilbenes was reported by Francisco and Resurreccion [23] and Yu, Ahmedna and Goktepe [14].

It is worth noting that proanthocyanidins from peanut skins have been studied by many authors. Proanthocyanidin dimers and trimers from peanut skins can interact with membrane phospholipids, presumably with their polar headgroup. Thus, they can provide protection against the attack of oxidants and other molecules that challenge the bilayer's integrity [8]. Phenolic compounds extracted from peanut skins presented a greater protective effect against the hemolysis of red blood cells than ascorbic acid under *in vitro* conditions [9]. Peanut skin extracts also presented inhibition ability against yeast growth [24].

Some studies reported optimized conditions for peanut skin extraction, but with different process from the current work, such as microwave-assisted extraction [21], using methanol as the solvent system [22] or studying the peanut skin particle size and number of extractions [25]. In the present study, ethanol and its mixtures with water were chosen because of their feasibility for use in the food industry. Moreover, ethanol has a low cost and it is recognized as an environment-friendly solvent. According to the literature [22] a lower solvent concentration is necessary to achieve similar yield of total polyphenols when ethanol is used instead of methanol, shorter time yielded the highest total polyphenol and oxygen radical absorbance capacity. In the current work shorter time of extraction and peanut skin/solvent ratio were also addressed. Since peanut skin is a low value by-product [26], the use of high temperatures, which could result in higher costs for the process was not considered.

The present study aimed in optimizing the extraction process of peanut skins from IAC-Runner 505, a high oleic cultivar, most likely used in the industrial blanching process because they are less susceptible to oxidative damage by the peanut skin removal, which involves heating. The focus was placed on the analysis of predicted responses achieved by response surface methodology (RSM) of the total phenolic content (TPC) and antioxidant evaluations by FRAP, DPPH, ABTS and ORAC assays, which is a combination of widely used methods for studies with this purpose. The predicted individual responses were used to achieve the most efficient extraction in terms of antioxidant properties along with the best independent variables.

2. Experimental Section

2.1. Materials

Peanut skin samples (cv. IAC-Runner 505) were kindly donated by CAP—Agroindustrial, Dumont, São Paulo State, Brazil.

2.2. Methods

2.2.1. Extraction Procedure

The extracts were obtained using 0, 20, 50, 80 and 100% ethanol in distilled water. First, 1.0; 1.6; 2.5; 3.4 or 4.0 g of peanut skins were added in a closed glass container with 100 mL of solvent at concentrations previously explained, and then were shaken for 20, 28, 40, 52 or 60 min in a water bath at 30 °C. The extract was then filtered, transferred to amber bottles and kept at −18 °C until analysis. Extractions were performed at once, except for runs 15-18 which represented the central point. All extraction combinations are summarized in Table 1.

2.2.2. Total Phenolic Contents

Total phenolic contents were determined using appropriate dilutions obtained from the extracts reported above (Table 1). The procedure was carried out according to the Folin-Ciocalteau method [27], with slight modifications as described by de Camargo et al. [28]. Briefly, the extracts with appropriate dilutions (0.5 mL), deionized water (4 mL), and Folin-Ciocalteau reagent (0.5 mL) were added into flasks and mixed thoroughly. After 3 min, 1 mL of a Na_2CO_3 saturated solution (20 g in 70 mL of water) was added, and the mixture was kept in the dark under at room temperature for 2 h. Finally, the absorbance was read at 760 nm using a Shimadzu UV-1800 spectrophotometer (Shimadzu Corporation, Kyoto, Japan). The results are expressed as milligram gallic acid equivalents/g dry weight.

2.2.3. Ferric Reducing Antioxidant Power (FRAP)

The FRAP assay was conducted according with the method of Benzie et al. [29] using appropriate dilutions obtained from the extracts reported above (Table 1). In acidic medium (pH 3.6), the FRAP method evaluates the ferric reducing power of antioxidants. The response is measured as the intensity of the blue color when the ferric tripyridyltriazine (Fe^{3+}-TPTZ) complex is reduced to the ferrous (Fe^{2+}) form. The FRAP reagent, which is a mixture [25 mL of acetate buffer (acetate 300 mM, pH = 3.6) + 2.5 mL of TPTZ 10 mM TPTZ in 40 mM HCl) + 2.5 mL of $FeCl_3$ (20 mM in aqueous solution)] was prepared at the time of analysis. The appropriate dilutions of extracts of peanut skins (0.1 mL) were added to 3 mL of FRAP reagent. The absorbance was read at 595 nm using a Shimadzu UV-1800 spectrophotometer (Shimadzu Corporation, Kyoto, Japan) after incubation in a water bath at 37 °C for 30 min. The calibration curve was prepared using ferrous sulfate and the results were expressed as mmol of Fe^{2+}/g dry weight.

2.2.4. DPPH Radical Scavenging Activity

Antioxidant activity was measured using the DPPH (2,2-diphenyl-1-picrylhydrazyl) radical assay [30] and appropriate dilutions obtained from the extracts reported above (Table 1). The diluted extracts (0.50 mL) were added to a 60 μmol ethanolic solution of DPPH (3 mL). The absorbance was determined at 517 nm using a Shimadzu UV-1800 spectrophotometer (Shimadzu Corporation; Japan), after 45 min in the dark. DPPH radical scavenging activity was calculated using the equation below:

$$\text{DPPH radical scavenging activity (\%)} = [(Abs_{control} - Abs_{sample})/(Abs_{control})] \times 100$$

where $Abs_{control}$ was the absorbance of DPPH radical + ethanol; Abs_{sample} is the absorbance of DPPH radical + peanut skin extract or trolox. The results were expressed as trolox equivalents/g dry weight.

2.2.5. ABTS Radical Scavenging Activity

In this assay from Re et al. [31] and described by de Camargo et al. [13] the ABTS radical [2,2'-azino-bis(3-ethylbenzothiazoline-6-sulfonic acid)], which is generated by oxidation with potassium persulfate, was utilized in ethanolic extracts with appropriate dilutions obtained from the extracts reported above (Table 1). A 7 mM stock solution of ABTS was prepared one day before the analysis, and the working solution was prepared by diluting the stock to reach absorbance of 0.70 ± 0.02 (734 nm). The diluted extracts (20 μL) were added of the ABTS radical solution (2 mL), and the absorbance was read at 734 nm after 6 min using a Shimadzu UV-1800 spectrophotometer (Shimadzu Corporation, Kyoto, Japan). ABTS radical scavenging activity was calculated using the following equation:

$$\text{ABTS radical scavenging activity (\%)} = [(\text{Abs}_{\text{control}} - \text{Abs}_{\text{sample}})/(\text{Abs}_{\text{control}})] \times 100$$

where $\text{Abs}_{\text{control}}$ was the absorbance of ABTS radical + ethanol; $\text{Abs}_{\text{sample}}$ is the absorbance of ABTS radical + peanut skin extract or trolox. The results are expressed as trolox equivalents/g dry weight.

2.2.6. Oxygen Radical Absorbance Capacity (ORAC)

The ORAC assay used was based on the method of Ou, Hampsch-Woodill and Prior [32] with minor modifications. The appropriate dilutions obtained from the extracts reported above (Table 1) were performed in 75 mM phosphate buffer (pH 7.0). Fluorescein (508.25 nM) and the AAPH [2,2′-azobis(2-methylpropionamidine) dihydrochloride] solution (76 mM) were also prepared in phosphate buffer (pH 7.0). The reaction was carried out by adding 30 μL of the sample, 60 μL of fluorescein as oxidizable substrate, and 110 μL of AAPH (76 mM). The procedure was performed in a Greiner Bio-One flat bottomed 96 well black microplates (Greiner Bio-One Gmbh, DE). Determination of ORAC was carried out using a plate reader (SpectraMax M3, Molecular Devices LLC,US). The incubation was conducted at 37 °C for 2h and the fluorescence was recorded every min. The excitation and emission wavelength was set to 485 and 528 nm, respectively. ORAC values were expressed as trolox equivalents/g dry weight.

2.2.7. Experimental Design and Statistical Analysis

A central composite design of three factor/five level was employed to investigate the total phenolic content and the antioxidant properties as evaluated by FRAP, DPPH, ABTS and ORAC methods. The explanatory variables were the percentage of ethanol in water (%, v/v), extraction time (min) and the percentage of peanut skin (%, w/v). The experimental design with the range and center point of three independent variables is given in Table 1. Experimental data were analyzed with the software Statistica 11.0. The effects were analyzed by response surface methodology and multiple regression analysis. Second-order mathematical model were adjusted, including linear and quadratic terms, and interactions between independent variables. The models were evaluated regarding the coefficient of determination (R^2) and F tests. The model formula is represented by the equation below:

$$Y = \beta_0 + \beta_1 x_1 + \beta_2 x_2 + \beta_3 x_3 + \beta_{11} x_1^2 + \beta_{22} x_2^2 + \beta_{33} x_3^2 + \beta_{12} x_1 x_2 + \beta_{13} x_1 x_3 + \beta_{23} x_2 x_3$$

In which Y is the predicted response, x_1, x_2, and x_3 represent the coded levels of independent variables, β_0 is the intercept coefficient and β*'s* are the coefficients estimated by the least squares method.

Table 1. Coded values and corresponding actual values used in the experimental design

	Independent variable	Simble	Coded Values				
			-1.68	**-1**	**0**	**1**	**1.68**
Actual Values	ethanol percentage (%, v/v)[1]	x_1	0	20	50	80	100
	extraction time (min)	x_2	20	28	40	52	60
	peanut skin percentage (%, w/v)	x_3	1.0	1.6	2.5	3.4	4.0

[1] v is volume in mL, min is extraction time in minutes, and w is weigh in grams.

To define the optimum conditions a standardized response was generated with further combination data of five predicted responses (TPC, FRAP, DPPH, ABTS, and ORAC) and, finally, the generated data was submitted to a second analysis by Tukey's test ($p < 0.05$) performed with SAS software. Correlation analyses ($p < 0.01$) and ($p < 0.05$) were carried out using the ASSISTAT 7.6 program.

3. Results and Discussion

3.1. Model Fitting

The observed responses for total phenolics and antioxidant activity evaluations of peanut skin extracts at different conditions are presented in Table 2. TPC ranged from 54.6 to 118.8 mg GAE/g, FRAP ranged from 85.58 to 167.1 mmol Fe^{2+}/g, and TEAC for DPPH, ABTS and ORAC ranged from 285.1 to 631.99, from 928.08 to 2675.7, and from 634.04 to 1897.11 μmol/g, respectively. The range between the lowest and the highest value for each assay was between two and three-fold. This demonstrated the positive effect in optimizing the extraction process at this stage, when methods that would take too much time and expensive materials are not cost effective.

All compounds may not be extracted at the optimized condition. Ballard et al. [22] were not able to identify resveratrol in water or ethanolic extracts of peanut skins, but they did it in the methanolic extract. However, it is expected that at optimized conditions one would be able to extract a reasonable spectrum of compounds with effective antioxidant properties.

Table 2. Central composite design (CCD) with observed response for total phenolic content (TPC) and antioxidant evaluations by FRAP, DPPH, ABTS, and ORAC methods

Run	Ethanol Percentage %, v/v[1]	Time min	Peanut Skin Percentage %, w/v	Observed Response[2]				
				TPC	FRAP	DPPH	ABTS	ORAC
				mg GAE/g[3,4]	mmol Fe^{2+}/g	µmol TE/g[5]	µmol TE/g	µmol TE/g
1	20	28	1.6	95.23	132.4	492.55	2028.72	1284.4
2	80	28	1.6	94.00	140.4	524.50	1906.98	1356.4
3	20	52	1.6	94.27	119.9	458.39	2563.88	1417.8
4	80	52	1.6	102.3	129.6	428.95	2288.12	1141.5
5	20	28	3.4	71.84	114.5	471.63	1472.60	634.04
6	80	28	3.4	79.52	106.1	480.80	1813.12	1095.9
7	20	52	3.4	72.65	107.1	285.12	928.08	950.43
8	80	52	3.4	79.89	85.58	347.52	1587.21	1125.2
9	0	40	2.5	54.60	99.61	314.38	1334.14	656.58
10	100	40	2.5	71.79	99.49	354.76	1583.38	965.76
11	50	20	2.5	91.87	135.1	585.61	2093.64	1206.9
12	50	60	2.5	92.50	90.57	372.31	2164.95	989.22
13	50	40	1	118.8	167.1	523.93	2675.72	1897.1
14	50	40	4	84.50	113.6	301.06	1768.19	1215.4
15	50	40	2.5	108.8	136.2	585.47	1858.41	1459.4
16	50	40	2.5	103.6	134.6	616.46	1716.88	1347.8
17	50	40	2.5	113.1	131.6	605.83	1788.05	1409.1
18	50	40	2.5	109.6	135.3	631.99	1788.86	1464.1

[1] v is volume in mL, min is time in minutes and w is weigh in grams;

[2] Data represent the means of triplicate analysis for each run;

[3] GAE is gallic acid equivalent;

[4] The mass is expressed in dry weigh;

[5] TE is trolox equivalents.

However, the purpose of the current work was not identification and quantification of individual compounds, but their further application. If one intends to proceed with the identification of bioactive compounds, it is recommended to search for the best extraction procedure in each case, which may require methods such as the extraction of soluble and insoluble bound forms of polyphenols as performed by Chandrasekara and Shahidi [3].

TPC, DPPH and ABTS results from the present work are in good agreement with a previous study [13]. ORAC values are also similar to the results reported by Ballard et al. [21]. Since ferric ions [33,34] are applied for catalyzing the oxidation of oil model systems it is worth paying attention to the ability of such antioxidant extracts in reducing ferric to ferrous ions.

The experimental data of the present work was used to fit the response surface regression models. The variance analysis of the quadratic regressions is shown in Table 3.

F calculated values were at least three-fold *F* tabulated, hence the models can be used to predict TPC, FRAP, DPPH, ABTS and ORAC values. In addition, the lack of fit was not significant ($p < 0.05$). Furthermore, both R^2 and adjusted R^2 were higher than 0.9000 in all adjusted models.

The second order mathematical models, neglecting insignificant terms, are shown in Table 4. They can be used both separately and as combination data as will be further explained in Section 3.2.

Table 3. Variance analysis (ANOVA) for total phenolic content (TPC) and antioxidant evaluations by FRAP, DPPH, ABTS, and ORAC methods

Source of variation (sum of squares)	Responses				
	TPC	FRAP	DPPH	ABTS	ORAC
Regression	4764.09	7247.31	213074.86	2879468.90	1466328.83
Residual	176.53	250.16	12512.24	129495.69	98574.39
Lack of fit	130.65	238.48	11367.88	119479.00	89751.00
Pure error	45.88	11.68	1144.36	10016.00	8823.00
Total	4940.62	7247.31	225587.10	3008965.00	1564903.00
F_{calc}*	87.71	51.28	31.22	31.77	27.27
F_{tab}	3.18	3.09	3.09	3.14	3.09
R^2	0.9643	0.9655	0.9445	0.9570	0.9370
Adjusted R^2	0.9533	0.9467	0.9143	0.9268	0.9027

* If *F* calculated is three-fold higher than *F* tabulated the model can be used for prediction purposes.

Table 4. Second order mathematical models of total phenolic content (TPC) and antioxidant activities by FRAP, DPPH, ABTS, and ORAC assays

TPC (mg GAE/g)[1] =	106.4080
	+ 7.4167 x (Ethanol Percentage)
	-30.5455 x (Ethanol Percentage^2)
	-10.0032 x (Extraction Time)
	-20.4381 x (Peanut Skin Percentage)
FRAP (mmol Fe^{2+}/g) =	134.4057
	-24.5255 x (Ethanol Percentage^2)
	-18.4525 x (Extraction Time)
	-15.1222 x (Extraction Time^2)
	-29.1402 x (Peanut Skin Percentage)
	4.3825 x (Peanut Skin Percentage^2)
	-11.9275 x (Ethanol Percentage x Peanut Skin Percentage)
DPPH (μmol TE/g) =	607.927 x
	-177.661 x (Ethanol Percentage^2)
	-118.410 x (Extraction Time)
	-75.343 x (Extraction Time^2)
	-101.686 x (Peanut Skin Percentage)
	-122.442 x (Peanut Skin Percentage^2)
	-47.520 x (Extraction Time x Peanut Skin Percentage)
ABTS (μmol TE/g) =	1794.180
	149.638 x (Ethanol Percentage)
	-286.585 x (Ethanol Percentage^2)
	188.564 x (Extraction Time^2)
	-661.254 x (Peanut Skin Percentage)
	254.228 x (Peanut Skin Percentage^2)
	349.289 x (Ethanol Percentage x Peanut Skin Percentage)
	-421.682 x (Extraction Time x Peanut Skin Percentage)
ORAC (μmol TE/g) =	1469.577
	139.501 x (Ethanol Percentage)
	-456.017 x Ethanol Percentage^2)
	-252.733 x (Extraction Time^2)
	-372.253 x (Peanut Skin Percentage)
	-158.845 x (Ethanol Percentage x Extraction Time)
	210.234 x (Ethanol Percentage x Peanut Skin Percentage)

[1] GAE is gallic acid equivalents;

[2] TE is trolox equivalents.

It is worth having all the models because a particular assay may be better correlated than others for an actual application (e.g., bulk oil or oil-in-water emulsion). This may due to the structure-antioxidant activity relationships already explained by Rice-Evans, Miller and Paganga [35]. This can be elucidated according to the different mechanisms that the target antioxidant is expected to follow.

The lack of correlation among antioxidant assays has also been reported [36]. This is the main reason for using several assays in the present study. While FRAP involves reduction of ferric to ferrous ions via electron transfer [37], DPPH involves hydrogen donation [30], ABTS focuses on electron transfer reactions [38], and ORAC stands from chain-breaking antioxidant capacity against peroxyl radicals [39]. Relationships of independent and dependent variables can be visualized in the three-dimensional response surfaces. The antioxidant evaluations correlated well with TPC. Thus, only its surface responses are shown (Figures 1-3).

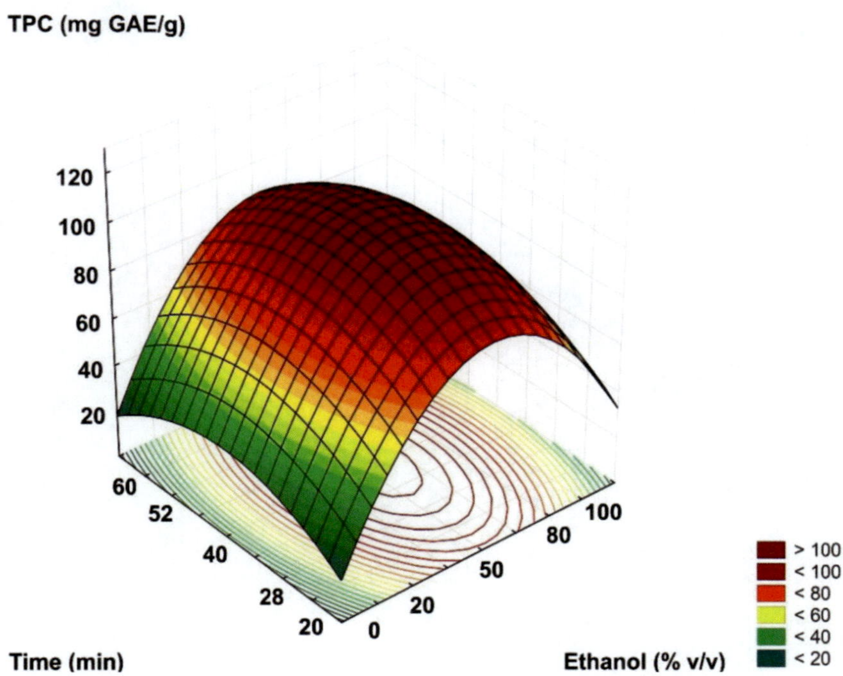

Figure 1. Interaction between extraction time and percentage of ethanol.

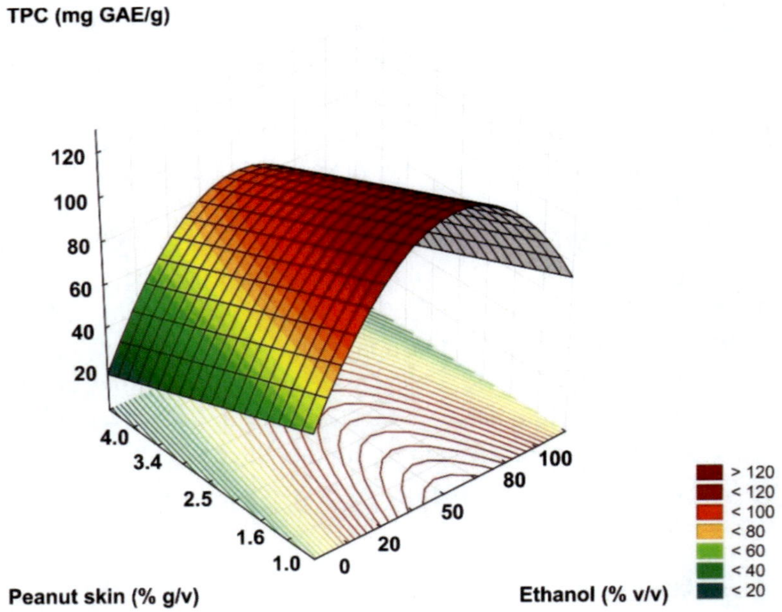

Figure 2. Interaction between ethanol and percentage of peanut skin.

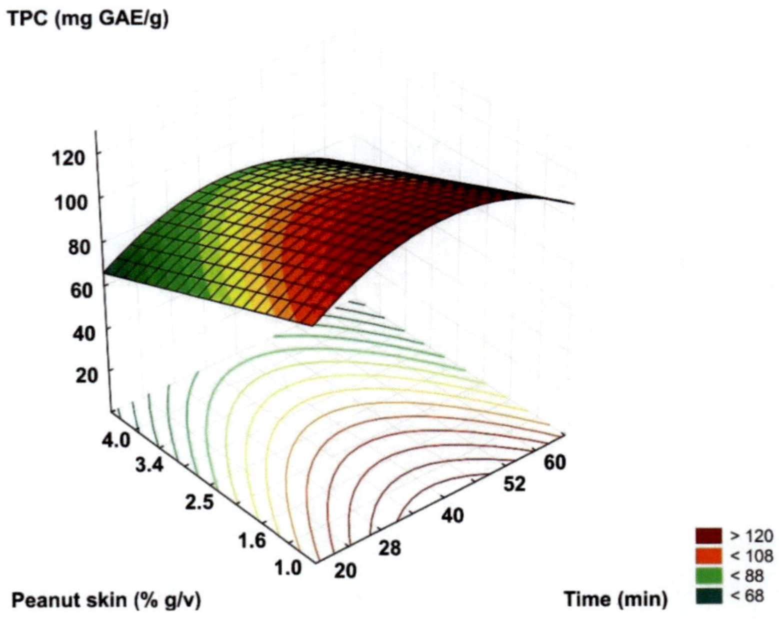

Figure 3. Interaction between percentage of peanut skin and time.

Figure 1 displays the interaction between extraction time and percentage of ethanol at a fixed peanut skin percentage (2.5%). It was noted that the best extraction conditions regarding the percentage of ethanol is close to the central point (50% ethanol in water). On the other hand, when the extraction time is analyzed there is a large range of extraction efficiency. The interaction between ethanol and peanut skin percentage when the extraction time is kept at 40 min is shown in Figure 2. The lower the peanut skin percentage the higher the TPC values. One could think that the best extraction conditions should be the lowest percentage of peanut skin, however this would significantly increase the amount of solvent required for the process. In addition, in Figure 3 it is worth noting the influence of the peanut skin percentage on TPC. Regarding the interaction of peanut skin percentage with time of extraction, the best extraction time was around 40 min (ethanol kept at 50%).

3.2. Combining Observed and Predicted Responses

In order to calculate the global standardized response of observed and predicted yields transformations were carried out according to the equation below:

$$GSR_i\,(\%) = \{\Sigma\,[(V_i/HV) \times 100]\}/n$$

Where GSR_i is either the global standardized observed or predicted response for the run_i.

V_i is the value either for the predicted or observed response for the run_i.

HV is the highest value found for either the predicted or observed response for the method in question.

n = number of methods used to fit individual models

High positive correlations ($p < 0.01$) between standardized observed and predicted yields for each assay are summarized in Figure 4. Pearson's correlation values were 0.9857, 0.9817, 0.9342, 0.9798, 0.9742, and 0.9921 for TPC, FRAP, DPPH, ABTS, ORAC, and GSR, respectively.

Since a high positive correlation ($p < 0.01$) between the standardized observed and the predicted yields matching all five assays was achieved (Figure 4), the proposed protocol can be used to improve the optimization of antioxidant extraction conditions using methods with different reaction mechanisms. With the standardized predicted response, it is expected to extract phytochemicals with antioxidant properties for different applications such as in pharmaceutical products, for improving shelf life of high lipid foods and development of dietary supplements, among others. This protocol can also be used when several responses are required to make a final decision such as for research and development of new food products that demand sensory evaluations of several attributes such as color, aroma, taste, and texture, among others.

Table 5. Standardized observed and the predicted observed yields

Run	Ethanol Percentage %, v/v[1]	Extration Time min	Peanut Skin Percentage %, w/v	Global Standardized Observed Yield[2] %	Global Standardized Predicted Yield %
1	20	28	1.6	76.18 ± 5.01abc	77.52 ± 5.12bcd
2	80	28	1.6	77.79 ± 6.13abc	79.68 ± 7.27ab
3	20	52	1.6	78.84 ± 9.94abc	77.85 ± 9.07abc
4	80	52	1.6	75.46 ± 11.3abc	76.45 ± 7.47bc
5	20	28	3.4	58.42 ± 15.8ab	59.46 ± 14.5cd
6	80	28	3.4	66.41 ± 6.68bcd	68.61 ± 5.16bcd
7	20	52	3.4	51.04 ± 12.0d	50.44 ± 8.50d
8	80	52	3.4	58.42 ± 5.99cd	56.02 ± 6.49d
9	0	40	2.5	47.96 ± 9.01d	50.37 ± 8.88d
10	100	40	2.5	57.24 ± 3.90cd	56.87 ± 2.88d
11	50	20	2.5	78.55 ± 10.4abc	77.99 ± 13.2abc
12	50	60	2.5	64.81 ± 13.6bcd	67.69 ± 7.46bcd
13	50	40	1	96.58 ± 7.65a	97.12 ± 6.43a
14	50	40	4	63.39 ± 9.19bcd	64.79 ± 6.56bcd
15	50	40	2.5	82.05 ± 11.35ab	83.25 ± 12.1ab

[1] v is volume in mL, min is extraction time in minutes and w is weigh in grams;
[2] Data obtained with GSR equation ± standard deviations.

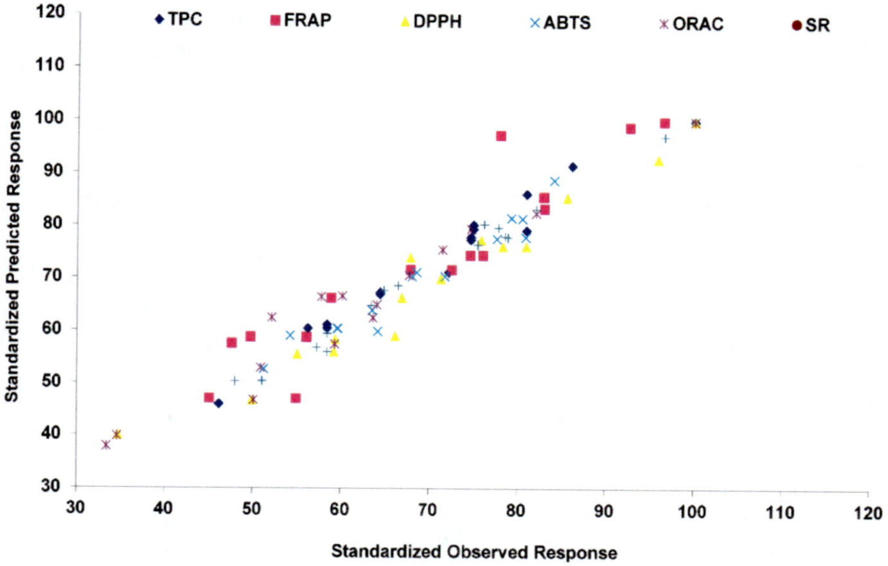

Figure 4. Correlations of observed and predicted yields of TPC, DPPH, ABTS, FRAP, ORAC and Global Standardized Response (GSR).

According to the Tukey's test ($p < 0.05$) no difference was found among runs number 2, 3, 11, 13, and 15 of the standardized predicted responses (Table 5), which presented the highest extraction yields. Runs number 2 and 13 were contrary to the purpose of extracting with the lowest ethanol and highest peanut skin mass as possible, thus they were not considered as further, remaining the runs number 3, 11 and 15. There was no significant difference between runs number 11 and 15, furthermore the run number 15 required 40 min of extraction over 20 min for number 11, thus the run number 15 was discontinued. Finally, between the remaining runs (3 and 11), number 11 showed to be the best choice because of lower extraction time and higher amount of peanut skin processed. Furthermore, increasing the percentage of ethanol from 20 to 50% using 5000 L batches, one could extract 375 kg/h while using just 20% ethanol the extraction capacity decreases to 92.5 kg/h. This way, it can be inferred that increasing 2.5-fold the ethanol percentage would result in a 4.0-fold increase in the processing capacity. Thus, the optimum extraction conditions are: 2.5% peanut skin extracted with 50.0% ethanol for 20 min. It is also remarkable that the ethanol concentration of the present study is lower than in several other works from the literature [13,14] which, in average, are in the range of 80 to 100%. Furthermore, the time required for the standardized predicted response is 20 min, which could be 40 min if only the TPC fitted model had been taken into account. The current work shows a promising tool for future studies on the extraction of antioxidant phytochemicals.

Conclusion

The optimization of individual responses as a preliminary screening tool for various effects can be useful for matching several responses and applying complementary statistical analysis that can improve results and serve to make final decisions. Using just one tool could lead to a misjudgment such as choosing extraction conditions of 1.0% peanut skin extracted with 50.0% ethanol for 40 min when in fact it was demonstrated that the optimum extraction conditions were 2.5% peanut skin extracted with 50.0% ethanol for 20 min. Furthermore, the present study highlighted the possibility of using a lower amount of solvent and process time to extract phytochemicals with antioxidant properties generated as by-products in the peanut industry. These results are of practical interest for recycling/reuse of low cost feedstock. Although analysis were conducted with peanut skins, the proposed protocol can be useful in future studies.

Acknowledgments

CAP—Agroindustrial (Peanut skin samples), and FAPESP—São Paulo Research Foundation (Ph.D. scholarship – Process 2012/17683-0).

References

[1] Deng, G. F., Lin, X., Xu, X. R., Gao, L. L., Xie, J. F. & Li, H. B. (2013). Antioxidant capacities and total phenolic contents of 56 vegetables. *Journal of Functional Foods*, *5*, 260-266.

[2] Prior, R. L., Lazarus, S. A., Cao, G. H., Muccitelli, H. & Hammerstone, J. F. (2001). Identification of procyanidins and anthocyanins in blueberries and cranberries (*Vaccinium* spp.) using high-performance liquid chromatography/mass spectrometry. *Journal of Agricultural and Food Chemistry*, *49*, 1270-1276.

[3] Chandrasekara, A. & Shahidi, F. (2011). Determination of antioxidant activity in free and hydrolyzed fractions of millet grains and characterization of their phenolic profiles by HPLC-DAD-ESI-MS^n. *Journal of Functional Foods*, *3*, 144-158.

[4] Racanicci, A. M. C., Danielsen, B., Menten, J. F. M., Regitano-d'Arce, M. A. B. & Skibsted, L. H. (2004). Antioxidant effect of dittany (*Origanum dictamnus*) in pre-cooked chicken meat balls during chill-storage in comparison to rosemary (*Rosmarinus officinalis*). *European Food Research and Technology*, *218*, 521-524.

[5] Shahidi, F. & Alexander, D. M. (1998). Green tea catechins as inhibitors of oxidation of meat lipids. *Journal of Food Lipids*, *5*, 125-133.

[6] Chandrasekara, N. & Shahidi, F. (2011). Antioxidative potential of cashew phenolics in food and biological model systems as affected by roasting. *Food Chemistry*, *129*, 1388-1396.

[7] Poiana, M. A. (2012). Enhancing oxidative stability of sunflower oil during convective and microwave heating using grape seed extract. *International Journal of Molecular Sciences*, *13*, 9240-9259.

[8] Francisco, M. L. D. & Resurreccion, A. V. A. (2012). Antioxidant capacity and sensory profiles of peanut skin infusions. *Lwt-Food Science and Technology*, *47*, 189-198.

[9] Nishihira, J., Sato-Ueshima, M., Kitadate, K., Wakame, K. & Fujii, H. (2009). Amelioration of abdominal obesity by low-molecular-weight polyphenol (Oligonol) from lychee. *Journal of Functional Foods*, *1*, 341-348.

[10] Terra, X., Valls, J., Vitrac, X., Merrillon, J. M., Arola, L., Ardevol, A., Blade, C., Fernandez-Larrea, J., Pujadas, G., Salvado, J., et al. (2007). Grape-seed procyanidins act as antiinflammatory agents in endotoxin-stimulated raw 264. 7 macrophages by inhibiting NFkB signaling pathway. *Journal of Agricultural and Food Chemistry*, *55*, 4357-4365.

[11] Seeram, N. P., Adams, L. S., Zhang, Y. J., Lee, R., Sand, D., Scheuller, H. S. & Heber, D. (2006). Blackberry, black raspberry, blueberry, cranberry, red raspberry, and strawberry extracts inhibit growth and stimulate apoptosis of human cancer cells in vitro. *Journal of Agricultural and Food Chemistry*, *54*, 9329-9339.

[12] Roopchand, D. E., Kuhn, P., Rojo, L. E., Lila, M. A. & Raskin, I. (2013). Blueberry polyphenol-enriched soybean flour reduces hyperglycemia, body weight gain and serum cholesterol in mice. *Pharmacological Research*, *68*, 59-67.

[13] de Camargo, A. C., Vieira, T. M. F. S., Regitano-D'Arce, M. A. B. & Calori-Domingues, M. A., Canniatti-Brazaca, S. G. (2012). Gamma radiation effects on peanut skin antioxidants. *International Journal of Molecular Sciences*, *13*, 3073-3084.

[14] Yu, J., Ahmedna, M. & Goktepe, P. (2005). Effects of processing methods and extraction solvents on concentration and antioxidant activity of peanut skin phenolics. *Food Chemistry*, *90*, 199-206.

[15] Yu, J., Ahmedna, M., Goktepe, I. & Dai, J. (2006). Peanut skin procyanidins: Composition and antioxidant activities as affected by processing. *Journal of Food Composition and Analysis*, *19*, 364-371.

[16] Lou, H. X., Yamazaki, Y., Sasaki, T., Uchida, M., Tanaka, H. & Oka, S. (1999). A-type proanthocyanidins from peanut skins. *Phytochemistry*, *51*, 297-308.

[17] Sarnoski, P. J., Johnson, J. V., Reed, K. A., Tanko, J. M. & O'Keefe, S. F. (2012). Separation and characterisation of proanthocyanidins in Virginia type peanut skins by LC-MS^n. *Food Chemistry*, *131*, 927-939.

[18] Monagas, M., Garrido, I., Lebron-Aguilar, R., Gomez-Cordoves, M., Rybarczyk, A., Amarowicz, R. & Bartolome, B. (2009). Comparative flavan-3-ol profile and antioxidant capacity of roasted peanut, hazelnut, and almond skins. *Journal of Agricultural and Food Chemistry*, *57*, 10590-10599.

[19] Appeldoorn, M. M., Sanders, M., Vincken, J. P., Cheynier, V., Le Guerneve, C., Hollman, P. C. H. & Gruppen, H. (2009). Efficient isolation of major procyanidin A-type dimers from peanut skins and B-type dimers from grape seeds. *Food Chemistry*, *117*, 713-720.

[20] Lou, H. X., Yuan, H. Q., Yamazaki, Y., Sasaki, T. & Oka, S. C. Alkaloids and flavonoids from peanut skins. *Planta Medica* (2001, *67*, 345-349.

[21] Ballard, T. S., Mallikarjunan, P., Zhou, K. Q. & O'Keefe, S. Microwave-assisted extraction of phenolic antioxidant compounds from peanut skins. (2010). *Food Chemistry*, *120*, 1185-1192.

[22] Ballard, T. S., Mallikarjunan, P., Zhou, K. & O'Keefe, S. F. (2009). Optimizing the extraction of phenolic antioxidants from peanut skins using response surface methodology. *Journal of Agricultural and Food Chemistry*, *57*, 3064-3072.

[23] Francisco, M. L. D. & Resurreccion, A. V. A. (2009). Development of a reversed-phase high performance liquid chromatography (RP-HPLC) procedure for the simultaneous determination of phenolic compounds in peanut skin extracts. *Food Chemistry*, *117*, 356-363.

[24] Sarnoski, P. J., Boyer, R. R. & O'Keefe, S. F. (2012). Application of proanthocyanidins from peanut skins as a natural yeast inhibitory agent. *Journal of Food Science*, *77*, M242-M249.

[25] Nepote, V., Grosso, N. R. & Guzman, C. A. (2005). Optimization of extraction of phenolic antioxidants from peanut skins. *Journal of the Science of Food and Agriculture*, *85*, 33-38.

[26] Sobolev, V. S. & Cole, R. J. (2004). Note on utilisation of peanut seed testa. *Journal of the Science of Food and Agriculture*, *84*, 105-111.

[27] Swain, T. & Hillis, W. E. (1959). The phenolic constituents of *Prunus domestica*. I. — The quantitative analysis of phenolic constituents. *Journal of the Science of Food and Agriculture*, *10*, 63-68.

[28] de Camargo, A., Vieira, T., Regitano-D'Arce, M., Calori-Domingues, M. & Canniatti-Brazaca, S. (2012). Gamma radiation effects on peanut skin antioxidants. *International Journal of Molecular Sciences*, *13*, 3073-3084.

[29] Benzie, I. F. F. & Strain, J. J. (1996). The ferric reducing ability of plasma (FRAP) as a measure of "antioxidant power": The frap assay. *Analytical Biochemistry*, *239*, 70-76.

[30] Brand-Williams, W., Cuvelier, M. E. & Berset, C. (1995). Use of a free radical method to evaluate antioxidant activity. *LWT Food Science and Technology*, *28*, 25-30.

[31] Re, R., Pellegrini, N., Proteggente, A., Pannala, A., Yang, M. & Rice-Evans, C. (1999). Antioxidant activity applying an improved ABTS radical cation decolorization assay. *Free Radical Biology and Medicine*, *26*, 1231-1237.

[32] Ou, B., Hampsch-Woodill, M. & Prior, R. L. (2001). Development and validation of an improved oxygen radical absorbance capacity assay using fluorescein as the fluorescent probe. *Journal of Agricultural and Food Chemistry*, *49*, 4619-4626.

[33] Paiva-Martins, F. & Gordon, M. H. (2002). Effects of pH and ferric ions on the antioxidant activity of olive polyphenols in oil-in-water emulsions. *Journal of the American Oil Chemists Society*, *79*, 571-576.

[34] Harrison, K. & Were, L. M. (2007). Effect of gamma irradiation on total phenolic content yield and antioxidant capacity of almond skin extracts. *Food Chemistry*, *102*, 932-937.

[35] Rice-Evans, C. A., Miller, N. J. & Paganga, G. (1996). Structure-antioxidant activity relationships of flavonoids and phenolic acids. *Free Radical Biology and Medicine*, *21*, 417-417.

[36] Ou, B. X., Huang, D. J., Hampsch-Woodill, M., Flanagan, J. A. & Deemer, E. K. (2002). Analysis of antioxidant activities of common vegetables employing oxygen radical absorbance capacity (ORAC) and ferric reducing antioxidant power (FRAP) assays: A comparative study. *Journal of Agricultural and Food Chemistry*, *50*, 3122-3128.

[37] Benzie, I. F., Chung, W. & Strain, J. J. (1999). "Antioxidant" (reducing) efficiency of ascorbate in plasma is not affected by concentration. *The Journal of Nutritional Biochemistry*, *10*, 146-150.

[38] Wolfenden, B. S. & Willson, R. L. (1982). Radical-cations as reference chromogens in kinetic studies of ono-electron transfer reactions: Pulse radiolysis studies of 2,2 [prime or minute]-azinobis-(3-ethylbenzthiazoline-6-sulphonate). *Journal of the Chemical Society, Perkin Transactions 2*, *0*, 805-812.

[39] Cao, G., Verdon, C. P., Wu, A. H. B., Wang, H. & Prior, R. L. (1995). Automated-assay of oxygen radical absorbency capacity with the COBAS FARA-II. *Clinical Chemistry*, *41*, 1738-1744.

In: Peanuts
Editor: Richard W. Cook

ISBN: 978-1-63321-013-4

Chapter 3

GAMMA IRRADIATION TO IMPROVE MICROBIOLOGICAL SAFETY OF PEANUTS: EFFECTS ON PEROXIDE VALUE, HS-SPME–GC/MS HEXANAL CONTENT AND SENSORY ACCEPTANCE

Adriano Costa de Camargo*[*], *Marisa Aparecida Bismara Regitano-d'Arce*, *Thais Maria Ferreira de Souza Vieira*, *Severino Matias de Alencar, Claudio Rosa Gallo*, *Marta Helena Fillet Spoto*, *Paula Porrelli Moreira da Silva* and *Solange Guidolin Canniatti-Brazaca

Department of Agri-Food Industry, Food & Nutrition, ''Luiz de Queiroz''
College of Agriculture (ESALQ/USP),
University of São Paulo, Brazil

[*] Corresponding author: E-Mail: adrianoesalq@gmail.com.

ABSTRACT

In-shell peanuts were submitted to gamma irradiation (2.5, 5.0, 7.5 and 10.0 kGy) and evaluated on their microbiological safety. Yeasts and molds were detected in non-irradiated samples but not in irradiated ones. 5.0 kGy was suitable in reducing the total coliform count by two log cycles, thus 5.0 kGy was chosen to be the highest dose for further analyses. Peroxide value and hexanal content significantly increased at 5.0 and 2.5 kGy, respectively. Taste was the only sensory attribute statistically different and this was noticed only at 5.0 kGy. However, there was no rejection in this sample. The purchase intent was not affected by any gamma irradiation dose. 2.5 kGy can be used to improve microbiological safety but better results are reached with 5.0 kGy. To the best of our knowledge there is no other publication that addresses the microbiological safety, oxidation status and their relation on sensory results of in-shell gamma irradiated peanuts. Also, it is not common to achieve sensory acceptance of nuts with doses as high as 5.0 kGy, therefore this report will be helpful for the peanut industry.

Keywords: Cobalt-60; microbiology, oxidation status; volatile compounds, sensory evaluation

1. INTRODUCTION

Highly unsaturated fatty acids have positive effects in reducing the risk of certain forms of cardiovascular and inflammatory diseases [1]. Also the role of food phenolics and polyphenolics in the prevention of cardiovascular disease and certain types of cancer is well recognized [2]. IAC-Runner 886 peanut cultivar has a high percentage of unsaturated fatty acids, proteins, tocopherols [3], and polyphenols [4]. However, there is a concern about peanut consumption since potential mycotoxigenic fungi in peanuts and peanut products are a problem for the peanut industry. Worldwide regulations for aflatoxins limit their levels in food to 20 μg/kg or less; however, it is difficult or even impossible to attain such low concentrations due to environmental conditions in most places where peanuts are produced and stored [5], creating an economical issue. As with other food products, peanuts and peanut products also need to fit other microbiological standards regarding *Escherichia coli* and *Salmonella*.

Gamma irradiation of peanuts at 5.0 kGy [6] has been found to be an effective treatment to completely eliminate mycotoxic fungi in peanuts. Insects are known to be vectors of mycotoxin-producing fungi [7]. Low doses of gamma irradiation (0.2–0.8 kGy) are also efficient for killing and sterilizing insects [8]. However, gamma irradiation induced oxidation has been an issue to be addressed. In a six month experiment [3], regarding the oxidation stability of peanuts we provided evidence indicating that, if gamma irradiation is considered an alternative for industrial-scale conservation, in-shell peanuts are the best feedstock. We also presented results [4] indicating that, during one year storage, no correlation was found between gamma irradiation and antioxidant activity, total phenolic content and fatty acid profile in in-shell peanuts. Furthermore, 5.0 kGy protected against mycotoxigenic fungi.

Mexis et al. [9] have been working on ways of improving the gamma irradiation treatment. One of their studies was performed on gamma irradiated almond kernels, taking into account active and modified atmosphere packaging, the container oxygen barrier, and storage conditions. Our research group has also been searching for improved ways of applying gamma irradiation, mostly with focus on decreasing gamma irradiation induced oxidation [3,4]. To the best of our knowledge there is no information in the literature on in-shell gamma irradiated peanuts regarding its sensory acceptance. Thus, based on previous reports [3,4] the present study aimed to investigate other natural microflora (microbiological safety), peroxide value (primary oxidation compounds), hexanal content (a secondary oxidation product that plays an important role in organoleptic properties of lipid foods), and most important, the sensory acceptance of in-shell gamma irradiated peanut samples (cv. IAC-Runner 886) subjected to doses selected on basis of microbiological safety. Our previous work has been performed with the minimum dose around 5.0 kGy. However, in order to understand the course of gamma irradiation effects, in the present study we also provided data about the effect of low gamma irradiation dose (2.5 kGy). The results presented here will be helpful for the peanut industry.

2. Experimental Section

2.1. Material

In-shell peanut samples (cv. IAC-Runner 886) were kindly donated by CAP—Agroindustrial, Dumont, São Paulo State, Brazil.

2.2. Methods

2.2.1. Irradiation Process

In-shell peanut samples (cv. IAC-Runner 886) were separated into 1.5-kg portions and placed in polyethylene plastic bags. The bags (excluding controls) were irradiated at tentative doses of 2.50, 5.00, 7.50, and 10.0 kGy, at a dose rate of 3.75 kGy/h. The minimum absorbed doses were 2.5, 5.10, 7.50, and 10.3, respectively. Dosimetric measurements were carried out with a Harwell Perspex polymethylmethacrylate Amber 3042 dosimeter (PMMA Instruments, Harwell, UK). The irradiation process was carried out in the city of São Paulo, São Paulo State, Brazil. A multipurpose Cobalt-60 γ-irradiation apparatus from the Nuclear Energy Research Institute (IPEN) was used. The samples were irradiated in air, at temperature of 20 °C, and stored at room temperature until the moment of microbiological, lipid and sensory analyses.

2.2.2. Safety evaluation

2.2.2.1. Sample preparation

Gamma irradiated in-shell peanuts were removed from their shells at the time of analysis. The samples (25 g) and 225 mL of peptone water 0.1% (Merck, Whitehouse Station, NJ, USA) were crushed in a sterilized blender to obtain the first dilution. Serial 10-fold dilutions using peptone water (0.1%) were prepared from the first one.

2.2.2.2. Salmonella spp

The TECRA Unique *Salmonella* Test (3M Microbiology Products, St. Paul, MN, USA) described by the method 2000.07 from AOAC [10] was used for detection of *Salmonella* spp. The TECRA Unique *Salmonella* Test is broken down into six stages: capturing, washing, replicating, conjugate binding, washing, and finally color development. All the steps were performed in accordance to the official method and the results were read as recommended by the supplier.

2.2.2.3. Yeasts and Molds

The samples (0.1 mL of each dilution) were analyzed in acidified Potato Dextrose Agar medium (Difco Laboratories, Detroit, MI, USA) followed by incubation at 25 °C for 3-5 days, according to the method described by Downes and Ito [11]

2.2.2.4. Coliform bacteria

The SimPlate Coliform and *Escherichia coli* Color Indicator (CEc-CI) medium, method 2005.03 from AOAC [12], was used for the detection and quantification of total coliform and *E. coli*. The SimPlate device (BioControl, Bellevue, WA, USA) was filled by 1 mL of each sample dilution and CEc-CI. The incubation was carried out at 35 ºC over 24 h. The wells that presented color changes from the background were counted for total coliforms. The wells with fluorescence color change (UV light, 366 nm) were counted for *E. coli.*

2.2.3. Chemical evaluation

2.2.3.1. Oil Extraction

For analysis of the lipid fraction of peanuts, samples were cold pressed with a Carver Press (Carver, Inc., Wabash, IN, USA). After pressing, crude peanut oil samples were filtered and transferred to amber bottles, nitrogen was injected and the oil samples were frozen (−18 °C) until analyses.

2.2.3.2. Peroxide value

The peroxide value, in terms of lipid hydroperoxide (LOOH) concentrations, was determined by ferric ion complex measurement spectrophotometry method, according to Shanta and Decker [13], with slight modifications reported by Branco and Castro [14]. The method is based on the ability of lipid hydroperoxides to oxidize ferrous ions (Fe^{+2}) to ferric ions (Fe^{+3}). The red-violet ferric thiocyanate complex presents strong absorption at the range of 500 to 510 nm. This method is more sensitive than iodometric titration assay, which is based on the oxidation of the iodide ion (I^-) by hydroperoxides present in the samples. For better comprehension, all solutions are described first. Solution 1: $BaCl_2$ (0.132M) was prepared in HCl (0.4 M). Solution 2: Fe^{+2} (0.072 M) was obtained from the mixture (1:1, v/v) of $FeSO_4$ (0.144) and $BaCl_2$ (0.132M). Solution 3: NH_4SCN:Fe^{2+} (1:1, v/v) was obtained by mixture of NH_4SCN (3.94 M) and Fe^{+2} (0.072 M). For analysis, cold pressed peanut oils were weighed (0.3 g) and mixed with 1.5 mL iso-octane/2-propanol solution (3:1, v/v). The mixture was vortexed three times for 10 seconds, and 200 μL of the resultant mixture was added to a 2.8 mL solution of methanol/n-butanol (2:1, v/v). Finally, 30 μL of NH_4SCN:Fe^{2+} (1:1, v/v) were added. The tubes were vortexed and incubated at room temperature for 20 minutes. The absorbance was read at 510 nm using a Shimadzu UV-1800 spectrophotometer (Shimadzu Corporation, Kyoto, Japan). The peroxide value (meq LOOH/kg oil) was calculated using a standard curve of cumene hydroperoxide.

2.2.3.3. Headspace solid-phase microextraction (HS-SPME) procedure

The standard curve was prepared by direct hexanal dissolution in non-irradiated cold-pressed peanut oil to eliminate the influence of the solvent presence in high concentrations compared to hexanal, and consequently its absorption on the fiber. The solid-phase microextraction was performed with a divinylbenzene (DVB)-carboxen-polydimethylsiloxane (PDMS), 50/30 cm, 2 cm long fiber assembly coupled to a SPME manual holder assembly (Supelco, Bellefonte, PA, USA). SPME fiber was preconditioned as recommended by the supplier (1 h at 270 ºC). 5 g of peanut oil sample, or peanut oil spiked with hexanal, was placed in a 20 mL headspace vial crimped with an aluminium seal containing a rubber septum and kept at 80 °C in water bath for 30 min. The polytetrafluoroethylene/silicone septum covering the vial was pierced with a SPME needle to expose the fiber to the oil headspace for 10 min. Finally, the fiber was retracted into the needle and was immediately injected into the gas chromatograph.

2.2.3.4. Determination of hexanal content by gas chromatography–mass spectrometry (GC-MS)

GC-MS analyses of the hexanal absorbed onto the SPME fibre was performed on a gas chromatograph GC 2010 (Shimadzu Corp., Kyoto, Japan) coupled to a mass spectrometer QP 2010 Plus (Shimadzu Corp., Kyoto, Japan). A capillary column (RTX-5MS 30 m × 0.25 mm × 0.25 μm, Restek, Bellefonte, PA, USA) was used. The temperature program started at 32 °C. After 3 min the temperature was raised to 60 °C at a rate of 5 °C/min. This temperature was kept for 3 min, and then was raised to 200 ºC at 8 °C/min, remaining at 200 °C for 10 min. Finally, the temperature was raised to 280 °C at 20 °C/min, remaining at this temperature for 5 min. Helium was used as the carrier gas at a flow rate of 1.0 mL/min. The injector (splitless mode) and the ion source were operated at 270 and 200 °C, respectively. The interface was kept at 200 °C and the detector was operated in single ion monitoring (SIM) mode with the following ions, *m/z*: 44, 56, 41, 100. Data integration was performed using the LabSolutions-GCMS software (Shimadzu Corp., Kyoto, Japan). Hexanal was identified by comparing its retention time and ion fragmentation with a coded and authentic standard (Sigma-Aldrich, St Louis, MO, USA) under the same conditions as well as with the Wiley Version 8 library.

2.2.4. Sensory Evaluation

Sensorial analyses were performed as soon as the samples were checked for their microbiological safety (within a week). An untrained panel (60 members), composed by students and employees from "Luiz de Queiroz" College of Agriculture (ESALQ/USP), aged between 18 and 60 years, participated of the acceptability test. 20 g of peanuts (removed from their shells) were placed in small plastic cups coded with three-digit random numbers and offered to the panel. All members were served by a set of three samples (control, 2.50 and 5.0 kGy) and water at room temperature. They were asked to rinse their mouth between each sample. Color, odor, taste, texture, and global impression were evaluated. Scores were recorded on a paper ballot using a five-point hedonic scale (5 = extremely like, 4 = like, 3 = neither like nor dislike, 2 = dislike, and 1 = extremely dislike). In addition, the purchase intent was evaluated (5 = definitely would buy, 4 = probably would buy, 3 = maybe buy/maybe not buy, 2 = probably would not buy, and 1 = definitely would not buy). Scores of ≥ 3 points were considered as acceptable.

2.2.5. Statistical Analysis

A completely randomized design with three replicates per treatment was used. Analyses of variance and Tukey's test ($p < 0.05$) were performed with SAS software.

3. Results and Discussion

3.1. Microbiological Evaluation

The effectiveness of gamma irradiation in inhibiting microbial growth is shown in Table 1. As can be noticed 5.0 kGy was able to reduce the total coliform count by two log cycles. No *Escherichia coli* was found in any sample, gamma irradiated or not. The present results agree with Wilson-Kakashita, Gerdes and Hall [15] whose study with English walnuts demonstrated that gamma irradiation at 5.0 kGy was efficient at inhibiting coliform bacteria growth.

Table 1. Gamma irradiation effects* on microbiological characteristics of in-shell peanuts

Microorganisms**	0.0 kGy	2.5 kGy	5.0 kGy	7.5 kGy	10.0 kGy
Yeasts and Molds (CFU/g)***	7.8 x 10^2	<10	<10	<10	<10
Total Coliform (MPN/g)****	4.8 x 10^3	<10	4 x 10	2 x 10	<10
Escherichia coli (MPN/g)	<10	<10	<10	<10	<10

*Mean values of duplicate samples for each test procedure;
***Salmonella* was absent in 25g in every sample
*** CFU = Colony Forming Unity;
**** MPN = Most Probable Number.

In the current study, yeast and molds were not detected in gamma irradiated samples. Yeast and molds analysis includes the mycotoxigenic fungi, an economical problem for the peanut industry. In a previous work [4] it was demonstrated that 5.0 kGy was efficient for the decontamination of mycotoxigenic fungi in blanched peanuts. Regarding fungal count, Al-Bachir [16] demonstrated that 2.0 kGy was the suitable dose for gamma irradiated walnuts, which are in good agreement with the present study.

Aziz and Mahrous [17] showed that no aflatoxin B1 was detected in inoculated seeds (10^6 *A. flavus* spores) after 30 days of incubation at 28ºC. According to the authors, this was due to 5.0 kGy gamma irradiation applied on those samples. Furthermore, control seeds were found having values as high as 280, 210, and 100 μg/kg for wheat, soybean and fababean, respectively. These values are higher than those tolerated by most countries [5] that have adopted regulations for aflatoxins in food to a max 20 μg/kg.

The present study also focused on sensory evaluation. To ensure the safety of the peanuts consumed by the panel, coagulase-positive *Staphylococcus aureus* and aflatoxins were also investigated (data not shown). No coagulase-positive *Staphylococcus aureus* was detected and aflatoxin was under the detection limit (detection limit for aflatoxins B1 and G1 = 0.5 μg/kg and for aflatoxins B2 e G2 = 0.3 μg/kg).

Although better results could be achieved with 5.0 kGy the data presented here shows that 2.5 kGy can be applied to improve the microbiological safety of in-shell peanuts with good results. *Salmonella* was absent in 25g of every sample. *E. coli* was also absent in all samples. Yeasts and molds in control samples satisfied the Brazilian food legislation [18], thus these samples were able to be served to the sensory panel. Matching results of our previous work

[4] with the microbiological characteristics evaluated on the present study, 5.0 kGy was chosen as the maximum dose for sensory evaluation. This data is helpful for the peanut industry because the higher the dose the larger the gamma irradiation induced oxidation.

3.2. Oxidation Status

3.2.1. Peroxide Value

Like other conservation methods, gamma irradiation may change the sensory attributes and the extent of that depends on several factors. For high lipid foods, lipid percentage, fatty acid composition, moisture content, presence of antioxidants, in addition to the surface structure and porosity of the food product, affect its stability [19]. In-shell IAC-Runner 886 peanuts have already been studied by our research group. Their proximate compositions percentages were: 2.1 (ash), 46.5 (lipid), 20.3 (protein), 25.9 (fiber), and 7.5 (carbohydrates). The major fatty acids (g/100 g of crude oil) were 13.3 (C16:0), 44.9 (C18:1, ω9) and 37.1 (C18:2, ω6), while saturated, monounsaturated and polyunsaturated fatty acids, accounted for 16.5, 37.1, and 46.4 (g/100 g of crude oil), respectively. Tocopherol contents (mg/100 g of crude oil) were 19.1 (α-Tocopherol), 0.6 (β-Tocopherol), 24.4 (γ-Tocopherol), and 1.1 (δ-Tocopherol) [3]. The total phenolic content was 4.6 mg gallic acid equivalent/g, with antioxidant activity (ABTS method) of 17.0 μmol TEAC/g [4]. This information is useful for the present study.

In a previous work [3] it was demonstrated that gamma irradiation was less harmful to the tocopherol content in in-shell peanuts than in peeled ones. Additionally, the lowest induction period evaluated by Oil Stability Index Rancimat method was found in the first one, which suggested that in-shell gamma irradiated peanuts were more stable to termoxidation than peeled peanuts. It was also demonstrated that gamma irradiated in-shell peanuts presented less secondary oxidation products than those of blanched and peeled samples.

The model proposed by Farmer et al. [20] shows the formation of free radicals as the initial step in the mechanism of lipid autoxidation. Ionizing radiation is sufficiently high in energy to remove an electron from water, which is the main component of foods and living organisms. It also generates reactive species, including free radicals such as the hydroxyl radical and hydrogen peroxide [21]. The higher the dose the larger the gamma irradiation induced free radical.

Hydroperoxides (primary oxidation compounds) decompose homolytically and generate alkoxyl radicals. These radicals suffer cleavage and form aldehydes and other breakdown products (secondary oxidation compounds) which contribute to oxidative and flavour deterioration in lipid foods [22]. The peroxide value, in terms of lipid hydroperoxide (LOOH) concentrations, is shown in Table 2. Gamma irradiation increased peroxide value at 5.0 kGy ($p < 0.05$). This trend is in accordance with the data from Gölge and Ova [23] in gamma irradiated (up to 5.0 kGy) pine nuts. Figure 1 suggests the gamma irradiation induced free radical pathway.

Fatty acids or acylglycerol can have their hydrogen atoms removed by gamma irradiation induced free radicals (1a), which are the initiators on the lipid oxidation chain (Figure 1) and the alkyl radical produced at this stage can react with oxygen, raising lipid peroxyl radical concentrations (2). Antioxidants can inhibit hydroperoxide formation (3), by scavenging free radicals present at the initiation step (1b). In this case, the antioxidant radical previously produced can undergo termination reaction generating the covalently linked tocopheryl dimer (1c). If this is not the case, which was assumed for the present work since peroxide value increased (Table 2), the reaction chain goes on and other fatty acids can have hydrogen atoms removed by the lipid peroxyl radical previously formed and produce hydroperoxide plus alkyl radicals (3). Hydroperoxides decompose to alkoxyl radical (4), which break into aldehydes and other breakdown products (5). Antioxidants can also act at this point by inhibiting reaction decompositions that would lead to flavour deterioration. According to Frankel and Meyer [22] these inhibitions can occur by hydrogen donation to form stable hydroxy compounds (6) or by the termination reactions (7). In a previous work [3] we demonstrated that the occurrence of gamma irradiation induced oxidation was dependent on tocopherol content in peanut samples, but not entirely prevented. At that time, it was assumed that in-shell gamma irradiated peanuts had less oxygen available, and light absence, thus these factors and the high tocopherol content could have interacted and might explain why in-shell gamma irradiated peanuts were the best feedstock for irradiation. While Mexis et al. [24] reported eight-fold increase in peroxide value for gamma irradiated raw peanuts (7.0 kGy) the current work found less than two-fold increase at 5.0 kGy. This difference can also be due to in-shell irradiation, low oxygen availability and light absence.

Table 2. Gamma irradiation effects[1] on oxidation status in-shell peanuts

Oxidation Status	0.0 kGy	2.5 kGy	5.0 kGy
Peroxide Value (meq LOOH/kg oil)[2]	23.41 ± 0.30a[3]	24.97 ± 1.34a	33.79 ± 2.04b
Hexanal Content (mg/kg oil)	0.16 ± 0.03a	0.26 ± 0.00b	0.71 ± 0.01c

[1]Data represent the means of triplicate analysis for each sample ± standard deviations;
[2] meq = miliequivalent; LOOH = Lipid hydroperoxide;
[3] means with the same letters within a row are not different according to Tukey's multiple test ($p > 0.05$).

3.2.2. Determination of Hexanal Content by Gas Chromatography–Mass Spectrometry (GC-MS)

There was an increase of hexanal concentration in in-shell gamma irradiated peanuts ($p < 0.05$). Hexanal concentrations presented here (Table 2) are in good agreement with those reported by Mexis et al. [9] in raw, unpeeled almond kernels submitted to doses up to 3.0 kGy. The greatest systematic variation of the relative levels of free radicals in peanuts were due to the light, whereas the oxygen availability had the largest influence on the formation of hexanal [19]. Secondary oxidation compounds (aldehydes, ketones, hydrocarbons, etc.) are the major sensory problem to be addressed in high lipid foods and hexanal is widely used as an indicator of flavour deterioration. Hexanal presents low threshold; values as low as 5 μg/kg were reported by Buttery, Turnbaugh and Ling [25] and more recently Cometto-Muñiz and Abraham [26] reported the value of 0.33 μg/kg. This aliphatic aldehyde is generated from linoleic acid oxidation, which is one of the major fatty acids from IAC-Runner 886 peanut cultivar [3]. The ratio of the oxidation rates of stearic, oleic and linoleic acids was 1:10:100 [27]. Thus, even when linoleic acid is in lower concentration in comparison to oleic acid, which is the case of IAC-Runner 886 peanut cultivar used in this work, hexanal is the most representative of secondary oxidation products.

3.2.3. Sensory Evaluation

Table 3 shows the sensory evaluation scores of in-shell gamma irradiated peanut samples. Color is most likely the first rejection factor experienced by consumers. Several works have demonstrated that gamma irradiation affects the color of nuts [9,24,28,29] and other food products. Peanut skin color varies from light brown to deep red, and most color pigments in plants, especially red, purple and blue, belong to the flavonoid class of anthocyanins, with other flavonoid compounds acting as co-pigments [30].

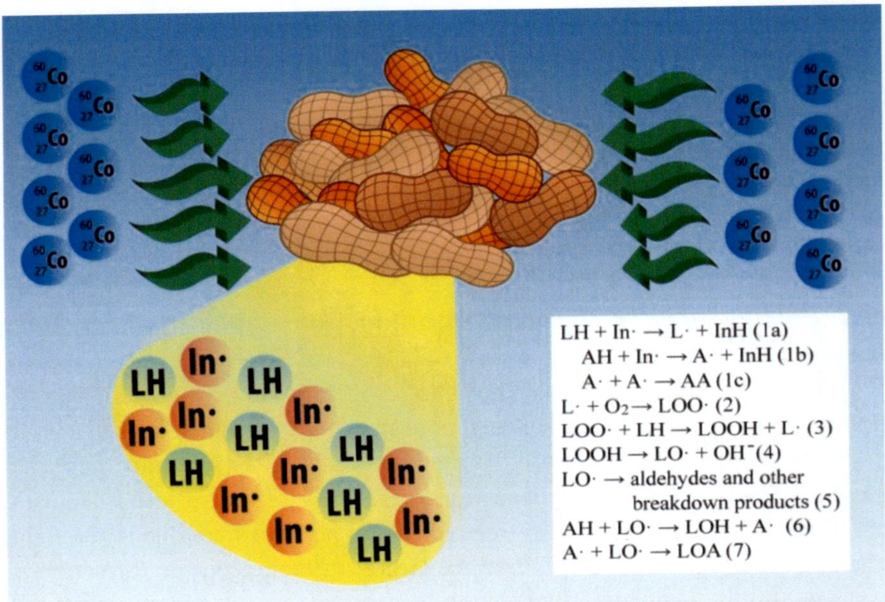

LH, Lipid alkyl; In·, Gamma irradiation induced free radicals; L·, Alkyl radical; AH, Antioxidant; A·, Antioxidant free radical; AA, Termination reaction product; LOO·, Lipid peroxyl radical; LOOH, Lipid hydroperoxide; LO·, Alcoxyl radical, LOH, Hydroxy compounds; LOA, Termination reaction product.

Figure 1. Gamma irradiation induced free radical oxidation pathway.

Table 3. Gamma irradiation effects[1] on sensory acceptance of in-shell peanuts

Dose (kGy)	Color	Odor	Taste	Texture	Global Impression	Purchase Intent
0.0	3.5 ± 1.0a[2]	3.3 ± 0.8a	3.7 ± 1.0a	3.8 ± 1.0a	3.7 ± 0.9a	3.4 ± 1.3a
2.5	3.6 ± 0.9a	3.3 ± 0.7a	3.4 ± 1.1ab	3.8 ± 1.0a	3.5 ± 1.1a	3.2 ± 1.3a
5.0	3.6 ± 1.0a	3.3 ± 0.8a	3.1 ± 1.3b	3.5 ± 1.0a	3.3 ± 1.1a	3.0 ± 1.4a

[1] Data represent the mean score ± standard deviation (n = 60);

[2] means with the same letters within a column are not different according to Tukey's multiple test ($p > 0.05$).

IAC-Runner 886 peanut skin has phenolic compounds such as condensed tannin (proanthocyanidins) and flavonoids [31]. Phenolic and antioxidant compounds are involved in redox reactions [32,33] leading to color changes. In this path gamma irradiation, which involves free radical reaction products [21], may cause color changes. In the present work the color was unaffected by gamma irradiation, which is in good agreement with our previous work [4]. We have found that, even during long term storage under room temperature, no correlation was found between gamma irradiation and objective color measurements (L*, Chroma, and °Hue).

In the present study the odor, texture and the global impression scores were also unaffected. The current results regarding texture attribute agree with those reported in the literature [24] for gamma irradiated (up to 7.0 kGy) raw peanuts. However, the odor results are different than those previously reported. This could be due to the lowest hexanal concentration in the present work (0.71 mg/kg oil) when compared with the values reported by Mexis et al. [24] (3.68 mg/kg of raw peanuts), both with doses of 5.0 kGy. Hexanal presents a low threshold [25,26] thus, few variations can affect sensory attributes.

Sensory differences were found in pine nuts irradiated with doses up to 5.0 kGy [23]. No correlation was revealed with the irradiation dose though. No significant differences were observed between irradiated (up to 2.0 kGy) and non-irradiated walnut samples in flavor and aroma immediately after irradiation [16]. Cashew nuts [28] remained sensory acceptable with doses < 3.0 kGy, while doses up to 1.5 kGy were acceptable for hazelnuts [29]. Almonds [34], peanuts, and pistachio nuts [24] can be treated with doses up to 3.0 kGy. For the authors, taste was the most gamma irradiation sensitive attribute.

In the present work, taste was the only attribute significantly influenced ($p < 0.05$) by gamma irradiation (5.0 kGy). This is supported by the peroxide values (Table 2). At 5.0 kGy in-shell gamma irradiated peanuts presented peroxide value of 33.79 meq LOOH/kg oil. Indeed it was expected that the sensory panel had noticed flavour alterations once the peroxide concentration was higher than 25 meq O_2/kg oil, which is the threshold for nut oils reported in the literature [35]. The taste scores decreased as the hydroperoxides and hexanal concentrations increased, meanwhile a score of $\geq$ 3 points was considered acceptable, thus none of the samples was rejected by the panel. This was confirmed by the purchase intent test, which demonstrated that gamma irradiation did not lead rejection by the consumers. No significant difference ($p < 0.05$) was observed regarding the purchase intent among the samples.

Although the panel (60 members) was constituted by volunteers (which means they came to the test on their own will), 85% of them reported taste as the major reason for peanuts consumption. Thus, the present results are representative. Still it is worth noting another statement from the panel. When asked which kind of peanuts they were used to consuming (blanched; without skin or peeled; with skin), most of them (67%) answered "I consume mostly blanched peanuts" and only 33% answered "I consume mostly peeled peanuts". Brazilian consumers also prefer consuming roasted, salted, spicy or sweet crusted peanuts. This probably influenced the final scores for purchase intent.

Conclusion

Gamma irradiation at 5.0 kGy can be applied to improve microbiological safety of in-shell peanuts. While hydroperoxides were statistically different at 5.0 kGy, hexanal content was increased at 2.5 kGy. Color, odor and texture were not affected by gamma irradiation. The sensory score for taste decreased at 5.0 kGy. However, since taste score was ≥ 3 points (considered as acceptable) this was not interpreted as a rejection issue. The purchase intent was not influenced by gamma irradiation treatment, thus in-shell gamma irradiation at 5.0 kGy are sensory and commercially viable. It is worth looking for post-harvest decontamination alternatives. Thus, the results presented here wil likely be helpful for the peanut industry.

Acknowledgments

Nuclear Energy Research Institute (Irradiation process), CAP—Agroindustrial (Peanut samples), and FAPESP—São Paulo Research Foundation (Ph.D. scholarship – Process 2012/17683-0 and Financial Support – Process 2009/18215-8).

REFERENCES

[1] Finley, J. W. & Shahidi, F. (2001). The chemistry, processing, and health benefits of highly unsaturated fatty acids: An overview. In *Omega-3 fatty acids*, American Chemical Society, Vol. *788*, 2-11.

[2] Shahidi, F. (2004). Functional foods: Their role in health promotion and disease prevention. *Journal of Food Science*, *69*, R146-R149.

[3] de Camargo, A. C., Vieira, T. M. F. S., Regitano-D'Arce, M. A. B., de Alencar, S. M., Calori-Domingues, M. A. & Canniatti-Brazaca, S. G. (2012). Gamma radiation induced oxidation and tocopherols decrease in in-shell, peeled and blanched peanuts. *International Journal of Molecular Sciences*, *13*, 2827-2845.

[4] de Camargo, A. C., Vieira, T. M. F. S., Regitano-d'Arce, M. A. B., de Alencar, S. M., Calori-Domingues, M. A., Spoto, M. H. F. & Canniatti-Brazaca, S. G. (2012). Gamma irradiation of in-shell and blanched peanuts protects against mycotoxic fungi and retains their nutraceutical components during long-term storage. *International Journal of Molecular Sciences*, *13*, 10935-10958.

[5] Dorner, J. W. (2008). Management and prevention of mycotoxins in peanuts. *Food Additives and Contaminants*, *25*, 203-208.

[6] Chiou, R. Y. Y., Lin, C. M. & Shyu, S. L. (1990). Property characterization of peanut kernels subjected to gamma irradiation and its effect on the outgrowth and aflatoxin production by *Aspergillus parasiticus*. *Journal of Food Science*, *55*, 210–213.

[7] Nesci, A., Montemarani, A. & Etcheverry, M. (2011). Assessment of mycoflora and infestation of insects, vector of *Aspergillus* section *flavi*, in stored peanut from Argentina. *Mycotoxin Research*, *27*, 5-12.

[8] Farkas, J. (2006). Irradiation for better foods. *Trends in Food Science & Technology*, *17*, 148-152.

[9] Mexis, S. F., Riganakos, K. A. & Kontominas, M. G. (2011). Effect of irradiation, active and modified atmosphere packaging, container oxygen barrier and storage conditions on the physicochemical and sensory properties of raw unpeeled almond kernels (*Prunus dulcis*). *Journal of the Science and Food Agriculture*, *91*, 634-649.

[10] AOAC. *Official methods of analysis of AOAC international*. 17th ed., AOAC International: Gaithersburg, MD, USA, 2002.

[11] Downes, F. P. & Ito, K. (2001). *Compendium of methods for the microbiological examination of food*. 4th ed., American Public Health Association: Washington, DC.

[12] AOAC. (2006). *Official methods of analysis of AOAC international*. 18th ed., Association of Official Analytical Chemists: Gaithersburg, MD.

[13] Shantha, N. C. & Decker, E. (1994). Rapid, sensitive, iron-based spectrophotometric methods for determination of peroxide values of food lipids. *Journal of AOAC International*, *77*, 421-424.

[14] Branco, G. & Castro, I. (2011). Optimization of oil oxidation by response surface methodology and the application of this model to evaluate antioxidants. *Journal of the American Oil Chemists Society*, *88*, 1747-1758.

[15] Wilson-Kakashita, G., Gerdes, D. L. & Hall, W. R. (1995). The effect of gamma-irradiation on the quality of english walnuts (*Juglans regia*). *Food Science and Technology-Lebensmittel-Wissenschaft & Technologie*, *28*, 17-20.

[16] Al-Bachir, M. (2004). Effect of gamma irradiation on fungal load, chemical and sensory characteristics of walnuts (*Juglans regia* L.). *Journal of Stored Products Research*, *40*, 355-362.

[17] Aziz, N. H. & Mahrous, S. R. (2004). Effect of γ-irradiation on aflatoxin B1 production by *Aspergillus flavus* and chemical composition of three crop seeds. *Food/Nahrung*, *48*, 234-238.

[18] Brasil. (2001). Resolução - RDC n° 12, de 2 de janeiro de 2001. Regulamento técnico sobre os padrões microbiológicos para alimentos. Agência Nacional de Vigilância Sanitária: Brasília, DF, Brasil.

[19] Jensen, P. N., Danielsen, B., Bertelsen, G., Skibsted, L. H. & Andersen, M. L. (2005). Storage stabilities of pork scratchings, peanuts, oatmeal and muesli: Comparison of ESR spectroscopy, headspace-GC and sensory evaluation for detection of oxidation in dry foods. *Food Chemistry*, *91*, 25 - 38.

[20] Farmer, E. H., Bloomfield, G. F., Sundralingam, A. & Sutton, D. A. (1942). The course and mechanism of autoxidation reactions in olefinic and polyolefinic substances, including rubber. *Transactions of the Faraday Society*, *38*, 348-356.

[21] Kilcast, D. (1995). Food irradiation: Current problems and future potential. *International Biodeterioration & Biodegradation*, *36*, 279-296.

[22] Frankel, E. N., Meyer, A. S. (2000). The problems of using one-dimensional methods to evaluate multifunctional food and biological antioxidants. *Journal of the Science of Food and Agriculture*, *80*, 1925-1941.

[23] Gölge, E. & Ova, G. (2008). The effects of food irradiation on quality of pine nut kernels. *Radiation Physics and Chemistry*, *77*, 365-369.

[24] Mexis, S. F. & Kontominas, M. G. (2009). Effect of gamma irradiation on the physico-chemical and sensory properties of raw shelled peanuts (*Arachis hypogaea* L.) and pistachio nuts (*Pistacia vera* L.). *Journal of the Science of Food and Agriculture*, *89*, 867-875.

[25] Buttery, R. G., Turnbaugh, J. G. & Ling, L. C. (1988). Contribution of volatiles to rice aroma. *Journal of Agricultural and Food Chemistry*, *36*, 1006-1009.

[26] Cometto-Muñiz, J. E. & Abraham, M. H. (2010). Odor detection by humans of lineal aliphatic aldehydes and helional as gauged by dose–response functions. *Chemical Senses*.

[27] O'Keefe, S., Wiley, V. & Knauft, D. (1993). Comparison of oxidative stability of high and normal-oleic peanut oils. *Journal of the American Oil Chemists' Society*, *70*, 482–489.

[28] Mexis, S. F. & Kontominas, M. G. (2009). Effect of γ-irradiation on the physicochemical and sensory properties of cashew nuts (*Anacardium occidentale L.*). *LWT - Food Science and Technology*, *42*, 1501-1507.

[29] Mexis, S. F. & Kontominas, M. G. (2009). Effect of γ-irradiation on the physicochemical and sensory properties of hazelnuts (*Corylus avellana* L.). *Radiation Physics and Chemistry*, *78*, 407-413.

[30] Chukwumah, Y., Walker, L. & Verghese, M. (2009). Peanut skin color: A biomarker for total polyphenolic content and antioxidative capacities of peanut cultivars. *International Journal of Molecular Sciences*, *10*, 4941-4952.

[31] de Camargo, A., Vieira, T., Regitano-D'Arce, M., Calori-Domingues, M. & Canniatti-Brazaca, S. (2012). Gamma radiation effects on peanut skin antioxidants. *International Journal of Molecular Sciences*, *13*, 3073-3084.

[32] Swain, T. & Hillis, W. E. (1959). The phenolic constituents of *Prunus domestica*. I. —The quantitative analysis of phenolic constituents. *Journal of the Science of Food and Agriculture*, *10*, 63-68.

[33] Re, R., Pellegrini, N., Proteggente, A., Pannala, A., Yang, M. & Rice-Evans, C. (1999). Antioxidant activity applying an improved ABTS radical cation decolorization assay. *Free Radical Biology and Medicine*, *26*, 1231-1237.

[34] Mexis, S. F., Badeka, A. V., Chouliara, E., Riganakos, K. A. & Kontominas, M. G. (2009). Effect of γ-irradiation on the physicochemical and sensory properties of raw unpeeled almond kernels

(*Prunus dulcis*). *Innovative food science & emerging technologies*, *10*, 87-92.

[35] Severini, C., Gomes, T., De Pilli, T., Romani, S. & Massini, R. (2000). Autoxidation of packed almonds as affected by Maillard reaction volatile compounds derived from roasting. *Journal of Agricultural and Food Chemistry*, *48*, 4635-4640.

In: Peanuts
Editor: Richard W. Cook
ISBN: 978-1-63321-013-4

Chapter 4

PEANUTS AS A SOURCE OF PROTEIN, UNSATURATED FATTY ACIDS, TOCOPHEROL AND POLYPHENOLS

Adriano Costa de Camargo [*]
and Solange Guidolin Canniatti-Brazaca
Department of Agri-Food Industry, Food & Nutrition,
"Luiz de Queiroz" College of Agriculture (ESALQ/USP),
University of São Paulo, Brazil

ABSTRACT

Peanuts are among the most popular oilseeds in the world. When their price is considered, they present a competitive advantage in comparison to other nuts such as macadamia, walnuts, hazelnuts, Brazil nuts and cashew nuts. Peanuts are a good source of protein, and, depending on the cultivar, may render amounts of up to 80% unsaturated fatty acids. Tocopherol, also known as vitamin E, is found in high concentration in peanuts. Furthermore, peanuts are recognized by their high polyphenol contents. Phenolic compounds from several classes, namely, phenolic acids, flavonoids, and stilbenes have been identified in peanuts. Polyphenols have antimicrobial, anti-inflammatory, anticarcinogenic, and antioxidant properties. As such, peanuts may be beneficial to consumers through the prevention of chronic diseases. This

[*] Author to whom correspondence should be addressed; E-Mail: adrianoesalq@gmail.com.

review summarizes information regarding the nutritional and possible nutraceutical potential of peanuts and peanut products, as well as the anticipated impacts of production of new cultivars and processing on their content. The value of peanuts as a source of nutrients and nutraceuticals is also highlighted and discussed.

Keywords: *Arachis hypogaea* L., nutrients, nutraceuticals, bioactivity

1. INTRODUCTION

Peanuts (*Arachis hypogaea* L.) and peanut products have an important space in human nutrition around the world. They are found in most of the grocery stores, can be consumed *in natura* as well as in traditional recipes [1]. A publication from the Food and Drug Administration (FDA) authorizes the following health claim for several nuts and peanuts: "Scientific evidence suggests but does not prove that eating 1.5 ounces per day of most nuts [, such as name of specific nut,] as part of a diet low in saturated fat and cholesterol may reduce the risk of heart disease. [See nutrition information for fat content.]" [2].

Due to their high lipid content peanuts are an important source of vegetable oil, being nowadays the third largest feedstock for vegetable oil extraction [3]. Oleic and linoleic acids are the major unsaturated fatty acids in peanuts, and their total content can be as high as 82 (C18:1) and 34% (C18:2) for high-oleic and normal-oleic cultivars, respectively. Furthermore, their protein percentage is also a factor that brings attention to peanuts. The lipid fraction of peanuts has a high tocopherol concentration, while peanut skins have high polyphenol contents. Their consumption has been regarded as beneficial to human health; however, only in the last few years studies addressing the use of peanut skins to increase the polyphenol content of foods such as peanut butter [4,5] or to produce beverages [6] has begun. Finally, the use of the protein meal, which is a by-product of the peanut oil extraction, has gained attention due to its amino acid profile [3]. In this regard, this chapter will focus on peanuts as a source of protein, unsaturated fatty acids, tocopherol and polyphenols, as well as examine the impact of production of new cultivars and processing on their content. Finally, future trends will be addressed.

2. Protein and Lipid Content and Their Health Importance

Lipid is the major component of peanuts, which is followed by protein, carbohydrate and ash. Peanuts lipid content influences the feeling in the mouth, the taste and flavour, which in turn affects their sensory attributes. The lipid content depends on the cultivar, with literature reporting values in the range of 23 to 47% [1,7]. The fatty acids found in peanuts is given in Table 1.

Table 1. Fatty acids of peanuts

Abreviation	Common name
C16:0	palmitic acid
C18:0	stearic acid
C18:1	oleic acid
C18:2	linoléico
C20:0	arachidic acid
C20:1	gondoic acid
C22:0	behenic acid
C24:0	lignoceric acid

Palmitic acid is one of the major fatty acids found in peanuts [8] and the oleic/linoleic ratio is a quality index that reflects their shelf-life, as a consequence of their oxidative quality [9]. Normal and mid-oleic peanuts are more susceptible to oxidative processes during storage at room temperature [10]. The oleic acid content is inversely proportional to the palmitic acid percentage [8]. Stearic, arachidic, eicosenoic, and lignoceric acids represent contents of up 4.0% of total fatty acid composition in peanuts. On the other hand, palmitic, oleic and linoleic acids are the major ones found in peanuts [8]. Their contents in peanut Runner types are in the range of 5.3-11.5%, 44.8-82.2%, and 2.8-33.9%, respectively [9]. Data from the literature demonstrate a high-unsaturated content in peanuts, in particular for high-oleic cultivars. High-unsaturated oil crop development has been procured to improve their nutritional benefits and shelf-life, which can be achieved with conventional breeding; however, climate conditions and soil properties also influence peanuts fatty acid profile. In a biological trial with postmenopausal, hypercholesterolemic women, participants were subjected to a low fat-monounsaturated rich diet from high- oleic peanuts and improved serum lipid and apolipoprotein profiles were detected [11]. Peanut oil high in oleic acid demonstrated a positive effect in enhancing insulin production in a biological model; moreover, type II diabetic mice fed with high-oleic acid from peanuts had their glucose levels decreased in comparison with animals administered a high fat diet with no oleic acid [12]. High-oleic acid peanut oil has also been demonstrated to suppress lung tumorigenesis in mice [13]. Diets high in unsaturated fatty acids and low in saturated fatty acids has also been associated with lower risk of cardiovascular risk [14].

Proteins from peanuts have digestibility comparable to that of animal protein [16]. Proteins are composed of non-essential and essential amino acids. The essential amino acids cannot be synthetized by the organism and must be provided via diet. Methionine, cysteine, valine, isoleucine, leucine, phenylalanine, tyrosine, histidine, lysine, threonine, and tryptophan are the essential amino acids found in peanuts. The non-essential amino acids are serine, arginine, glutamic acid, aspartic acid, proline, glycine, and alanine [3]. The protein content in the kernels range from 22 to 32% [1,15]. Additionally, the meal remaining after the oil extraction may render a protein content of up to 50%. The amino acid profile in the meal is dependent of the extraction process, e.g., enzyme-assisted aqueous extraction, solvent extraction, or cold pressing. The best amino acid profile has been found in the meal obtained by the enzyme-assisted aqueous extraction [3].

3. ANTIOXIDANTS

3.1. Tocopherols

The oxidation process can be delayed by the presence of natural or synthetic antioxidants; however, natural antioxidants may be lost during industrial process and/or storage. Phenolic compounds such as tocopherol, phenolic acids, monomeric flavonoids and proanthocyanidins are natural antioxidants found in peanuts. Tocopherol is well known as vitamin E. Four isomers of tocopherols are found in peanuts. Tocopherols are monophenols because they have only one phenolic ring. The difference among the isomeric forms of tocopherol is due to the content and position of methyl groups in each one. Other than being responsible for the antioxidant activity of the peanut lipid fraction, tocopherols are also beneficial to peanut consumers. Peanut skins are also regarded as sources of antioxidants, however, their tocopherol content is negligible when compared to the content of the kernel lipid fraction [17].

As well as for other nutrients, the tocopherol content can be different among cultivars. However, their concentration can be summarized as: alpha < gamma < delta < beta-tocopherol. Tocopherol isomers have different antioxidant capacities and sensitivities. According to the literature [1], alpha-tocopherol is the most sensitive to gamma-irradiation. On the other hand, the thermal sensitivity between 80 and 120 °C was delta > gamma > alpha > beta-tocopherol, and between 20 and 60 °C was alpha > gamma > beta > delta-tocopherol [18]. Since the blanching process (skin removal) involves heating, a loss of tocopherol is also expected and alpha-tocopherol has been demonstrated the most sensitive. Furthermore, the concentration of delta and beta-tocopherols is negligible. Although the blanching process has been found detrimental to tocopherol content in peanuts right after processing, recent findings [1] demonstrated that blanched peanuts were less sensitive to tocopherol losses during long term storage. This may be due to formation of Maillard compounds, which are formed during the heating process in the presence of amino acid and reducing sugar. Maillard compounds have antioxidant properties and can influence the oxidative stability of blanched peanuts, which in turn affects the oxidative stability of tocopherols.

In a recent study [19], the low intake and low serum concentration of alpha-tocopherol was associated with a higher rate of fractures in elderly women and men. Peanut consumption has also been associated with a higher intake of vitamin E. Furthermore, lower low-density lipoprotein and cholesterol levels have also been revealed. Finally, the consumption of peanut butter has been inversely associated with type 2 diabetes [20].

3.2. Polyphenols

Polyphenols from several classes have been reported in peanuts and peanut products. Polyphenols concentration depends on the cultivar, harvest period, and growing conditions of peanuts [21,22]. Some studies have been focused on the increasing content of polyphenols using UV radiation and ultrasound technology [23,24]. Germination has also been studied with the same purpose [25]. Changes in polyphenol concentrations and antioxidant activities due to roasting, storage, and gamma-irradiation have also been studied [10,26,27].

The roasting process has different effects in phenolic compounds from peanuts. While the blanching process, which involves heating, decreases tocopherol concentrations in the lipid fraction [1], the roasting induces the opposite effect in relation to the peanuts polyphenol content. Mild temperatures (< 135 °C) were able to enhance the total phenolic content of heat treated peanut skin [28]. Undetected compounds such as trans-resveratrol were also quantified after the germination process, furthermore, they presented *in-vitro* anti-inflammatory activities [29].

Peanuts, peanut products and their by-products have different polyphenol concentration. Peanut skins have 145 mg gallic acid equivalent/g for total phenolic content [30], peanuts and peanut butter have 3.96 and 5.36 mg/g, respectively [31], and peanut oil has 0.08 mg/g [32]. Such phenolic compounds were evaluated by spectrophotometric methods. As only gallic acid is used as standard, such values should be interpreted with caution, bearing in mind the limitations of this kind of assay which are much higher than evaluations carried out with HPLC, at which, limits of detection and quantification are lower and the response factor for each polyphenol, e.g., catechin, epicatechin, procyanidins, are taken into account. Although limited, the data aforementioned clearly demonstrates that phenolic compounds are mainly concentrated in peanut skins rather than in kernels.

Table 2 summarizes the major phenolic compounds in peanuts and peanut products. Although phenolic acids and stilbenes have been reported [33], the major compounds are monomeric flavonoids as well as dimers to oligomers of proanthocyanidins.

In consequence of different polyphenol concentrations, each peanut product has its own antioxidant activity. Their antioxidant activity can be ranked as follows: peanut skins > peanut butter > peanut kernels [30,31]. Although peanut skins represent only 2.6% of the total weight of peanuts [39], its contents have great health benefits to consumers. A recent study reported a total phenolic loss of 45% when peanuts were submitted to the blanching process (skin removal) [40]. Furthermore, several studies reported a higher antioxidant activity of peanut skins when compared to BHA (terc-butil-4-hidroxianisol), BHT (butylated hydroxytoluene), green tea, and vitamin C [27,41,42].

The anti-inflammatory and antimicrobial potential of phenolic compounds extracted from peanut skins have also been reported. Concentrations of 2.5 to 5.0% were able to inhibit the COX-2 protein expression, suggesting the anti-inflammatory action of polyphenols from peanut skins [43]. The antimicrobial activity of phenolic compounds from peanut skins was tested against *Saccharomyces cerevisiae*, *Zygosaccharomyces bailii*, and *Zygosaccharomyces bisporus* in a beverage model system. According to the authors, a concentration of 1 mg/mL extended the lag fase of all microorganisms and 10 mg/mL totally inhibited the yeast growth [44].

Table 2. Major polyphenols in peanuts and peanut products

Protocatechuic acid	Francisco and Resurreccion [33]
Caffeic acid	Francisco and Resurreccion [33]
p-Coumaric acid	Francisco and Resurreccion [33]
Epigallocatechin	Francisco and Resurreccion [33]
Catechin	Francisco and Resurreccion [33], Sarnoski et al. [34]
Epicatechin	Francisco and Resurreccion [33], Sarnoski et al. [34]
Quercetin	Francisco and Resurreccion [33]
Resveratrol	Francisco and Resurreccion [33]
Proanthocyanidin dimer A1	Lou et al. [35], Appeldoorn et al. [36]
Proanthocyanidin dimer A2	Lou et al. [35], Appeldoorn et al. [36]
Proanthocyanidin dimer B2	Lou et al. [37], Francisco and Resurreccion [33]
Proanthocyanidin dimer B3	Lou et al. [37],
Proanthocyanidin dimer B4	Lou et al. [37],
Proanthocyanidin dimer B7	Appeldoorn et al. [36]
Proanthocyanidin trimer A	YU et al. [38], Sarnoski et al. [34]
Proanthocyanidin trimer B	YU et al. [38]
Proanthocyanidin trimer C1	Sarnoski et al. [34]
Proanthocyanidin tetramer A	YU et al. [38], Sarnoski et al. [34]
Proanthocyanidin tetramer B	YU et al. [38]

4. Future Trends

Although some studies related to peanut skin polyphenols have started in the nineties, to date their practical application as a source of nutraceutical compounds in the diet is limited to academic research. Few studies have been published recently, but some limitations need to be addressed. Francisco and Resurreccion [6] reported the development of a peanut skin beverage, however, the sensory attributes need to be improved. Another study carried out by Ma et al. [5] examined the fortification of peanut butter with peanut skins. The authors reported a significant increase in the antioxidant activity of the product. Hathorn and Sanders [4] published a similar study and reported a significant change in the sensory descriptors when a concentration of 5% was added, however, a 1% addition has been demonstrated as sensory accepted. Peanut skins have a strong astringent taste due to the high content of condensed tannins (proanthocianidins), thus, the sensory acceptance might be the most relevant issue to be addressed. Spray-dried peanut skin extracts presented higher antioxidant activity and total phenolic content [45], which suggests that the food industry may consider using such process to produce a functional ingredient. Finally, peanut skins still have some protein content and the threshold to provoke allergic symptoms is as low as 100 μg [46]. Thus, the use of peanut skins as a functional ingredient, even at low concentration, should come with proper identification to protect allergenic people from accidental consumption. Still, in the field of by-products, the protein fraction remaining after oil extraction has shown to be a good source of essential amino acids. Future research in this field should further examine the use this low cost by-product, which has a potential to improve the health of consumers. Finally, the production of new peanut cultivars should address both shelf-life and nutritional quality.

REFERENCES

[1] de Camargo, A.C.; Vieira, T.M.F.S.; Regitano-D'Arce, M.A.B.; de Alencar, S.M.; Calori-Domingues, M.A.; Canniatti-Brazaca, S.G. Gamma radiation induced oxidation and tocopherols decrease in in-shell, peeled and blanched peanuts. *International Journal of Molecular Sciences* 2012, *13*, 2827-2845.

[2] Soetaert, D.J. Qualified health claims: Letter of enforcement discretion - nuts and coronary heart disease (docket no 02p-0505).

[3] Latif, S.; Pfannstiel, J.; Makkar, H.P.S.; Becker, K. Amino acid composition, antinutrients and allergens in the peanut protein fraction obtained by an aqueous enzymatic process. *Food Chemistry* 2013, *136*, 213-217.

[4] Hathorn, C.S.; Sanders, T.H. Flavor and antioxidant capacity of peanut paste and peanut butter supplemented with peanut skins. *Journal of Food Science* 2012, *77*, S407-S411.

[5] Ma, Y.Y.; Kerr, W.L.; Swanson, R.B.; Hargrove, J.L.; Pegg, R.B. Peanut skins-fortified peanut butters: Effect of processing on the phenolics content, fibre content and antioxidant activity. *Food Chemistry* 2014, *145*, 883-891.

[6] Francisco, M.L.D.; Resurreccion, A.V.A. Antioxidant capacity and sensory profiles of peanut skin infusions. *Lwt-Food Science and Technology* 2012, *47*, 189-198.

[7] Davis, J.P.; Dean, L.O.; Faircloth, W.H.; Sanders, T.H. Physical and chemical characterizations of normal and high-oleic oils from nine commercial cultivars of peanut. *Journal of the American Oil Chemists Society* 2008, *85*, 235-243.

[8] Andersen, P.C.; Gorbet, D.W. Influence of year and planting date on fatty acid chemistry of high oleic acid and normal peanut genotypes. *Journal of Agricultural and Food Chemistry* 2002, *50*, 1298-1305.

[9] Shin, E.-C.; Craft, B.D.; Pegg, R.B.; Phillips, R.D.; Eitenmiller, R.R. Chemometric approach to fatty acid profiles in Runner-type peanut cultivars by principal component analysis (PCA). *Food Chemistry* 2010, *119*, 1262-1270.

[10] Talcott, S.T.; Duncan, C.E.; Del Pozo-Insfran, D.; Gorbet, D.W. Polyphenolic and antioxidant changes during storage of normal, mid, and high oleic acid peanuts. *Food Chemistry* 2005, *89*, 77-84.

[11] O'Byrne, D.; Knauft, D.; Shireman, R. Low fat-monounsaturated rich diets containing high-oleic peanuts improve serum lipoprotein profiles. *Lipids* 1997, 37, 687-695.

[12] Vassiliou, E.K.; Gonzalez, A.; Garcia, C.; Tadros, J.H.; Chakraborty, G.; Toney, J.H. Oleic acid and peanut oil high in oleic acid reverse the inhibitory effect of insulin production of the inflammatory cytokine TNF-alpha both *in vitro* and *in vivo* systems. *Lipids Health and Disease* 2009, *8*, 25. doi: 10.1186/1476-511X-8-25.

[13] Yamaki, T.; Yano, T.; Satoh, H.; Endo, T.; Matsuyama, C.; Kumagai, H.; Miyahara, M.; Sakurai, H.; Pokorny, J.; Shin, S., et al. High oleic acid oil suppresses lung tumorigenesis in mice through the modulation of extracellular signal-regulated kinase cascade. *Lipids* 2002, 37, 783-788.

[14] Dariush Mozaffarian; Renata Micha; Wallace, S. Effects on coronary heart disease of increasing polyunsaturated fat in place of saturated fat: A systematic review and meta-analysis of randomized controlled trials. *PLoS medicine* 2010, *7*. DOI: 10.1371/journal.pmed.1000252.

[15] Ng, E.C.; Dunford, N.T.; Chenault, K. Chemical characteristics and volatile profile of genetically modified peanut cultivars. *Journal of Bioscience and Bioengineering* 2008, *106*, 350-356.

[16] Singh, B.; Singh, U. Peanut as a source of protein for human foods. *Plant Foods for Human Nutrition* 1991, *41*, 165-177.

[17] Van Ha, H.; Pokorny, J.; Sakurai, H. Peanut skin antioxidants. *Journal of Food Lipids* 2007, *14*, 298-314.

[18] Telegdy Kováts, L.; Berndorfer-Kraszner, E. Über den antioxydationsmechanismus der tocopherole (α, β, γ, δ) in schweinefett. *Food / Nahrung* 1968, *12*, 407-414.

[19] Michaëlsson, K.; Wolk, A.; Byberg, L.; Ärnlöv, J.; Melhus, H. Intake and serum concentrations of α-tocopherol in relation to fractures in elderly women and men: 2 cohort studies. *The American Journal of Clinical Nutrition* 2014, *99*, 107-114.

[20] Jiang, R.; Manson, J.E.; Stampfer, M.J.; Liu, S.M.; Willett, W.C.; Hu, F.B. Nut and peanut butter consumption and risk of type 2 diabetes in women. *Journal of the American Medical Association* 2002, *288*, 2554-2560.

[21] Chukwumah, Y.; Walker, L.; Verghese, M. Peanut skin color: A biomarker for total polyphenolic ontent and antioxidative capacities of peanut cultivars. *International Journal of Molecular Sciences* 2009, *10*, 4941-4952.

[22] Alasalvar, C.; Karamac, M.; Kosinska, A.; Rybarczyk, A.; Shahidi, F.; Amarowicz, R. Antioxidant activity of hazelnut skin phenolics. *Journal of Agricultural and Food Chemistry* 2009, *57*, 4645-4650.

[23] Rudolf, J.R.; Resurreccion, A.V.A. Elicitation of resveratrol in peanut kernels by application of abiotic stresses. *Journal of Agricultural and Food Chemistry* 2005, *53*, 10186-10192.

[24] Sales, J.M.; Resurreccion, A.V.A. Maximising resveratrol and piceid contents in UV and ultrasound treated peanuts. *Food Chemistry* 2009, *117*, 674-680.

[25] Wang, K.H.; Lai, Y.H.; Chang, J.C.; Ko, T.F.; Shyu, S.L.; Chiou, R.Y.Y. Germination of peanut kernels to enhance resveratrol biosynthesis and prepare sprouts as a functional vegetable. *Journal of Agricultural and Food Chemistry* 2005, *53*, 242-246.

[26] Caemmerer, B.; Kroh, L.W. Shelf life of linseeds and peanuts in relation to roasting. *Lwt-Food Science and Technology* 2009, *42*, 545-549.

[27] de Camargo, A.; Vieira, T.M.F.S.; Regitano-D'Arce, M.; Calori-Domingues, M.; Canniatti-Brazaca, S. Gamma radiation effects on peanut skin antioxidants. *International Journal of Molecular Sciences* 2012, *13*, 3073-3084.

[28] Francisco, M.; Resurreccion, A. Total phenolics and antioxidant capacity of heat-treated peanut skins. *Journal of Food Composition and Analysis* 2009, *22*, 16-24.

[29] Chang, J.C.; Lai, Y.H.; Djoko, B.; Wu, P.L.; Liu, C.D.; Liu, Y.W.; Chiou, R.Y.Y. Biosynthesis enhancement and antioxidant and anti-inflammatory activities of peanut (*Arachis hypogaea* L.) arachidin-1, arachidin-3, and isopentadienylresveratrol. *Journal of Agricultural and Food Chemistry* 2006, *54*, 10281-10287.

[30] Ballard, T.S.; Mallikarjunan, P.; Zhou, K.Q.; O'Keefe, S. Microwave-assisted extraction of phenolic antioxidant compounds from peanut skins. *Food Chemistry* 2010, *120*, 1185-1192.

[31] Wu, X.L.; Beecher, G.R.; Holden, J.M.; Haytowitz, D.B.; Gebhardt, S.E.; Prior, R.L. Lipophilic and hydrophilic antioxidant capacities of common foods in the United States. *Journal of Agricultural and Food Chemistry* 2004, *52*, 4026-4037.

[32] Arranz, S.; Cert, R.; Perez-Jimenez, J.; Cert, A.; Saura-Calixto, F. Comparison between free radical scavenging capacity and oxidative stability of nut oils. *Food Chemistry* 2008, *110*, 985-990.

[33] Francisco, M.L.D.; Resurreccion, A.V.A. Development of a reversed-phase high performance liquid chromatography (RP-HPLC) procedure for the simultaneous determination of phenolic compounds in peanut skin extracts. *Food Chemistry* 2009, *117*, 356-363.

[34] Sarnoski, P.J.; Johnson, J.V.; Reed, K.A.; Tanko, J.M.; O'Keefe, S.F. Separation and characterisation of proanthocyanidins in Virginia type peanut skins by LC-MS^n. *Food Chemistry* 2012, *131*, 927-939.

[35] Lou, H.X.; Yamazaki, Y.; Sasaki, T.; Uchida, M.; Tanaka, H.; Oka, S. A-type proanthocyanidins from peanut skins. *Phytochemistry* 1999, *51*, 297-308.

[36] Appeldoorn, M.M.; Sanders, M.; Vincken, J.P.; Cheynier, V.; Le Guerneve, C.; Hollman, P.C.H.; Gruppen, H. Efficient isolation of major procyanidin A-type dimers from peanut skins and B-type dimers from grape seeds. *Food Chemistry* 2009, *117*, 713-720.

[37] Lou, H.X.; Yuan, H.Q.; Ma, B.; Ren, D.M.; Ji, M.; Oka, S. Polyphenols from peanut skins and their free radical-scavenging effects. *Phytochemistry* 2004, *65*, 2391-2399.

[38] Yu, J.M.; Ahmedna, M.; Goktepe, I.; Dai, J.A. Peanut skin procyanidins: Composition and antioxidant activities as affected by processing. *Journal of Food Composition and Analysis* 2006, *19*, 364-371.

[39] Sobolev, V.S.; Cole, R.J. Note on utilisation of peanut seed testa. *Journal of the Science of Food and Agriculture* 2004, *84*, 105-111.

[40] de Camargo, A.C.; Vieira, T.M.F.S.; Regitano-d'Arce, M.A.B.; de Alencar, S.M.; Calori-Domingues, M.A.; Spoto, M.H.F.; Canniatti-

Brazaca, S.G. Gamma irradiation of in-shell and blanched peanuts protects against mycotoxic fungi and retains their nutraceutical components during long-term storage. *International Journal of Molecular Sciences* 2012, *13*, 10935-10958.

[41] Wang, J.; Yuan, X.P.; Jin, Z.Y.; Tian, Y.; Song, H.L. Free radical and reactive oxygen species scavenging activities of peanut skins extract. *Food Chemistry* 2007, *104*, 242-250.

[42] Yu, J.; Ahmedna, M.; Goktepe, P. Effects of processing methods and extraction solvents on concentration and antioxidant activity of peanut skin phenolics. *Food Chemistry* 2005, *90*, 199-206.

[43] Lewis, W.E.; Harris, G.K.; Sanders, T.H.; White, B.L.; Dean, L.L. Antioxidant and anti-inflammatory effects of peanut skin extracts. *Food and Nutrition Sciences* 2013, *4*, 22-32.

[44] Sarnoski, P.J.; Boyer, R.R.; O'Keefe, S.F. Application of proanthocyanidins from peanut skins as a natural yeast inhibitory agent. *Journal of Food Science* 2012, *77*, M242-M249.

[45] Constanza, K.E.; White, B.L.; Davis, J.P.; Sanders, T.H.; Dean, L.L. Value-added processing of peanut skins: Antioxidant capacity, total phenolics, and procyanidin content of spray-dried extracts. *Journal of Agricultural and Food Chemistry* 2012, *60*, 10776-10783.

[46] Hourihane, J.O.; Kilburn, S.A.; Nordlee, J.A.; Hefle, S.L.; Taylor, S.L.; Warner, J.O. An evaluation of the sensitivity of subjects with peanut allergy to very low doses of peanut protein: A randomized, double-blind, placebo-controlled food challenge study. *Journal of Allergy and Clinical Immunology* 1997, *100*, 596-600.

In: Peanuts
Editor: Richard W. Cook
ISBN: 978-1-63321-013-4

Chapter 5

A NON-TOXIGENIC STRAIN OF *ASPERGILLUS FLAVUS* AS A BIOLOGICAL CONTROL AGAINST AFLATOXIN PRODUCTION IN PEANUTS

Maria Antonia Calori-Domingues[1,*], Deborah Teles[1], Giancarlo Hercoton Ponce[1], Adriano Costa de Camargo[1], Carlos Tadeu dos Santos Dias[1], Eduardo Micotti da Gloria[1], Lília Sichmann Heiffig-del Aguila[2] and Ignácio José de Godoy[2]

[1]Department of Agri-Food Industry, Food & Nutrition, "Luiz de Queiroz" College of Agriculture (ESALQ/USP), University of São Paulo, Brazil

[2]Agronomic Institute of Campinas (IAC), Campinas, Brazil

ABSTRACT

Peanuts, as a groundnut, are in constant contact with soil population of aflatoxigenic fungi from section *Flavi*, thus they may be infected by *A. flavus* before harvesting. Aflatoxins are recognized as carcinogens

---

* Author to whom correspondence should be addressed; Email: macdomin@usp.br

produced mostly by *A. flavus* and *A. parasiticus*. As such, their concentrations in peanuts and peanut products are limited to 20 μg/kg in Brazil or less in other countries. In the present study, a commercial product containing a non-toxigenic strain of *A. flavus* was evaluated as a biological control to avoid production of aflatoxin B1 (AFB1). The competitive effect of *A. flavus* NRRL 21882 (Afla-guard®) for the reduction of AFB1 contamination was evaluated under field conditions in peanuts of Valencia type (cv. IAC Tatu ST) at a low rainfall condition. Planting and crop management for aerial pest and disease control followed Brazilian recommended practices. The field was irrigated to induce germination and plant growth until 72 days after planting; after which, irrigation was suppressed to impose drought stress until harvesting for 34 days. The product containing *A. flavus* NRRL 21882 was applied 60 days after planting (22.4 kg/ha). Peanuts from four large plots (two treated and two devoid of the product) were evaluated for AFB1 contamination. A total of 20 samples per plot was evaluated. Pod samples were mechanically shelled and two subsamples were taken: subsample A (8 – 10 kg) denominated field kernel sample (FK), whose kernels were not segregated; subsample B (2 kg) denominated edible grade kernel (EK), comprising hand-picked kernels, free of damages and commercially graded. Peanuts grown in soil devoid of the product containing *A. flavus* NRRL 21882 were contaminated by AFB1 in concentrations of 1444 and 41 μg/kg in FK and EK, respectively. On the other hand, peanuts grown in soil treated with the product contained AFB1 in concentrations of 248 and 5.6 μg/kg in FK and EK, respectively. In both FK and EK, a highly significant ($p < 0.0001$) reduction of AFB1 concentration (84 and 83%, respectively) was observed for peanuts grown in soil with the product containing non-toxigenic strains of *A. flavus*.

Keywords: *Aspergillus flavus*, aflatoxin, biological control, peanuts

1. Introduction

Peanuts (*Arachis hypogaea* L.) are very popular around the world and can be consumed *in natura* as well as in many homemade recipes [1]. The food industry also uses peanuts to produce several types of candies, which makes children one of the most important target consumers. Peanuts have a high lipid content, which is composed mainly of unsaturated fatty acids [2], and is a source of proteins of high biological value as they are composed of non-essential and essential amino acids [3]. Peanuts are also a good source of minerals [4]. Vitamin E and polyphenols [1, 5], which have antioxidant properties, are highlighted as the future trend for increasing peanut consumption.

China is the first world producer of peanuts, followed by India, and the US. In 2013, Brazil produced 346 thousand tons [6], and is considered one of the countries with the highest potential to increase its production, which will place Brazil in a better position in the international market.

Although peanuts are well recognized as a good source of nutrients and phytochemicals their potential contamination is a concern of their producers and consumers [7]. Due to their production and post harvest conditions, peanuts might be contaminated with aflatoxigenic fungi [8,9]. Aflatoxin contamination is one of the most important issues to be addressed by peanut producers around the world. Aflatoxins are recognized as carcinogens produced mostly by *A. flavus* and *A. parasiticus*. Consumption of aflatoxin contaminated food is related to hepatic cancer incidence [10]. Aflatoxins can be produced by *A. flavus*, *A. parasiticus*, *A. nomius, and A. pseudotamarii*. However, *A. flavus and A. parasiticus* are the most important [11]. These fungi grow and reproduce in the soil [12] and may not cause any damage to the plant itself. In fact, the problem stands from their toxin production, which may cause health issues for humans and animals [13, 14].

In accordance with the world marked trend the Brazilian rules of production and commercialization had become stricter in the last few years. In Brazil, the aflatoxin tolerance for peanuts and peanut products for human consumption is 20 μg/kg. This limit refers to the total concentration of aflatoxin B1, B_2, G_1 and G_2 [15]. To achieve such low concentrations producers need to follow good agricultural practices during production and post-havest [16, 17]. However, some biotic and abiotic stress in the field are out of human control, which makes difficult to avoid the peanut contamination; among this drought conditions are the most important factor [18]. Equipments can be used to segregate contaminated peanuts and reduce the total contamination. However, it is not possible to ensure 100% safety. In fact, some samples that appear to be safe may test positive for aflatoxin [19].

The application of biological control to avoid the growth and reproduction of aflatoxigenic fungi is an important tool for the producer [20]. Afla-guard® is a commercial product composted of non-toxigenic strains of *Aspergillus flavus* (NRRL 21882). It is regarded as highly competitive in the soil, which may afford the biological control of toxin producing strains [21, 22]. Thus, the aim of the present study was to evaluate the effect of Afla-guard® application, on the reduction of aflatoxin contamination, in field conditions.

2. Material and Methods

2.1. Field Experiment

The field experiment was carried out in the city of Petrolina, Pernambuco State, Brazil. This location was chosen to expose the production to drought conditions, which is well recognized as a factor that induces aflatoxin production. The most traditional peanut cultivar (IAC Tatu ST) from Brazil was used in the experiment. This cultivar has faced a long history of aflatoxin contamination. The whole cycle from planting to harvesting took about 100-110 days. The experiment was conducted on a total area of 3.75 ha. Plants were cultivated according to common practices currently used for peanut production [17]. A fitossanitary control was carried out to prevent pests and diseases that would affect the aerial parts of the plant. Herbicides were used for weed control.

A set of moderated stress was induced in the plants as soon as they achieved maturity: a) suspension of fungicide application; b) suppression of irrigation to impose drought stress until harvesting; and c) late harvest by some days to induce sprouting. Such conditions facilitated the fungi infection and toxin production without severe impact to plant development.

2.2. Experimental Design, Non-Aflatoxigenic Strain Application, and Sample Harvesting

A completely randomized design with two replications per treatment was used. Peanuts from the IAC Tatu ST cultivar were grown in four plots of 5049 m^2 each. 60 days after planting, the product (Afla-guard®) was applied by hand to the surface field with a dose of 22.4 kg/ha. Two plots were not treated with the product to create a representative control sample. The harvest was carried out at day 115, which was followed by natural drying of the samples for four days. The final grain moisture was 8%.

20 samples of in-shell peanuts (30 kg each) were obtained from each plot. The harvest was carried out in 60 different places for each plot to ensure a representative sampling. This is important because the distribution of aflatoxins can have a great variance. The samples were sent to the Agronomic Institute of Campinas (IAC), Campinas, São Paulo State, Brazil, where they were mechanically shelled. A second verification was carried out

to evaluate the actual moisture of the samples. The moisture content was ≤ 8%, and no change was noted in comparison with the harvest day.

2.3. Sample Preparation

Peanut samples (removed from their shells) were divided in two subsamples. The first (subsample A), contained 10 kg, and the second (subsample B), contained 2 kg. Subsample A and B, hereafter will be referred to as field kernel (FK) and edible kernel (EK), respectively. FK did not go through any type of segregation and EK was previously segregated to remove grains that did not fit the required size (<6.7 mm or 17/64 inch) and had no apparent damage.

All experimental steps are shown in the figure 1. 160 samples (80 from FK and 80 from EK) were analyzed. Peanuts were blended with water (1:1, w/v) for 3 min to obtain a homogeneous paste. One analytical sample was taken from each subsample which was subjeted to extration and evaluated for their aflatoxin content.

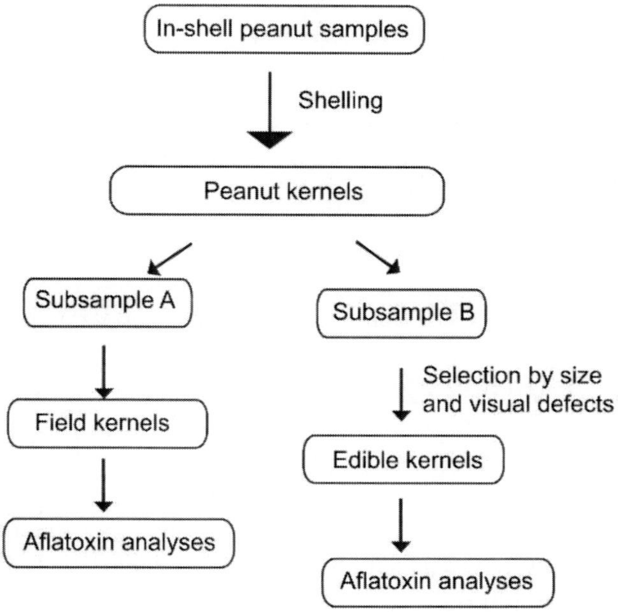

Figure 1. Post-harvest experimental steps for aflatoxin evaluation.

2.4. Aflatoxin Analysis

Aflatoxin B1 was identified and quantified using thin-layer chromatographic (TLC) according to the method 968.22 [23]. The detection and quantification limits were 0.5 and 1.0 μg/kg, respectively. In order to compare results, some samples were also investigated using high-performance liquid chromatography (HPLC). Analyses were performed using a Shimadzu equipment consisting of a LC-10AT pump, RF-10AXL fluorescence detector (λexc 365 nm, λem 435 nm), SIL-20A autosampler, CTO-20A oven at 35 °C, DGU-20A5 degasser, and LCsolution software. Aflatoxins were separated using a X-Terra Waters RP18 column (4.6 x 150 mm, 5 μm). A water:methanol:acetonitrile mixture (60:25:15) was used as the mobile phase and the system was operated in isocratic mode. The flow rate and injection volume were set at 1.0 mL/min and 20μL, respectively.

The method accuracy was evaluated by recovery tests using known AFB1 concentrations (1.3, 2.6 and 6.0 μg/kg). Non-contaminated peanut samples were spiked with the previously mentioned concentrations of AFB1 and subjected to the whole analytical process in a total of 5 replicates.

2.5. Statistical Analysis

Data was analyzed by ANOVA and the average comparison was carried out using the Tukey's test ($p < 0.05$) with SAS software (Statistical Analysis System, 2004).

3. Results and Discussion

3.1. Analytical Quality Control

TLC method had limits of detection and quantification of 0.5 and 1.0 μg/kg, respectively. The relative standard deviation for repeatability (RSDr) of the limit of quantification was 8% and the average recuperation was 90%. These values are in accordance with those recommended by the commission regulation 401/2006 [24].

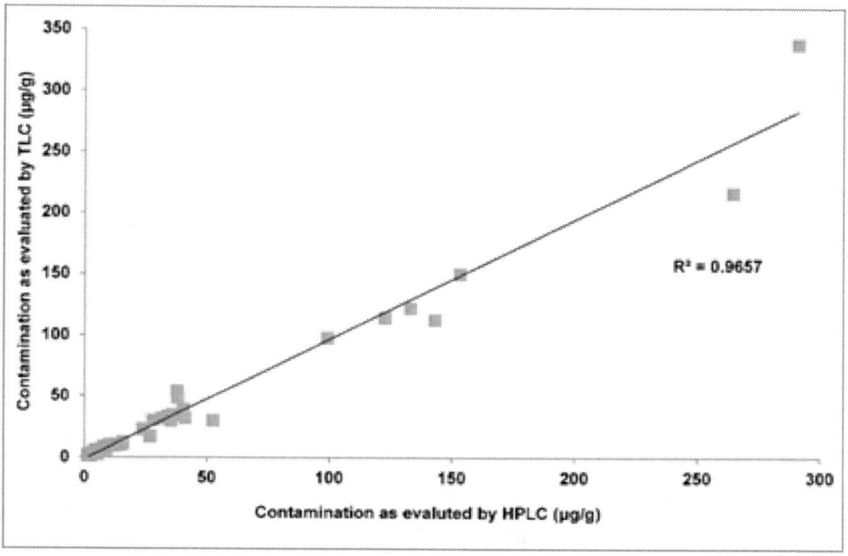

Figure 2. Correlation between results obtained by TLC and HPLC.

The recovery of samples artificially contaminated with AFB1 in concentrations of 1.3, 2.6, and 6.0 µg/kg were 74.6, 85.4, and 92.4%, respectively. A linear calibration curve was used for HPLC quantification. AFB1 concentrations for the standard curve were in the range of 0.255-12.07 µg/mL. The correlation coefficient (R^2) was 0.9986. The limit of quantification was 0.4 µg/kg. There was a significant positive correlation between results obtained by TLC and HPLC (R = 0.9827). Correlation analysis was carried out in the range of 1.5-300 µg/kg (Figure 2). Results from the present study show that TLC can be used for AFB1 determination. Shundo and Sabino [25] also reported no significant difference for determination of aflatoxin M1 in contaminated milk using TLC and HPLC.

3.2. Aflatoxin B1 Concentrations

The contamination of aflatoxin in samples obtained from soil treated and untreated with Afla-guard® are given in table 1 and figures 3 and 4. The total aflatoxin was also evaluated (data not shown), however, since aflatoxin B1 was the most representative, accounting for more than 90% of the total contamination, the present work is focused only in AFB1. Due to non-normal distribution results were transformed as follow: FK = log of concentration and

EK = (concentration)$^{-0.1}$. Statistical analysis demonstrated that FK and EK samples treated with Afla-guard® had a lower AFB1 contamination (p<0.0001). A decrease of 84 and 83% was noted in FK and EK samples, respectively. A similar result was obtained by Dorner and Lamb [21] in treated peanuts from US, however fungi growth and aflatoxin contamination differ depending on environmental conditions and field location, thus the present work addressed the efficiency of Afla-guard® in Brazilian conditions. Comparisons of contamination between samples from treated and untreated soil are shown in Figures 3 and 4.

Table 1. Average[1,2] and range of aflatoxin B1 contamination (µg/kg) in field and edible kernel

	Average of contamination		Range of contamination	
Sample	Field kernel	Edible Kernel	Field kernel	Edible Kernel
Treated	248a	5.6a	15-952	ND-99.2
Untreated	1444b	41b	272-4987	ND-291

[1] Means followed by different letters within a column are not significantly different (p>0.0001). ND = non detected (Limit of detection for AFB1 = 0.5 µg/kg). [2] Actual values, without any mathematical transformation.

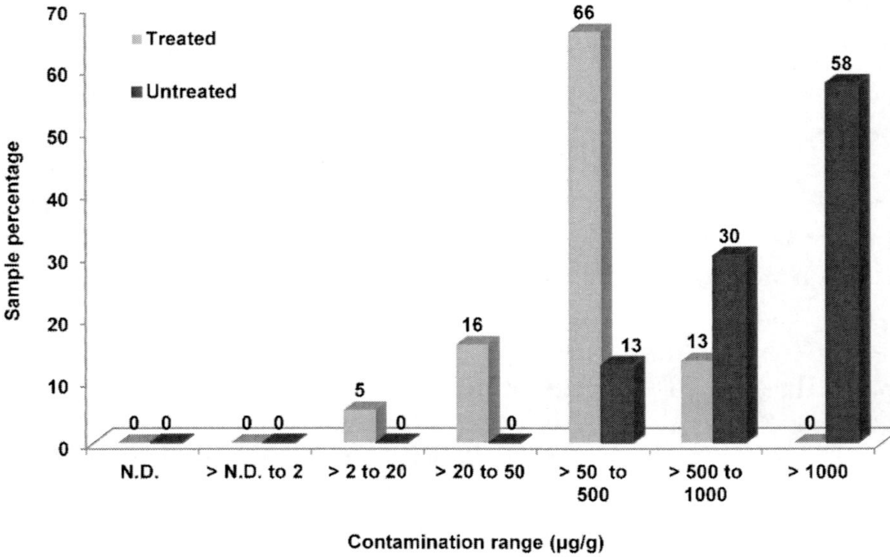

Figure 3. Concentration of AFB1 of samples from treated and untreated soil.

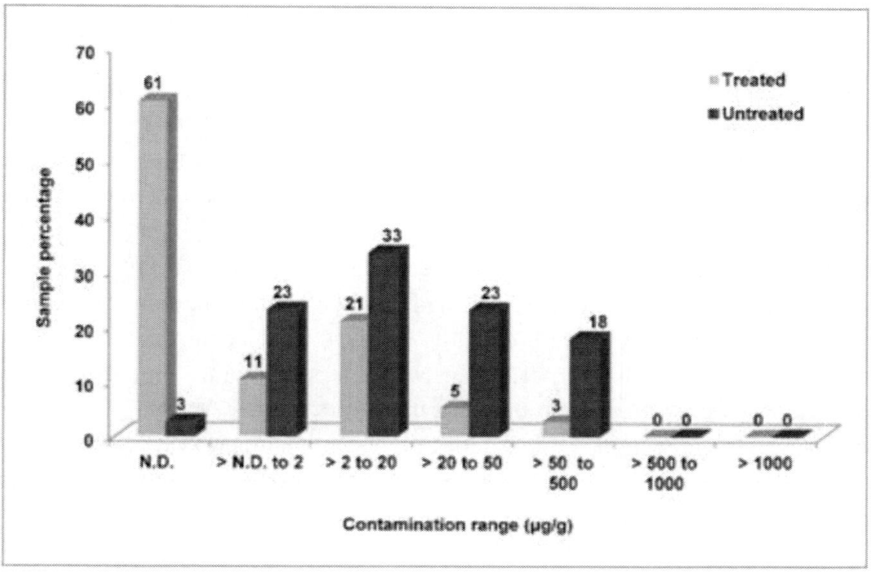

Figure 4. Concentration of AFB1 of samples from treated and untreated soil.

A non-detectable level of contamination was found in 60% of the treated EK samples, while only 3% of the untreated samples presented the same result. EK is the peanut that went through a previous selection. This step is mandatory because immature, broken, undersized, loose-shelled, rancid and discolored peanut kernels are more susceptible to aflatoxin contamination [26]. As such, after this step, aflatoxin contamination decreases. However, depending on the initial aflatoxin contamination, the product will likely not satisfy the present regulations. It is noteworthy that 58% of untreated FK samples were contaminated in concentrations higher than 1000 µg/kg (Figure 3). On the other hand, 66% of the treated samples had contamination in the range of 50-500 µg/kg. After sieving and visual selection the average concentration of AFB1 of EK samples was 41 and 5.6 µg/kg in samples from untreated and treated soil, respectively, which represented a decrease of 86%. The present results are in good agreement with those reported by Dorner and Lamb [21].

92% of EK samples from treated field fit the Brazilian regulation, which tolerates a total aflatoxin contamination of up to 20 µg/kg[15]. Moreover, 71% satisfied European Community regulations [24], that has a tolerance of 2 µg/kg for AFB1 and 4 µg/kg for total aflatoxins in peanuts intend for direct human consumption or use as an ingredient in foodstuffs. Oppositely, only 59 and 26% of EK samples from untreated soil satisfied the same requirements; respectively.

This is important because the European Community is regarded as an important importer of peanuts from countries like US, China, and Brazil. Finally, a great variance of AFB1 contamination was noted in samples harvested in different places. FK samples from treated soil of the first and second harvest plot had average contaminations of 238 and 317 μg/kg, respectively, with a respective variance coefficient of 102 and 108%. In contrast, samples from untreated soil had average contaminations of 1487 and 1791 μg/kg, respectively, and both had a variance coefficient of 85%.

In the present study, peanut growing was submitted to an induced contamination process. Because of this, their infection by AFB1 was high, and consequently such samples presented a higher contamination level than those worldwide tolerated. However, the current results demonstrated a significant reduction on their contamination when treated with Afla-guard®.

Conclusion

Aspergillus spp growing and aflatoxin induced contamination were successfully achieved as the initial experimental step. The application of Afla-guard® reduced AFB1 contamination in FK and EK samples. The use of non-toxigenic strain of *Aspergillus flavus* (Afla-guard®) will likely be an efficient tool to fit regulations regarding aflatoxin contamination. Consequently, a high quality peanut can be produced, which is beneficial to consumers.

Acknowledgments

We are grateful to João Bosco Ferreira for supporting the field experiment.

References

[1] de Camargo, A. C.; Vieira, T. M. F. S.; Regitano-D'Arce, M. A. B.; de Alencar, S. M.; Calori-Domingues, M. A.; Canniatti-Brazaca, S. G., Gamma radiation induced oxidation and tocopherols decrease in in-shell,

peeled and blanched peanuts. *International Journal of Molecular Sciences* 2012, 13, 2827-2845.

[2] de Camargo, A. C.; Canniatti-Brazaca, S. G.; Mansi, D. N.; Domingues, M. A. C.; Arthur, V., Efeitos da radiação gama na cor, capacidade antioxidante e perfil de ácidos graxos em amendoim (*Arachis hypogaea* L.). *Ciencia e Tecnologia de Alimentos* 2011, 31, 11-15.

[3] Latif, S.; Pfannstiel, J.; Makkar, H. P. S.; Becker, K., Amino acid composition, antinutrients and allergens in the peanut protein fraction obtained by an aqueous enzymatic process. *Food Chemistry* 2013, 136, 213-217.

[4] Phan-Thien, K. Y.; Wright, G. C.; Lee, N. A., Genotype-by-Environment Interaction Affects the Essential Mineral Composition of Peanut (Arachis hypogaea L.) Kernels. Journal of Agricultural and Food Chemistry 2010, *58*, 9204-9213.

[5] de Camargo, A.; Vieira, T.; Regitano-D'Arce, M.; Calori-Domingues, M.; Canniatti-Brazaca, S., Gamma radiation effects on peanut skin antioxidants. *International Journal of Molecular Sciences* 2012, 13, 3073-3084.

[6] IBGE, Pesquisa mensal de previsão e acompanhamento das safras agrícolas no ano civil. *Levantamento Sistemático da Produção Agrícola* 2014, 27, 1-85.

[7] de Camargo, A. C.; Vieira, T. M. F. S.; Regitano-d'Arce, M. A. B.; de Alencar, S. M.; Calori-Domingues, M. A.; Spoto, M. H. F.; Canniatti-Brazaca, S. G., Gamma irradiation of in-shell and blanched peanuts protects against mycotoxic fungi and retains their nutraceutical components during long-term storage. *International Journal of Molecular Sciences* 2012, 13, 10935-10958.

[8] Dorner, J. W., Management and prevention of mycotoxins in peanuts. *Food Additives and Contaminants* 2008, 25, 203-208.

[9] Nesci, A.; Montemarani, A.; Etcheverry, M., Assessment of mycoflora and infestation of insects, vector of *Aspergillus* section *Flavi*, in stored peanut from Argentina. *Mycotoxin Research* 2011, 27, 5-12.

[10] Miranda, D. D. C.; Arçari, D. P.; Ladeira, M. S. P.; Calori-Domingues, M. A.; Romero, A. C.; Salvadori, D. M. F.; Gloria, E. M.; Pedrazzoli, J., Jr.; Ribeiro, M. L., Analysis of DNA damage induced by aflatoxin B1 in Dunkin–Hartley guinea pigs. *Mycopathologia* 2007, 163, 275-280.

[11] CAST, Mycotoxins: Risks in Plant, Animal and Human Systems. Task Force Report N°139. In Mycotoxins: Risks in plant, animal, and human systems 2003; pp 48–57.

[12] Horn, B. W.; Dorner, J. W., Effect of nontoxigenic Aspergillus flavus and A. parasiticus on aflatoxin contamination of wounded peanut seeds inoculated with agricultural soil containing natural fungal populations. *Biocontrol Science and Technology* 2009, 19, 249-262.

[13] Bakirdere, S.; Bora, S.; Bakirdere, E. G.; Aydin, F.; Arslan, Y.; Komesli, O. T.; Aydin, I.; Yildirim, E., Aflatoxin species: their health effects and determination methods in different foodstuffs. *Central European Journal of Chemistry* 2012, 10, 675-685.

[14] Zychowski, K. E.; Pohlenz, C.; Mays, T.; Romoser, A.; Hume, M.; Buentello, A.; Gatlin, D. M.; Phillips, T. D., The effect of NovaSil dietary supplementation on the growth and health performance of Nile tilapia (Oreochromis niloticus) fed aflatoxin-B1 contaminated feed. Aquaculture 2013, *376*, 117-123.

[15] Brasil, Resolução RDC Nº 7, de 18 de fevereiro de 2011. Dispõe sobre limites máximos tolerados (LMT) para micotoxinas em alimentos. Ministério da Saúde. In 2011; pp 66-67

[16] Zorzete, P.; Baquiao, A. C.; Atayde, D. D.; Reis, T. A.; Goncalez, E.; Correa, B., Mycobiota, aflatoxins and cyclopiazonic acid in stored peanut cultivars. *Food Research International* 2013, 52, 380-386.

[17] Godoy, I. J.; Minotti, D.; Rezende, P., Produção de amendoim com qualidade. In CPT Produções Técnicas: Viçosa, MG, Brasil, 2005.

[18] Hamidou, F.; Rathore, A.; Waliyar, F.; Vadez, V., Although drought intensity increases aflatoxin contamination, drought tolerance does not lead to less aflatoxin contamination. *Field Crops Research* 2014, 156, 103–110.

[19] Zovico, C.; Fonseca, H.; Calori-Domingues, M. A.; Glória, E. M.; Borguini, R. G.; Silveira, V. P.; Piedade, S. S.; Barbin, D., Avaliação da seleção eletrônica pela cor na descontaminação de amendoim contaminado com aflatoxinas. *Scientia Agricola* 1999, 56, 371-376.

[20] Horn, B. W.; Dorner, J. W., Evaluation of different genotypes of nontoxigenic Aspergillus flavus for their ability to reduce aflatoxin contamination in peanuts. *Biocontrol Science and Technology* 2011, 21, 865-876.

[21] Dorner, J. W.; Lamb, M. C., Development and commercial use of afla-Guard® an aflatoxin biocontrol agent. *Mycotoxin Research* 2006, 22, 33-38.

[22] Dorner, J. W.; Cole, R. J., Effect of application of nontoxigenic strains of Aspergillus flavus and A-parasiticus on subsequent aflatoxin

contamination of peanuts in storage. *Journal of Stored Products Research* 2002, 38, 329-339.

[23] AOAC, Official Methods of Analysis of AOAC International. 18th ed.; AOAC International: Gaithersburg, MD, USA, 2006.

[24] European Commission, Regulation (EU) No. 165/2010. Off. J. European Union L50 2010 8-12.

[25] Shundo, L.; Sabino, M., Aflatoxin M1 in milk by immunoaffinity column cleanup with TLC/HPLC determination. *Brazilian Journal of Microbiology* 2006, 37, 164-167.

[26] Rustom, I. Y. S., Aflatoxin in food and feed: Occurrence, legislation and inactivation by physical methods. *Food Chemistry* 1997, 59, 57-67.

In: Peanuts
Editor: Richard W. Cook

ISBN: 978-1-63321-013-4

Chapter 6

GENETIC IMPROVEMENT IN OLEATE CONTENT IN PEANUTS

***Chuan Tang Wang*[1,*]*, Xiu Zhen Wang*[1]*, Yue Yi Tang*[1]*, Qi Wu*[1]*, Quan Xi Sun*[1]*, Qing Xuan Gong*[1]*, Zhen Yang*[1]*, Dong Qing Hu*[2]*, Zheng Jia Xu*[3]*, Wan Li Ni*[4]*, Xiao Ling Zhai*[5]*, Hua Yuan Gao*[6]*, Rong Hua Chen*[7]*, Xiao Lin Wang*[8]*, Shu Tao Yu*[9] *and Lang Qian*[10]**

[1]Shandong Peanut Research Institute, Qingdao, P R China
[2]Qingdao Entry-Exit Inspection and Quarantine Bureau, Qingdao, P R China
[3]Anhui Provincial Seed Association, Hefei, P R China
[4]Institute of Crop Plants, Anhui Academy of Agricultural Sciences, Hefei, P R China
[5]Qingdao Academy of Agricultural Sciences, Qingdao, P R China
[6]Institute of Peanut, Jilin Academy of Agricultural Sciences, Gongzhuling, P R China
[7]South Jiangxi Academy of Sciences, Ganzhou, P R China
[8]Zhumadian Academy of Agricultural Sciences, Zhumadian, P R China
[9]Institute of Peanut, Liaoning Academy of Agricultural Sciences, Fuxin, P R China
[10]Dalian Academy of Agricultural Sciences, Dalian, P R China

---

[*] Author for correspondence. chinapeanut@126.com.

ABSTRACT

Seed crops with high oleate content proved to have better keeping quality. High oleate diet helps to lower the harmful low density lipoprotein cholesterol level. Other health benefits of high oleate peanut include, increased sensitivity to insulin, amelioration in some inflammatory diseases, and preventive effects on tumorigenesis. In addition, high oleate peanut genotypes are considered more suitable for biodiesel production than their normal oleate counterparts. Significant progress in the genetic improvement of the cultivated peanut for high oleate has been made since the identification of the natural mutant F435 in University of Florida. The present chapter reviews recent technical advances in peanut fatty acid determination, genetics of oleate content, molecular basis of the high oleate phenotype, factors affecting oleate content, and peanut germplasm enhancement in high oleate content.

Keywords: Peanut, oleate, breeding, genetics, influential factor, analytical method

INTRODUCTION

In literature, there were 3 types of groundnut. Potato bean (*Apios americana*) was termed as American groundnut, and bambara nut (syncronyms: *Voandzeia sunterranea*, *Vigna subterranean*, hog-peanut) was called bambara groundnut or Madagascar groundnut, but the term 'groundnut' generally refers to peanut (*Arachis hypogaea* L.) (Rathnakumar, 2012).

Peanut Production and Uses

According to the US Department of Agriculture database (USDA/FAS, 2014), in 2011/2012, globally 23.06 million hectares (MH) were planted to peanut, with a total production of 37.87 million tons (MT) and an average yield of 1.64 tons per hectare (TH). Major peanut producers were China (16.05 MT), India (5.5 MT), Nigeria (2.96 MT), USA (1.66 MT), Burma (1.39 MT) and Indonesia (1.17 MT). India took the lead in area (5.30 MH). Of the main peanut producing countries, USA (3.80 TH) ranked first in yield, followed by China (3.50 TH).

In developing nations including China and India, more than half peanut produce is crushed for oil. In developed countries, however, most of the peanut goes to food uses. It is reported that in USA only 21.5% of the crop is processed for oil (Wilkin et al., 2014).

Why High Oleate?

Extended Shelf Life

Irrespective of the uses, fatty acid profiles of oilseed crops including peanut are considered relevant to the shelf life of food product and the health of consumers. Generally, oleate (C18:1) and linoleate (C18:2) together constitute about 80% of the total fatty acids in peanut seeds. Increase in oleic acid content will inevitably result in decrease in linoleic acid content in peanut. Oleic acid is less reactive with oxygen and hence more stable. Linoleate, however, is prone to oxidization, and may result in unpleasant odor. Indeed, several studies have demonstrated that high oleate (HO) peanut products have greater oxidative stability. O'Keefe et al. (1993) noted oil from a HO runner type peanut line (75.6% oleate, 4.7% linoleate) was more oxidation stable than that from the isogenic sister line with normal fatty acid composition (56.1% oleate, 24.2% linoleate). In the Schall oven test (80°C), the induction times were 682 and 47 hours for high and normal oils ($P<0.01$); for AOM (active oxygen method), the induction time were 69 and 7.3 hours for high and normal oils ($P<0.01$), respectively. It took 847 and 247 minutes to reach 50% loss in triglyceride area on TLC-FID (thin-layer chromatography-fame ionization detector) for high and normal oils ($P<0.01$). Braddock et al. (1995) found that peroxide values (PV) were lower for roasted HO peanut than normal peanut during storage at 25°C and 40°C and that peanutty flavor was more stable for HO than normal after 6 weeks of storage. They concluded that shelf life estimated from sensory data was two times longer in HO peanut. Mugendi et al. (1998) reported that two HO peanut lines (80% and 81% oleate) obtained from the University of Florida, F1250 and BC93Q10, when shelled, sized and dry-roasted to a medium roast and stored at 40℃at 18% relative humidity (r. h.), showed better flavor quality and stability than normal oleate peanut (Florunner, 53% oleate). At 10-week storage, peroxide values were 47 meq/kg for Florunner, and <3 meq/kg for high oleic peanut lines. The slopes of the PV-time curves were 4.2, 0.25 and 0.38 for Florunner, BC93Q10 and F1250, respectively, showing that the increases in PV were 16.8 and 11.1 times greater for normal oleate Florunner than for BC93Q10 and F1250, respectively. Similarly, according to Nepote et al. (2006), who used shelled fried-salted runner type peanut cultivars, high oleic Granoleico reached a PV of 20 meq/kg after 125 days of storage; however, normal oleate (NO) Tegua attained this value only after 19 days. Based on the study of Braddock et al. (1995), Mozingo et al. (2004) used a PV of 20 meq/kg as the arbitrary point to indicate unacceptable oxidation during storage. In contrast to previous studies where runner type peanut genotypes were used, Mozingo and his coworkers (2004) exploited Virginia types instead. They detected marked difference in shelf life of 2 Virginia type peanut cultivars with contrasting oleate content, viz. HO cultivar AgraTech VC-2 (80% oleate) and NO variety VA98R (50% oleate). For roasted inshell peanuts, VA98R reached a PV of 20 meq/kg by the end of 4 weeks of storage, whereas AgraTech VC-2 did not reach 20 meq/kg until approximately 32 weeks. For salted inshell peanuts, while VA98R exceeded a value of 20 meq/kg before the 2nd week, AgraTech VC-2 did not reach 20 meq/kg after 40 weeks of storage (Mozingo et al., 2004). Wilkin et al. (2014) found that HO whole peanut seeds, when packed into gas and light impermeable foil lined polyethylene bags, flushed with N_2 and stored at 30°C, showed a lag phase of at least 12 weeks before PV began to increase, while HO nibbed seeds showed an increase from week 1. Under such conditions, HO whole peanut seeds did not reach a PV of 15 even after 20 weeks of storage, whereas conventional whole peanut seeds reached a PV of 20 at 6-7 weeks.

Health Benefits for Humans

Increase in stability of peanut oil also makes partial hydrogenation unnecessary, thereby avoiding additional cost and introduction of *trans* fatty acids, compounds that exacerbate heart disease and diabetics (Chong et al., 2006; Chu et al., 2007). Higher *trans* fat intake is reported to be associated with an increased risk of all-cause mortality (Kiage et al., 2013).

O'Byrne et al. (1997) compared the serum lipid profiles of postmenopausal hypercholesterolemic women, previously with high-fat diets but then with a low fat–monounsaturated rich (LFMR) diet containing HO peanut, and women already eating low fat (LF) diets. After 6 months of following the LFMR diet, in the LFMR group, serum cholesterol and low density lipoprotein cholesterol (LDL-C) dropped by 10% and 12%, respectively, but did not change in the LF group. Only the LFMR group exhibited a trend toward beneficial changes in LDL-C/HDL-C (high density lipoprotein cholesterol) and apo (apolipoprotein) A-I/apo B ratios.

In the report of Vassiliou et al. (2009), oleic acid and peanut oil high in oleic acid enhanced insulin production in the rat pancreatic β cell line INS-1.

Pre-treatment with oleic acid reversed the inhibitory effect of the inflammatory cytokine TNF-α on insulin production. In type II diabetic mice, glucose level was lower in the peanut oil derived high oleic acid diet group than in other treatments with a high fat diet without oleic acid. The study of Yamaki et al. (2005) suggested the suppressive effects of dietary HO peanut oil on lung tunorigenesis (promotion stage) in mice treated with methyl nitrosourea (MNU). Data collected 30 days after MNU treatment showed that dietary HO peanut oil inhibited ornithine decarboxylase activity, induced the inactivation of Mek, and reduced proliferating cell nuclear antigen level in lungs more than did high linoleic safflower oil. A parallel effect was also noted in prostaglandin E_2 (PGE_2) level in the lungs.

Better Feed for Swine

Myer et al. (1992) observed a high incidence of off-flavor for bacon from pigs fed canola oil (CO) and to a lesser extent from pigs fed regular commercial peanuts (RP), but not from HO peanut or control pigs.

Good for Biodiesel Production

As cetane number (CN) is a diesel quality parameter which measures combustion quality during compression ignition, diesel fuel with a higher CN has better ignition properties (Wilson et al., 2013). Highly unsaturated fatty acids including linoleate are associated with low CN (Wilson et al., 2013). HO peanut genotypes are therefore considered more suitable for biodiesel production than their NO counterparts. In addition, the oleochemicals business sectors are investigating the use of HO vegetable oils as feedstock for producing numerous products including cosmetics and machine lubricants (Butzen and Schnebly, 2007; Koilkonda et al., 2013). Considering the above-mentioned advantages of HO peanut over NO peanut, increasing oleate content and in the meantime decreasing linoleate content has therefore become one of the major breeding objectives of peanut.

Analysis of Fatty Acids

Chromatography

Traditional FAMEs (fatty acid methyl esters) preparation procedure for peanut seeds consisted of crude fat extraction with Soxlet apparatus and subsequent esterization of fatty acids, which was tedious and time-consuming. A large portion of seed tissues and 2-14 hours were generally needed. Zeile et al. (1993) reported a method for sampling and direct transmethylation, where 15 mg of peanut cotyledonary tissues were adequate to prepare FAMEs for gas chromatography (GC) using N_2 and an 80°C water bath; the transmethylation step took longer than an hour. Kaveri et al. (2009) described a new protocol to prepare FAMEs, which only took 30 minutes, but required half portion of single seeds and heating apparatus (60°C for 20 min). They used gas liquid chromatography (GLC) to analyze FAMEs. Based on Fan (1991), Gao and Zhang (2010) developed a modified procedure for FAMEs preparation at room temperature (r. t.) using 20 mg peanut seed tissue distal to embryo end; yet the method was not optimized for GC autosampler.

Recently, Yang et al. (2012) described a protocol for analyzing 8 fatty acids using 5-20 mg of peanut seed tissues distal to embryo ends, which required only 35 minutes for preparation at r. t. and 18 minutes for GC analysis. The results proved to be accurate and reproducible, irrespective of sampling amount and fatty acid content. Effect of sampling on seed germinability was minimal. Optimized for GC autosampler, the protocol may cater the need for nondestructive sampling and gene pyramiding in genetic and breeding studies in peanut, and may facilitate genetic improvement in fatty acid composition of the peanut crop.

Though near infrared spectroscopy (NIRS) calibration equations for major fatty acids in peanut seeds are currently available for screening of a large number of breeding materials (Wang et al., 2014; Wang et al., 2012), final confirmatory studies with chromatography are still necessary. As NIRS calibration equations are developed for well-filled seeds, to determine fatty acids in shriveled seeds, chromatography might be the sole option in addition to capillary electrophoresis (CE).

Capillary Electrophoresis

Using 100 accessions of peanut materials of 3 market types (Virginia, runner and Spanish type), Chamberlin et al. (2011) studied the utility of CE in determination of the ratio of oleate to linoleate (O/L), in comparison with the results from GC analysis. The Pearson's correlation coefficient was as high as 0.96, statistically significant at 0.01 level. Similar to the GC analysis conducted by them, the CE method needed 5-6 hours.

NIRS

As mentioned above, traditionally, fatty acids in peanut were determined by chromatography. Nondestructive GC methods using part of peanut seed have already been reported (Yang et al., 2012), but they are still time-consuming, unsuitable for screening of large populations for quality segregants. NIRS, on the other hand, provides a fast, accurate, green and low cost alternative.

In Australia, Fox and Cruickshank (2005) reported NIRS models for bulk peanut seed samples for predicting oleic, linoleic, palmitic and stearic acids. In USA, Tillman et al. (2006) reported NIRS calibration equations suitable for predicting oleic and linoleic acid content in single peanut seeds. Sundaram et al. (2010) studied the possible application of NIRS method for determination of in-shell peanut (Virginia and Valencia types) fatty acids, and concluded that for both types fatty acid prediction could be used for initial screening purpose. Sundaram et al. (2011) established a NIR (near infrared) reflectance spectroscopic method for analyzing main fatty acids contents in larger seed samples. The NIR method saved a lot of time. It only took 5-10 minutes for analysis, compared to GC procedure which required 2-4 hours (Sundaram et al., 2011). In China, Wang (2010) and Wang et al. (2012, 2014) developed NIRS calibration equations predictive of main fatty acids [oleic, linoleic and palmitic acids, and the 4 potentially harmful fatty acids (FPHFA), including palmitic, arachidic, behenic and lignoceric acid] content in sun-dried bulk peanut seed samples and in individual single peanut seeds. NIRS models for bulk peanut seed samples can be used for selection in F_2, M_3 or later generations as long as seed quantity is adequate.

Apart from the utility in breeding, for seed companies, the NIRS models may also be used in purity control when HO peanut seeds are multiplied, and for oil/food processing sectors, these models can be utilized in quality evaluation of HO peanut raw materials (Wang et al., 2014).

Refractive Index (RI)

The RI is the ratio of speed of light in a vacuum to the speed of light in a given material (Davis et al., 2013). Holley and Hammons (1968) found a positive and significantly high correlation coefficient (r=0.779) between RI and the iodine number of 67 peanut strains. Khan et al. (1974) pointed out that the Bausch and Lomb oil grading precision refractometer had several advantages over GC equipment. The refractometer was cheap and virtually had no cost while in operation. Its efficiency was also high: what could be indexed in an hour with a refractometer essentially equaled 8-hour's work with chromatographic techniques (Khan et al. 1974). Peanut with an O/L (oleic acid to linoleic acid ratio) of ≥9 are generally regarded as high oleate by US peanut industry, whereas NO peanut has an O/L lower than 9 (Davis et al., 2013). Gu et al. (2006) used a RI threshold of 1.468 to study the genetics of HO. When RI≤1.468, the seeds were classified as high oleic; a RI greater than1.468 indicated NO phenotype. Davis et al. (2013) studied the potential of RI and density measurement of peanut oil to determine oleic and linoleic acids contents. Oleic acid content, linoleic acid content, density and RI were all strongly linearly correlated for oil blends with O/L ratios of ~2 to 16 (R^2>0.98). Threshold density or RI values indicated high potential for rapid differentiating samples with an O/L ≥9. Density measurements took less than 1 min after oil injection for samples first equilibrated at r. t. But the major limitation for single peanut seeds is that a density meter requires a minimum of ~2 ml of oil for each measurement. RI measurements were rapid (<30 s) for samples held at r. t. prior to measurement at 20°C. The microliters of oil needed for RI assay, however, can be collected from a single seed. According to Davis et al. (2013), using a RI cutoff of 1.46985, all but 2/200 seeds with an O/L less than 9 would be correctly classified as either normal or high oleic. Since RI measurements are highly temperature sensitive, to differentiate peanut oils according to oleic and linoleic acids contents, a temperature control of at least 0.1°C is recommended, and RI measurements accurate to at least four decimal points seems necessary. In RI measurements, care must be taken to minimize solid content of expressed oil, as such particulates are a potential source of variation. D. S. Sweigart was one of the co-authors of the paper by Davis et al. (2013). Prior to this report, in an American Peanut Research and Education Society (APRES) annual meeting, Sweigart et al. (2011) reported that they were able to differentiate HO single peanut seeds from regular peanut seeds, using a multi-cell press to avoid cross-contamination of oils, a device capable of reading to the 5th decimal place (0.00001 RI) in the measurement of oil RI (Bellingham & Stanley RFM 340+) [but different from the machine used by Davis et al. (2013)], and a temperature control to +/- 0.1°C. In a patented invention document and the Ph.D thesis, Lei et al. (2009) and Lei (2010) described the use of RI to differentiate HO peanut (≥70% oleic acid content) from NO peanut (<70% oleic acid content). Analysis can be performed with a half peanut seed and oleic acid content can be calculated from the RI value. If the RI value at 25°C is equal to or less than 1.4667, then the peanut material tested is predicted as high oleic (Lei, 2010).

GENETICS OF OLEIC AND LINOLEIC ACID CONTENT AND O/L

Inferences from Crosses Only Involving Normal Oleate Peanut

Before the identification of the world first HO peanut genotype F435 by Norden et al. (1987), Sykes and Michaels (1986) used NO peanut materials to study the genetics of fatty acid content, and reported that for oleic, linoleic acid and O/L, general combination ability (GCA) was significant only for Virginia type (male) parents. Specific combination ability (SCA) was significant for oleic acid and O/L. GCA for Virginia type parents significantly exceeded SCA for all fatty acids except arachidic, and also for O/L. GCA for Valencia type parents significantly exceeded SCA only for oil content. Significant SCA estimates were found for oil content, palmitic and oleic acids and O/L. Even after 1987, there were still some genetic studies using NO peanut. Mercer at al. (1990) crossed 8 parents in diallel, and found that GCA was important than SCA in F_1 and F_2 generations, indicating the importance of additive effects in the inheritance of fatty acid composition. Maternal effects were significant in F_1 but not in F_2. Reciprocal effects were significant in both generations indicating an interaction between nuclear and extranuclear factors. Xu et al. (1995) noted that for oleic, linoleic an palmitic acid content, GCA and SCA were significant, suggesting that the 3 traits were affected by additive and nonadditive effects with additive effects being predominant. Wan and Tan (1995) showed that oleic, linoleic acid and O/L were mainly controlled by additive genes, having a broad sense heritability of >90%. Wan et al. (2002) showed that O/L, oleic, linoleic, palmitic, stearic and behenic acid contents were conformed to the additive-dominant genetic model, with predominant additive effects and incomplete dominance. Upadhyaya and Nigam (1999) detected additive × additive epistasis for oleic acid in 2 environments studied. Aruna and Nigam (2009) indicated oleic acid and O/L were predominantly under the control of additive gene action. Using the major gene plus polygene mixed genetic models for quantitative traits (Gai et al., 2003) to investigate the inheritance of fatty acid contents in peanut, Han et al. (2011) crossed *hirsuta* type peanut genotypes having an O/L ratio of 4.4 or 5.8

with Spanish type cultivar Yueyou 13 (O/L=1.5). They found that the genetics of oleic and linoleic acid content was in agreement with the one-pair-of-major-gene additive-dorminant model, and that the genetics of O/L was in line with the two-pair-of-major-gene additive-dorminant model. Ding et al. (2007) found O/L in the crosses Qingmiaodou/Quanzhoumake (with an O/L of 5.49 and 1.92, respectively) and Fuchuandahuash/Longanbaowanhuasheng (with an O/L of 5.83 and 1.53, respectively) was controlled by one major gene with negative dominance effect plus polygenes. Heritability of major genes (HMG) in the 2 crosses was 61.27% and 64.09%, and heritability for polygenes (HPG) was 33.85% and 34.52%, respectively. Zhang et al. (2011) also used Gai's models and found that oleic, linoleic and palmitic acid content was under the control of two major genes, HMG being 75.11%, 75.00% and 60.95%, respectively. O/L was controlled by three major genes with HMG of 70.65%.

Inferences from Crosses Involving High Oleate Peanut

To study the genetics of oleic acid content, Moore and Knauft (1989) used F435 (~80% oleic acid) as male and female parent in crosses involving Virginia market type cultivar F78114 (40% oleic acid) and a component line from Sunrunner, F519-9 (54% oleic acid), and the resulted F_1s were backcrossed. In the crosses with F78114, F_1 seed had 40%-44% oleic acid. F_2 seeds from 4 families displayed bimodal distribution and were classified as normal oleic acid (30%-60%) or high oleic acid (70%-80%). The number of seeds in the two categories was consistent with a 15:1 ratio. F_1 plants were used as male or female parent in the backcrosses with F78114, only producing NO seeds. Backcross to F435, however, gave the expected 3:1 ratio of NO to HO seeds. The results supported the hypothesis that two recessive genes control the high oleic acid trait in the crosses. In the crosses with F519-9, F_1 seeds were normal oleic, and there was no reciprocal cross difference. F_2 seeds also showed a bimodal distribution, with seeds containing between 45%-70% and between 70%-85% oleic acid classified as NO and HO, respectively. The number of seeds in the two categories was consistent with a 3:1 ratio. Backcross of F_1 to F519-9 produced NO seeds. Backcross to F435 resulted in offspring fitting in a 1:1 ratio, confirming the single gene hypothesis in the crosses. They proposed gene symbols *ol1* and *ol2* to designate the duplicate recessive alleles in F435 that condition the high oleic acid trait. Further studies by Knauft et al. (1993) showed monogenic inheritance of the high oleic trait in 12 parental backgrounds and digenic inheritance in 1 background, suggesting that either of the two recessive genes may be common in peanut germplasm. Isleib et al. (1996) studied the fatty acid genotypes of 5 Virginia-type peanut cultivars. $F_{4:5}$ progenies were assayed for fatty acid content by GC. Segregation ratios in NC 7, NC 9, NC 10C or VA-C 92R derived populations were consistent with a monogenic model, suggesting that these cultivars have genotype $Ol_1Ol_1ol_2ol_2$ or $ol_1ol_1Ol_2Ol_2$. Progeny of NC-V 11/F435 were consistent with the digenic model, indicating that NC-V 11 has genotype $Ol_1Ol_1Ol_2Ol_2$. Gu et al. (2006) studied the genetics of HO in 2 crosses, k8834/Kaixuan 03-1 and k9069-1/ Kaixuan 03-1. The NO:HO ratio in F_2 generations was 3:1 and 15:1, in accordance with the monogenic and digenic model, respectively. Oleate phenotypes in F_2s from the cross Kainong 30/Kaixuan 01-6 fit the 3(normal):1(high) ratio (Gu et al., 2013). In the study of López et al. (2001), 6 Spanish type peanut cultivars with low O/L ratios were hybridized as females to F435-2-3, the high O/L line. Segregation in F_2 and BC_1F_1 progenies showed that high oleic acid content in Spanish type peanut is digenic inherited. The presence of low-intermediate O/L genotypes indicated that other genetic modifiers may be involved in determining the precise O/L ratio. Muitia et al. (2006) noted the presence of mid-oleic progeny in F_2 generations in 2 crosses. An epistatic model of action was consistent with the data from the cross Tamrun OL01/Nema TAM, fitting a digenic 9(low oleic):6(mid-oleic):1(high oleic) ratio; an additive gene action model was consistent with the data from the cross Nema TAM/OLin, fitting a 5(low oleic):10(mid-oleic):1(high oleic) ratio (Muitia et al., 2006). Isleib et al. (2006) demonstrated partial dominance, pleiotropism and epistasis in the inheritance of the high oleate trait in peanut.

Singkham et al. (2011) found significant GCA effects for oleate and O/L in F_2 and F_3 generations. In the study, SCA and reciprocal effects were also significant, but their relative contributions to variations among crosses were much smaller than those of GCA effects, suggesting the importance of additive gene action in the inheritance of oleate content in peanut (Singkham et al., 2011). Singkham et al. (2012) detected significant additive, dominance and epistasis gene effects for oleate, linoleate and O/L. Barkley et al. (2013) studied genotypic effect of *ahFAD2* on fatty acid profiles in 6 segregating populations. The results showed that dominance was incomplete for the wild type allele of *ahFAD2*, and that both loci exhibited significant additive effects. The *ahFAD2* loci showed pleiotropic interactions with palmitic, oleic, linoleic acids and the O/L ratio. Fatty acid levels in these progeny were affected by the parental genotype, which suggested that other genes also influence fatty acid composition of peanut. Singkham et al. (2010a) estimated the narrow-sense heritability for oleate and linoleate in 3 crosses, namely, Georgia-02C (HO phenotype)/KKU 1(NO phenotype), SunOleic 97R(HO phenotype)/KKU 1 and SunOleic 97R/Georgia 02C. The narrow-sense heritability for oleate and linoleate was intermediate to high for oleate (63%-72%) and linoleate (57%-72%), indicating that selection for high oleate would be effective in F_2 generation.

Several workers studied the genetics of oleic acid or O/L using Gai's models and high oleic parents. Ding et al. (2007) reported that O/L in the cross Shanyou 162/SunOleic 95R was controlled by 2 major genes with additive-dominant-epistatic effects. Estimates of HMG and HPG were 64.66% and 33.45%, respectively. Han et al. (2010) crossed 8-153 (with an O/L ratio of ~40), a stable derivative of Yueyou 162/SunOleic 95R, with NO Yueyou 13, and oleate and linoleate contents of P_1, P_2, F_1, F_2 generations and $F_{2:3}$ families were determined. Oleate content in this cross was found to be controlled by 2 major genes with additive-dorminant effects (E-2 mode). For F_2 generation and $F_{2:3}$ families, HMG was 77.28% and 55.00%, and HPG was 13.34% and 32.13%, respectively. The first major gene (8.8172) had additive effects much higher than did the second major gene (4.0387). The dominant effect of 2 major genes was -10.2475 and -9.0420, respectively. Linoleate content in the cross was controlled by 2 major genes with additive-dominant-epistatic effects (B-1 mode). For F_2 generation and $F_{2:3}$ families, HMG was 88.30% and 79.84%, respectively. The estimates of additive effects of the 2 major genes, *da* and *db*, were -7.3949 and -6.9568, respectively. The estimates of dominant effects of the 2 major genes, *ha* and *hb*, were 1.3879 and 1.5438, respectively. The interactive effects between *da* and *db, da* and *hb, db* and *ha*, *ha* and *hb* were -4.5216, -1.7688, -1.9808 and -1.1172, respectively. Huang et al. (2012) crossed HO peanut introductions wt08-0932 and wt08-0934 with NO peanuts, and obtained F_2 seeds. The results showed that oleate and linoleate contents were controlled by 2 major genes with additive-dominant-epistatic effects. HMG was 66%-89% for oleate and 70%-85% for linoleate, respectively, indicating the presence of polygenic effects. Negative dominant effects were observed for both major genes conditioning oleate content, whereas positive dominant effects were detected for linoleate content. Both the additive and dominant effects of the first major gene were much higher than those of the second major gene. Two mutated major genes result in HO phenotype. The difference in additive and dominant effects between the 2 major genes leads to medium-low and medium-high oleate phenotype when only one major gene is of mutant type.

MOLECULAR BASIS OF THE HIGH OLEATE PHENOTYPE IN PEANUT

FAD2 (*Fatty Acid Desaturese 2*) is a well-known gene coding for oleate/ω-6-/Δ^{12}- desaturase or dehydrogenase that converts oleate into linoleate in crop plants. Elevated oleate content and reduced linoleate content in oilseeds caused by dysfunctional *FAD2* have been reported. Hence, *FAD2* and Δ^{12} desaturase were considered the logical candidate gene for high oleate studies in peanut.

Reduced Microsomal Δ^{12}- Desaturase Activity in F435

Ray et al. (1993) found that the Δ^{12}- desaturase activity in microsomes of developing seeds of F435 (HO natural mutant) was less than 1/10 of that in the NO wild type parent, F78-1339. Wheeler et al. (1994) compared the microsomal polypeptide patterns between high (F435) and normal oleate (F78-1339) isogenic peanut lines using 2-D gel electrophoresis. F435 was unique in that it had a pair of 18 kDa polypeptides focusing at about pH 9.3 at stage 1 maturity, instead of a 20 kDa polypeptide pair focusing at pH 6.8 and 7.3. They postulated that the 20 kDa polypeptides could be components of the Δ^{12}- desaturase complex.

Low Activity of Microsomal Oleoyl-PC Desaturase Encoded by *AhFAD2A* with 448G>A Coupled with Severely Reduced Transcript of *AhFAD2B*

Using 2 HO peanut materials, M2-225(an AT108 DES mutant) and 8-2122 (a hybrid derivative of F435 and GK7), and 3 NO genotypes, F78-1339, AT108 and GK7, Jung et al. (2000a) isolated 2 microsomal oleoyl-PC (phosphatidychloline) desaturase genes. Screening a cDNA library constructed with RNAs extracted from F78-1339 developing seeds with the *Arabiodopsis FAD2* cDNA as a probe resulted in a cDNA clone with an ORF (open reading frame) of 1140 bp, encoding a putative polypeptide of 379 amino acids. The deduced amino acid sequence showed 82%, 74% and 70% identity to that of soybean *FAD2-1*, soybean *FAD2-2* and *Arabiodopsis FAD2*, respectively. The gene was then termed as *ahFAD2A*, as in later studies it grouped together with the corresponding sequence from *A. duranensis,* the putative A-genome donor of the cultivated peanut (*Arachis hypogaea* L.), when both of the coding sequence and 5' UTR (5'-untranslated region) were included in analysis. Since the cultivated peanut is an allotetraploid, there might be multiple genes coding for microsomal oleoyl-PC desaturases in peanut. Using positive plaques obtained from the above cDNA screen and primers generated from *ahFAD2A*, PCR products were obtained and sequenced. Sequences of the PCR products fell into 2 categories: one corresponded to *ahFAD2A*, and the other represented a new sequence, which was named as *ahFAD2B*, considering the fact that it grouped together with the corresponding sequence from *A. ipaënsis*, the most possible B-genome donor of the cultivated peanut. Several positive clones were obtained after screening of the λ FIXII genomic library of F78-1339 with the *ahFAD2A* cDNA probe. Using PCR primers designed based on the sequence of *ahFAD2B* 5'-UTR, clones that containing 5' end regions of oleoyl-PC desaturase genes were identified. Digested purified λ DNA, after electrophoresis, was subjected to Southern analysis using *ahFAD2B* 5'-UTR sequences as a probe. A 5-kb *Eco*R I fragment that hybridized to the probe was subcloned and a ~600-bp region of the insert containing the putative "promoter region", 5'-UTR and 5' reading frame region was characterized by sequencing (Jung et al. 2000a) [Note: López et al. (2000) proposed a putative intron of 1,564 bp upstream of the Δ^{12} Fad coding sequence in NO Tamspan 90]. Sequence comparison of the reading frames of the genomic clone and cDNA clones showed that this genomic clone corresponded to *ahFAD2A*. The promoter region of *ahFAD2B* was obtained by PCR using genomic DNA as template. A 1067-bp region containing the putative "promoter region", 5'-UTR and 5' reading frame region was amplified. Clones that corresponded to *ahFAD2B* were identified by sequencing the reading frame of the inserts. There is a 19-bp insertion in *ahFAD2A*, or a 19-bp deletion in *ahFAD2B*, in the 5'-UTR. Digestion of RT-PCR products showed that in developing seeds (stage 2) of HO materials (M2-225 and 8-2122) the amount of *ahFAD2B* transcript was severely reduced, while the transcription of *ahFAD2A* was not affected [Note: Regarding the reduction in *ahFAD2B* transcript, López et al. (2002) questioned if it was just an artifact in transcription analysis when primers downstream the insertion site were used]. Jung et al. (2000b) further studied the molecular mechanism underlying the HO phenotype in peanut using Virugard (NO, $ol_1ol_1OL_2OL_2$), 59-4144[HO, hybrid derivative of AT108(NO, $ol_1ol_1OL_2OL_2$) and F1250(HO, =SunOleic 95R, developed from a cross between Sunrunner and F435), 91-1718(NO, $OL_1OL_1OL_2OL_2$) and F_2

hybrids between Virugard and 59-4144. Enzyme digestion of RT-PCR products using RNA extracted from seeds of F_2 and parental lines showed that severely reduced level of *ahFAD2B* transcription correlated absolutely with the HO phenotype in the cross. Yeast expression analysis demonstrated that the protein product of *ahFAD2A* from HO peanut and NO peanut with $ol_1ol_1OL_2OL_2$ genotype showed significantly low oleoyl-PC desaturase activity. Amino acid sequence comparison strongly supported the possibility of the D150N (D=aspartic acid, N=asparagine) change in *ahFAD2A* near the highly conserved histidine-rich motif of membrane desaturases responsible for the reduced activity of the enzyme. Another *ahFAD2A* allele cloned from 91-1718 (NO) does not have the D150N change.

Bruner et al. (2001) studied the effect of amino acid change at position 150 caused by A→G or G→A (448A>G or 448G>A) on the oleoyl-PC desaturase activity, using the *ahFAD2A* (encoding a protein with reduced oleoyl-PC desaturase activity) and *ahFAD2B* (functional) genes isolated by Jung et al. (2000a). As expected, N150D led to the recovery of the enzyme activity, whereas D150N led to severely reduced enzyme activity.

As stated above, the reason for low activity of oleoyl-PC desaturase encoded by *ahFAD2A* was elucidated. As for *ahFAD2B*, Patel et al. (2004) discovered an insertion of MITE (minature incerted-repeat transposable element) (at 988 position) towards the 3' end of the coding region in the gene in M2-225. They speculated that nonsense-mediated decay (NMD) may play a role in reduction of *ahFAD2B* transcript in the seeds of M2-225. As Patel et al. (2004) did not find any differences in the *ahFAD2B* of 8-2122 and that of the normal, they were unable to explain the HO phenotype of the mutant. López et al. (2002) indicated that F435 plants appear to display heterogeneity in the 441_442insA mutation in *ahFAD2B*. 8-2122, as a hybrid derivative of F435, may not have this frameshift mutation (Patel et al., 2004). This allows for the possibility that there exist other genes or regulatory factors that influence the expression of the HO trait (López et al., 2002).

Dysfunctional Δ^{12} Fad Caused by 441_442insA or 448G>A in the Coding Region

López et al. (2000) studied the gene sequences of Δ^{12} *Fad* in F435 (HO) and Tamspan 90 (NO), and identified 2 polymorphisms in Δ^{12} *Fad* appear to be associated with high O/L. In F435, there is an "A" insertion 442 bp after the start codon (441_442insA), which may result in a truncated, inactive protein and the loss of one of the histidine boxes believed to be important to the enzyme activity. In F435, there is a second type of Δ^{12} *Fad*, which lacks the "A" insertion but has a base change from G to A at the 448 bp from the start codon (448G>A), which causes an amino acid substitution. López et al. (2002) showed that the "A" insertion and the amino acid change were expresses in both leaf and seed tissue of the high and low-intermediate O/L genotypes. They postulated that several copies of Δ^{12} *Fad* are present in the cultivated peanut genome, and concluded that O/L is dependent on the number of functional copies. Zhou et al. (2011) reported 3 kinds of *ahFAD2* transcripts (*ahFAD2A*, *ahFAD2B* and pseudogene) in 13 peanut accessions.

Later, Yu et al. (2008) also identified "A" insertion 442 bp after the start codon (441_442insA) in Δ^{12} *Fad* from several hybrid derivatives (E11, E12, E16 and E18) of a γ-ray irradiation induced HO peanut mutant SPI098. Yeast expression analysis demonstrated the frameshift 441_442insA mutation results in low activity or deactivation of theΔ^{12} fatty acid desaturase in HO genotypes.

MITE Insertion in *ahFAD2B* of Mycogen-Flavo

Patel et al. (2004) identified MITE insertion in the center of the coding region of *ahFAD2B* in Mycogen-Flavo. The insertion site is different from that found in M2-225. No significant decrease in gene transcript was noted (Patel et al., 2004).

Novel *ahFAD2* Mutations in Peanut Mutants with Elevated Oleate Content

Base alterations were identified in *ahFAD2A* from TGM121M, a mutant with elevated oleic acid content resulting from γ-ray irradiation and sodium azide (NaN_3) treatment (Mondal et al., 2011). 485T>C led to an amino acid change from tryptophan to arginine at position 133, and 536G>A caused an amino acid substitution of aspartic acid by asparagine at position 150 (Mondal et al., 2011).

Novel mutations in *ahFAD2B* were detected in NaN_3-treated Huayu 22 (Wang et al., 2011a) or EMS (Ethyl methanesulfonate) -treated LF 2 (Fang et al., 2012). Both mutants had elevated oleate content compared with their wild types. A C to T mutation at position 281 of coding region of *ahFAD2B* resulted in an isoleucine to threonine change at position 94 of amino acid sequence in the NaN_3 mutant (Wang et al., 2011a). As to the EMS mutant, the 448G>A mutation in *ahFAD2A* was the same as in previous reports, and the 906A>G mutation in *ahFAD2A* did cause amino acid change; the 313C>T mutation in *ahFAD2A* led to an amino acid alteration from histidine to tyrosine at position 105, which was located in the first histindine box (Fang et al., 2012). Yeast expression analysis showed that the enzyme encoded by the mutant type *ahFAD2B* from the EMS mutant had lost its oleate desaturase activity (Fang et al., 2012).

Role of *ahFAD2A/ahFAD2B* in Peanut Oleate Content as Evidenced by Marker-Phenotype Relationship Analysis

Sarvamangala et al. (2011) reported 3 quantitative trait loci (QTL) (TC6H03-TC11A04, TC5A07-IPAHM395 and TC3A12-PM433) for oleic acid and linoleic acid, with lower than 10% contributions to phenotypic variance of oleic acid, linoleic acid or O/L. They used simple sequence repeat (SSR) markers in this study, with no attempt to explore the relationship between *ahFAD2* alleles and the oleate phenotype.

Chu et al. (2007) reported that the *ahFAD2A* mutant allele (with 448G>A mutation) was present in 31.6% of the accessions from the mini-core of the US peanut germplasm collection. This mutant allele was frequent in subspecies *hypogaea*. However, it is absent from subspecies *fastigiata* and the putative A-genome donor, *A. duranensis*. Lei et al. (2010) studied the distribution frequencies of individual *ahFAD2A* alleles in Chinese peanut mini-core collection, and found a close relationship with oleate content. Barkley et al. (2011) detected that oleate contents differed significantly among 3 genotype groups, Ol_2Ol_2, Ol_2ol_2 and ol_2ol_2. Wang et al. (2011c) tested the oleate content in 55 breeding lines, and found the 4 genotype groups, Ol_1Ol_1 Ol_2Ol_2, ol_1ol_1 Ol_2Ol_2, Ol_1Ol_1 ol_2ol_2 and ol_1ol_1 ol_2ol_2, exhibited a marked difference in oleate content. Wang et al. (2011d) conducted association analyses using US peanut mini-core collection, and verified that the functional SNP from the *FAD2A* gene was significantly associated with oleic acid, linoleic acid, and O/L.

Shirasawa et al. (2012) found that phenotype variation in O/L ratio explained by *ahFAD2A/ahFAD2B* genes was 89.5%. Wang et al. (2013a) used a multiple linear regression approach to quantify the contribution of *FAD2* to fatty acid profile in peanut. Fatty acid contents in single peanut seeds of two

F_2 populations derived from normal oleate × high oleate crosses were determined by gas chromatography and *FAD2A/FAD2B* genotype was analyzed by allele-specific PCR (AS-PCR) assay (Yu et al., 2013). According to the multiple linear regression models, 60% of the variation in oleic or linoleic acid content, about 50% of the variation in palmitic acid and lower than 25% of the variation in eicosenoic acid could be explained by the genotypic effect of *FAD2A* and *FAD2B*. Mutant type *FAD2B* generally had absolute values of regression coefficients higher than mutant type *FAD2A*, suggesting that *FAD2B* might be more important than *FAD2A* in conditioning fatty acid biosynthesis/accumulation. The study indicated that factors other than *FAD2A/FAD2B* might also affect fatty acid profiles in peanut. Two reports support the hypothesis. Chamberlin et al. (2011) found NO seeds from seed lots of the HO peanut cultivar Brantley. According to Wang et al. (2013b), despite selection in F_2 single plants (F_3 seeds) for HO bulk seeds, NO seeds were found in later generations. Wang et al. (2013b) underlined the necessity of additional selection(s) for the HO trait, preferably seed by seed, during breeding process prior to bulk harvest for a yield trial, to exclude possible off-types (NO seed within the HO seed lot) in cultivar releases. It is important that the HO phenotype of a cultivar should be stable.

Use BSA (Bulk Segregants Analysis) coupled with NGS (next generation sequencing), we were able to isolate 20 SNPs (Single Nucleotide Polymorphism) potentially related to genes conditioning oleate content in peanut (Chuan Tang Wang and Yue Yi Tang, unpublished data). These candidates need further verification in populations.

Chen et al. (2013) grew 29 entries of varieties and advanced breeding lines in 2 locations in 3 years with 3 replications to estimate the effects of G × E interaction on fatty acid composition of cultivated peanuts. They used real-time PCR and functional SNP markers to genotype the lines tested, and Additive Main Effects and Multiplicative Interaction (AMMI) model to estimate additive effects of *FAD2A* and *FAD2B* genes and G × E interaction. The results showed significant G × E interactions for oleic acid and a larger additive effect of *FAD2B* than *FAD2A*.

Pandey et al. (2014) used 2 recombinant inbred line (RIL) mapping populations derived from SunOleic 97R × NC94022 and Tifrunner × GT-C20, and mapped *FAD2A* and *FAD2B* on AhIX and AhV linkage groups, respectively. They found 2 marker intervals representing mutant alleles *FAD2A* and *FAD2B* contributing up to 23.46% and 39.3% phenotypic variance (PVE), respectively for oleic acid, up to 26.1% and 41.2% PVE, respectively for linoleic acid, and up to 10.8% and 30.5% -74% PVE, respectively for O/L ratio (Pandey et al., 2014). They concluded that the contribution of *FAD2B* is higher than *FAD2A*.

The study of Barkley et al. (2013) suggested that there is a dosage effect for the oleic and linoleic phenotypes in that as the number of mutant *ahFAD2* alleles increases the oleic acid content increases and the linoleic acid content decreases. In contrast to the conclusions from Wang et al. (2013a), Chen et al. (2013) and Pandey et al. (2014), Barkley et al. (2013) asserted that mutant *ahFAD2* alleles in the A genome do not have a bigger effect on oleic acid accumulation than the mutant alleles in the B genome or *vice versa*.

FACTORS AFFECTING FATTY ACID PROFILE

Singkham et al. (2010b) studied the effects of genotype, environmental factors and G × E interaction on the fatty acids composition of peanut seeds using 21 peanut materials of 3 categories: high oleate, intermediate oleate and low oleate. Significant G × E interaction was detected in oleate, linoleate and O/L, but its importance was lower than genotypic main effects. For oleate content, significant G × E interaction was only found in intermediate oleate and low oleate groups.

Genotype

In the 4 botanical varieties of the cultivated peanut, Virginian and *hirsuta* types generally have an O/L ratio higher than do Spanish and Valencia types. Mukri et al. (2012) analyzed the oleate content of peanuts from ICRISAT (International Crops Research Institute for the Semi-Arid Tropics) peanut mini-core collection, and the variation ranged from 33.60%-73.54%, with ICG2381 (73.54%) from *hypogaea* variety being the highest. Oleate content in GM4-3 from *vulgaris* variety was also higher than 70% (71% oleate). Shin et al. (2010) reported fatty acid composition of US runner type peanut cultivars. Normal oleate varieties Georgia Green, Tamrun 96, C-99R, Georgia-01R, Georgia-03L and AP-3 had an O/L ratio of 1.79-1.94, 1.64-1.73, 2.04-2.16, 2.50, 2.40 and 2.01, respectively. Intermediate oleate peanut cultivar Tamrun OL01 had an O/L ratio of 4.36-5.38. O/L for high oleate peanut cultivars Tamrun OL02, Flavorunner-458 and Georgia-02C was 14.90-19.34, 2.50-15.15 and 16.38-16.78, respectively. Anderson and Gorbet (2002) reported the results from an experiment using high, intermediate and normal oleate peanut materials in 3 years and 3 seeding dates. The oleate content of high oleate SunOleic 97R, UF98326, UF99621 and 88x1B-OLBC1-6-1-3-1-b2-B averaged 77.8%-82.5%, and O/L was 18-51. Intermediate oleate material Florida MDR98 contained 59.8%-68% oleate. Normal oleate materials Georgia Greene, Andru 93, Florunner, 86x13A-4-2-3-2-b3-B and UF97102 had an O/L ratio of 1.7-3.5.

Seed Market Grade and Maturity

There are controversial research results about whether kernel grade affects fatty acid composition in peanut. Mozingo et al. (1988) found a similar tendency in 5 US Virginia type peanut cultivars, where oleic acid content and the O/L ratio of a specific variety consistently increased as the kernels became larger in size (Extra large > Medium >No. 1). Significant inter-grade difference was detected in palmitic, stearic, oleic, linoleic, arachidic, eicosenoic and behenic acid content and O/L (Mozingo et al., 1988). Hashim et al. (1993) studied the fatty acid composition in 3 market grades (No.1, medium and Jumbo) of Florunner (a runner type peanut cultivar), and found a decrease trend in long-chain saturated fatty acids, eicosenoic acid and O/L with the increase in seed size. But there was no marked difference in oleic acid content of the 3 market grades. In China, Zhang et al. (2009a) reported results from a study on the effects of grading on the main quality attributes of peanut kernels using film mulching cultivation. No significant differences in oleic, linoleic acid content and O/L were detected among the No. 1, No. 2 and No. 3 grade peanut kernels of a given peanut genotype.

The indeterminant fruiting pattern of peanut dictates that at any harvest dates fruit of a wide range of maturity are harvested (Sanders, 1989). The maturity distribution in commercially sized China peanuts has not been studied; yet according to Sanders (1989), sized Florunner seeds had different maturity groups, and the largest seed size contained the high percentage of mature peanuts. Effect of market grade on nutritional quality of peanut seeds in a large part reflects the effect of seed maturity. Sanders et al. (1982) found that O/L increased with the increasing maturity (as determined by hull-scrape method) from 2 to 6 (O/L did not significantly differ between maturity group 7 and 6), and that free fatty acids and Iodine Value (IV) decreased with the increasing maturity from 2 to 7. Yu and Min (1997) reported that with the increase in maturity, O/L increased gradually and remained essentially unchanged when seeds approached full maturity.

Temperature and Soil Moisture Content

Holladay and Pearson (1974) observed that high temperature at 4 weeks before harvest led to elevated oleic acid content and O/L in peanut seeds. Golombek et al. (1995) reported increase in O/L of 3 Spanish type peanut cultivars under elevated soil temperature treatments (20/14, 26/20 and 32/26°C). In Tai'an, China, Wan et al. (1995) studied the relationship between O/L of well-filled seeds of 3 peanut materials (Haihua 1, Hua 17 and 814) and average air temperature (Ta) or soil temperature (5 cm depth) (Ts) during pod development stage. They found that O/L was positively correlated with Ta at 0.01 or 0.05 level, and that O/L was positively correlated with Ts at 0.01 level. O/L showed stronger correlation with Ts than with Ta. In order to determine the key climatic factors affecting peanut quality, Li et al. (2010) used correlation analysis, path analysis and stepwise regression analysis, based on peanut quality data and meteorological data during peanut season from the 18 main peanut producing provinces in China in 2008. Significant correlation (at 0.01 level) was detected between O/L and individual climatic factors. O/L showed significant positive correlation at 0.01 level with >15°C accumulated temperature and rainfall during peanut season, and significant negative correlation at 0.01 level with sunshine hours and day and night temperature difference during peanut season. Stepwise regression analysis revealed that day and night temperature difference was the main factor affecting peanut O/L ratio.

Dwivedi et al. (1996) studied the effect of drought on quality of post-rainy season peanut. They found that mid-season [40-80 days after sowing(DAS)]drought had no significant effect on fatty acids other than eicosenoic acid, and that end-of-season (80DAS till harvest) drought significantly reduced linoleic and behenic acid content, and significantly increased stearic and oleic acid content. Reduced activity of oleate desaturases caused by high soil temperature resulting from drought is believed to be the reason for elevated O/L.

Sowing Date

Chiou et al. (1995) pointed out that spring crops of peanut had higher oleate content than did fall crops. Mondal and Badigannavar (2010) reported that rainy season peanut contained more oleate than did summer season peanut in India. In Tai'an, China, Wan et al. (1995) found significant correlation between O/L ratio of well-filled peanut seeds (Haihua 1, Hua 17 and 814) and seeding dates. In the 1990 experiment, with the delay of seeding date between April 13 and July 6, the O/L ratio dropped constantly. O/L of summer peanut was lower than that of spring peanut. In USA, Anderson and Gorbet (2002) observed a trend that oleic acid decreased and linoleic acid increased with the increasingly later planting date (mid-April, mid-May, early-June), which was in accordance with the common sense that relatively low temperature in podding zone was conducive to enzyme activity of oleate desaturases, thereby resulting in more linoleic acid.

Polyethylene Film Mulch

Wan et al. (1995) studied if polyethylene film mulch cultivation affected peanut O/L, and found that film mulch raised soil temperature, thereby increasing the O/L ratio.

Location

The same peanut genotype, when planted in different locations, may have significantly different O/L ratios, which may be the reflection of the compound effect of soil and climatic factors. For an instance, Shiyouhong No. 4, when planted in Guangzhou, contained higher than 70% oleate; however, when planted in Shandong, the oleate content was much lower. Several peanut materials with relatively high oleate identified in the eighth five-year-plan period of China were planted in Nanning (Guangxi province), Wuhan (Hubei province) and Laixi (Shandong province). O/L ratios were consistently higher in Nanning than in Wuhan or Laixi (Yu et al., 2011). In USA, Brown et al. (1975) pointed that from south to north (29°18'-36°43'N), oleic and palmitic acid tended to decrease while polyunsaturated fatty acids tended to increase. In Argentina, Grosso et al. (1996) reached a similar conclusion. Peanut produced in southeast regions contained more oleic acid than did other regions. Hinds et al. (1995) found peanut grown in volcanic clay loam had more stearic acid and total fatty acids and less linoleic acid and unsaturated fatty acids than did peanut grown in volcanic sandy loam.

BREEDING METHODOLOGIES FOR HIGH OLEATE PEANUTS

Use of Mutagenesis

Natural Mutants

Norden et al. (1987) analyzed 494 accessions of peanut breeding materials for fatty acid composition in sound mature kernels (SMKs) by GC, and identified 2 high oleic acid natural mutants, 435-2-1 and 435-2-2, both of which originated from F78-1339 and were also named as F435, UF435 or F435HO. The mutants had 79.91% and 79.71% oleate, about 2% linoleic acid, and an O/L ratio of 37.34 and 34.81, respectively. Many peanut cultivar releases in USA were derived from F435. In China, Wang et al. (2011) reported a natural mutant with high oleic acid (FB4). Its HO phenotype was first identified with NIRS and later on confirmed by GC.

Irradiation Mutants

A high oleic mutant was obtained fromγ-ray treated populations of Georgia Runner in US (Table 1). Yu et al. (2003) identified 4 peanut mutants with an O/L ratio of over 15 from γ-ray induced mutants derived progenies, SPI 087 (79.01% oleate, O/L= 25.48), SPI 098(81.59% oleate, O/L=37.25), SPI184 (81.19% oleate, O/L=25.29) and SPI 214(80.67% oleate, O/L=17.89). Wang et al. (2011b) reported a HO γ-ray induced mutant, CTWE. Mondal and Badigannavar (2010) analyzed 69 selections obtained from 200-300Gyγ-ray treated populations of TPG 41 (57% oleate in rainy season crop, 66.7% oleate in summer season crop), and identified 6 mutants with >60% oleate in rainy season crop and >70% oleate in summer season crop.

Chemical Mutants

Among the high oleic peanut cultivar released in US, FlavoRunner 458 was an EMS mutant, and AT225 High Oleic was a DES (Diethylsulfate) mutant. With the help of NIRS models for bulk seed samples and single seeds, Wang et al. (2011a) identified a single M_3 plant with >60% oleate from the mutagenized populations Huayu 22 treated with 0.39% sodium azide solution, which was later confirmed by GC analysis. Similarly, E2-4-83-12, an EMS mutant of LF 2 (Virginia type peanut cultivar), was identified by Fang et al.

(2012). The mutant contained 64.2% oleate, in contrast to 44.2% in its wild type.

Mutants Resulting from Irradiation and Chemical Mutagen Treatment

Using 200-300Gy γray and 1-3 mM sodium azide to treat TFDRG5, Mondal et al. (2011) obtained 47 morphological mutants in M_3 population. Fatty acid composition was analyzed in M_8 and M_9. TGM192M had 70.67% and 70.89% oleate, and 12.61% and 12.97% linoleate, whereas the wild type TFDRG5 only had 55.50% and 55.16% oleate, and 25.68% and 26.41% linoleate. With poor agronomic characters, TGM192M may be used as parental material for breeding new peanut cultivars.

Intra-Specific Hybridization and Backcrossing

Most of the HO mutants have not been used directly as cultivars. Through hybridization with high-yielding peanut cultivars or further backcrossing, more than 30 HO peanut cultivars have been released in USA (Table 1). TSWV resistance was not incorporated into earlier HO peanut cultivar releases; that is the reason why these varieties only had limited planting area. Recent HO peanut cultivar releases have acceptable TSWV resistance.

Georgia Hi-O/L and Georgia 02C, 2 HO peanut cultivars developed in USA, were hybrid derivatives of a γ -ray mutant of Georgia Runner. The HO peanut cultivar Georgia-08V was derived from the cross C-99R/Georgia Hi-O/L (Table 1).

In China, several HO peanut varieties have been released. Huayu 32, a HO hybrid derivative of S17/SPI 098, was released for commercial production in 2009 in Shandong province. H03-3, a HO peanut cultivar derived from K9508-1/Kaixuan 01-6, was released for cultivation in 2007 in Anhui province. Kainong 61, a HO peanut hybrid derivative of Kainong 31/ Kaixuan 01-6, was released for cultivation in 2012 in Henan province (Gu et al., 2013). Jihua 11 is a peanut cultivar with 56.44% oil and 80.70% oleate released in 2013 in Hebei province. This cultivar was derived from the cross Jihua 5/Kainong 01-6 (Chen et al., 2013). A large number of new HO lines are now under productivity evaluation at multi-locations at provincial or national level. These lines were mostly derived from crosses using high oleic peanuts as male parents and local adapted cultivars as female parents, and have even higher yield levels compared with earlier varietal releases (Wang et al., 2013b).

In 2005, South Africa released SA Juweel, a HO high-yielding Spanish type cultivar derived from the cross Akwa (an adapted peanut cultivar)/UF85-1241(a HO breeding line from USA) (Pretorius et al., 2010).

Breeding for adapted peanut cultivars with HO kernels has been one of the major objectives of the projects supported by Queensland Department of Primary Industries (QDPI) since 1994 (Cruickshank et al., personal communication). HO F_2 individuals were used in backcrossing, 3-way crosses and as a starting point for selection following the pedigree method. Wheeler and Middleton, 2 cultivars with high oleate, were released in 2003. Wheeler is a Virginia type peanut cultivar developed from a backcross to Conder, a high yielding Nut-IN-Shell variety. Middleton, also a Virginia type peanut cultivar, was a pedigree selection from a 3-way cross using Streeton (a drought tolerant cultivar) as the 50% parent (Cruickshank et al., personal communication). As an outcome of the joint breeding effort of Peanut Company of Australia Limited (PCA), Qld Department of Employment, Economic Development and Innovation (DEEDI), Kingaroy and the Grains Research and Development Corporation (GRDC), Tingoora, a HO peanut cultivar that matures in 105-110 days, was derived from a cross between Walter (with drought tolerance) and D45-p37-102 (with foliar disease tolerance) in 2003. Pedigree selection for yield, grade and disease tolerance was practiced during the period 2003-2009.

Use of Wild Peanut Relatives

Jiang et al. (2009) identified 2 accessions of wild peanut materials as with high oleate. 19-6 (*A.duranensis*) contained 60.9% oleate, and 23-1 (*A.* sp.) had 60.0% oleate. Tang et al. (2013) identified 6 accessions of wild *Arachis* species as with an O/L ratio of higher than 1.5. Among them, A14-3 (*A.correntina*) had 67.91% oleate, and its O/L was 4.91 (Table 2).

Table 1. Main high oleic peanut cultivars released in the USA

Cultivars	Other names	Type	Origin	Year of release	PVP		
					Certificate No.	Year expired	Applicants
SunOleic 95R	F1250	R	[F435-2-3-B-2-1-b4-B-B-3-b3—b3-1-B×F591-9(a Sunrunner component line)]F_1s were backcrossed to F591-9. HO seeds were selected for further backcrossing. BC_3F_2 were planted in field. Pedigree selection method was followed. BC_3F_4s were harvested and pooled for yield evaluation. O/L=23	1995	9400148	9.30.2012	Florida Agricultural Experiment Station, University of Florida
FlavoRunner 458	458, Flavorunner 458, C458, Mycogen-Flavorunner	R	EMS treated Florunner seeds were sown in May 1992. M_2 seeds were sown in Puerto Rico in winter. A single M_2 plant was selected. M_3 seeds with >80% oleate were identified. O/L=24.1 US patent 5948954	1997	9600242	7.31.2017	James Sutton, Mycogen Corporation Gordon Patterson, Hershey Foods Corporation
SunOleic 97R	F1334	R	The cross was the same as SunOleic 95R. BC_4F_2s were planted in field and selected following the pedigree method. BC_4F_8s were harvested and pooled for yield evaluation. O/L=24.6	1997	9700181	7.31.2017	Univ. of Fla. Agric. Expt. Sta.
GK-7 High Oleic	AgraTech GK-7 High Oleic	R	HO peanut F_2 seeds were selected from the cross between GK-7 and F435, and backcrossed to GK-7. Selection was made for 4 years following the pedigree method.	1997	9800019	Application Abandoned	Golden Peanut Company, LLC
AT225 High Oleic	M2-225	R	AT108 DES mutant. US patent 5945578.	1997	9700010	Application Abandoned	Golden Peanut Company, LLC

Cultivars	Other names	Type	Origin	Year of release	PVP		
					Certificate No.	Year expired	Applicants
AgraTech 1-1	AT 1-1	R	High oleic F_2 hybrids of F435 x GK-7 were selected and backcrossed to GK-7. High oleic BC_1F_2s were backcrossed to GK-7. High oleic BC_2F_1s were backcrossed to GK-7. BC_3F_2, BC_4F_1 and BC_4F_2: high oleate selection. BC_4F_2s were sown in field and selected for yield and resistance. O/L=20	1999	200000134	11.15.2022	Golden Peanut Company, LLC
AgraTech 201	AT 201, 97-2556	R	High oleic F_2 hybrids of F435 x GK-7 were selected and backcrossed to GK-7. High oleic BC_1F_2s were backcrossed to GK-7. High oleic BC_2F_1s were backcrossed to GK-7. BC_2F_2: high oleate selection. Selfed progenies were under continuous selection for seed shape, plant type and TSWV resistance. High oleic single plants were selected from BC_2F_4. O/L=20	1999	200000135	11.15.2022	Golden Peanut Company, LLC
Georgia Hi-O/L	GA 942007	V	Pedigree: GC-C330A x GA-T2636M(Georgia Runner γ ray mutant). F_2-F_4: single plant selection. F_6-F8: Multi-location yield test. O/L=41.8	1999	200000255	11.15.2022	University of Georgia Research Foundation, Inc.
Olin	Tx962120	S	Backcross derivative of (Tamspan 90 x UF435-1), and Tamspan 90. BC_1F_2 single seeds were analyzed for O/L. O/L=22.4	2002	200200149	3.3.2024	Texas Agricultural Experiment Station
Tamrun OL 01	Tx977006	R	Backcross derivative from the cross between Tamrun 96(Tx896100) and SunOleic 95R. O/L=13.0	2002	200200150	5.10.2024	Texas Agricultural Experiment Station

Table 1. (Continued)

Cultivars	Other names	Type	Origin	Year of release	PVP		
					Certificate No.	Year expired	Applicants
Georgia-02C	GA982508	R	Derived from the cross between Southern Runner and Georgia Runner γ ray mutant. F_2-F_4: Single plants selection for O/L and resistance to TSWV and CBR. F_6-F_8: yield test. O/L=32.4	2002	200300050	3.24.2025	University of Georgia Research Foundation, Inc.
Tamrun OL 02	Tx977053	R	Backcross derivative from the cross between Tamrun 96（Tx896100）and SunOleic 95R. O/L=29	2002	200300170	11.10.2024	Texas Agricultural Experiment Station
Andru II	UF98614	R	Pedigree: (F627B x Andru 93)F_1 x Sunrunner HO BC_3(backcross derivative from the cross between Sunrunner and F435-HO. O/L=32.3	2002	200300179	8.25.2025	Florida Agricultural Experiment Station
ANorden	UF98511	R	Pedigree：72x84B- [breeding line from Florunner x F427B-3-1-7-4(sister line of Altika) x F1218 (backcross derivative from the cross between Sunrunner and F435HO). O/L=27.5	2002	200300205	8.25.2025	Florida Agricultural Experiment Station
Hull	UF98326	R	Pedigree: (Southern Runner x F435-HO)F_1 x UF81206. O/L=36.5	2002	200300207	8.25.2025	Florida Agricultural Experiment Station
GP-1	UF98604	R	Pedigree : (MarcI x F435-HO)F_1 x MarcI. Breeding method : Pedigree method. O/L=28.0	2002	200300321	8.25.2025	Florida Agricultural Experiment Station
AT-215	AT Exp 215	R	Derived from a cross between Viruguard and AT108 HO. Breeding method: Pedigree selection. O/L=25.1	2007	200700261	7.30.2028	Golden Peanut Company, LLC

Cultivars	Other names	Type	Origin	Year of release	PVP		
					Certificate No.	Year expired	Applicants
Georgia 04S		S	Derived from the cross between(Georgia Browne x UF 435-O/L-2)F_4 and Georgia Browne. 87.79%Oleate, 2.59%linoleate. O/L=34.25.	2004	200500121	7.26.2025	University of Georgia Research Foundation, Inc.
Georgia-05E		V	Developed from the cross between Georgia-01R (derived from a cross between PI 203395 and Georgia Browne) and GA942010 (a high oleate breeding line derived from the cross between 2 Georgia Hi-O/L sister lines). F_2-F_4: Pedigree selection. $F_{4:6}$: performance test. O/L=37.32	2005	200600059	5.3.2027	University of Georgia Research Foundation, Inc.
Florida-07	UF04327	R	Pedigree : 89xOL14-11-1-1-1-b2-B（HO phenotype came from F435-HO1） x C-99R. Breeding method : Pedigree method. O/L=30.4	2006	200800069	6.5.2028	Florida Foundation Seed Producers, Inc.
Tamrun OL06	TX034342, Reg. no. CV-91, PI 642850	R	Derived from a fourth backcross between Tamspan 90 and a BC_3 progeny developed from the crosses between Tamspan 90 and UF 435–2–1. O/L=18.1	2006	200800279	9.14.2032	Texas AgriLife Research
Tamrun OL07	TX033630	R	Pedigree : Tamrun 96 x (Tx901639-3 x SunOleic 95R)F_2. O/L=34.4	2006	200800280	2.20.2033	Texas AgriLife Research
Florida Fancy	UF003618	V	Pedigree : 87x8-2-1 x [UF85410x93Q10 (sister line of SunOleic 97R)]F_1. O/L=21.4	2007	200800231	9.14.2032	Florida Agricultural Experiment Station
McCloud	UF03326	R	-	2006	-	Application Abandoned	Florida Agricultural Experiment Station
York	UF0432,Reg. No. CV-114, PI 653717	R	Derived from a cross between a backcross HO selection breeding line of UF81206(89xOL24-3-1-2-2-b2-B) (female) and C-99R. ~80%Oleate. O/L=22.7	2006	200800186	9.14.2032	Florida Agricultural Experiment Station

Table 1. (Continued)

Cultivars	Other names	Type	Origin	Year of release	PVP		
					Certificate No.	Year expired	Applicants
Georgia-08V	GA 012535	V	Pedigree: C-99R x Georgia Hi-O/L. O/L=38.14	2008	200900238	9.14.2032	University of Georgia Research Foundation, Inc.
Georgia-09B	GA 032902, Reg. No. CV-110, PI 658595	R	Originated from the first backcross (BC_1) made between 'Georgia Green' and $F_{2:3}$ (Georgia Green x GA 942004). Pedigree selection was followed in the early segregating generations. Performance testing began in the $BC_1F_{4:6}$ generation. O/L=29.3	2009	201000075	2.20.2033	University of Georgia Research Foundation, Inc.
Georgia-11J	-	V	Pedigree: Georgia-05E (HO donor) x Georgia-03L. 82.87% oleate, 2.69% linoleate. O/L= 34.33	2011	201200100	6.19.2033	University of Georgia Research Foundation, Inc.
107	FloRun™ '107', UF08301	R	Pedigree: (89x 0L14-11-1-1-I-b2-B) x C-99R O/L=29.3		201100459	9.14.2032	Florida Foundation Seed Producers, Inc.
Red River Runner	TX994313	R	Derived from three-way cross among Tamrun 96, breeding line TX901639-3 and Sunoleic 95R. O/L =21.3.	2010	201200244	7.30.2033	Texas AgriLife Research
Spain		V	Pedigree: VA-C 92RJ89 x OL28. A single HO F_2 seed was identified using NIRS (Tillman et al., 2006). From the F_2-F_4, a modified SSD (single seed descent) advancement program was followed. From the F_5-F_7, pedigree selection was used to identify plants with large seeds and pods. O/L=54	2011	201200394	7.30.2033	Florida Foundation Seed Producers, Inc.

Cultivars	Other names	Type	Origin	Year of release	PVP		
					Certificate No.	Year expired	Applicants
Tamrun OL 11	Tx055308, Reg. No. CV-118, PI 665017	R	Derived from the cross between Tx977116 $F_{2:8}$ (HO, resistant to TSWV) and Tamrun 98 [NO]. Early selections following the pedigree selection method. Initial yield testing began in the $F_{3:5}$ in 2006 and continued through 2009. O/L=22.9	2011	201300196	9.30.2033	Texas AgriLife Research, State of Texas Research Agency
727	UF 10302, TUFRunner™ '727'	R	Pedigree: (90xOL61-H02-1-1-b2-B) x (86x43-23-2-1-1-). Individual F_2 seeds were screened with NIRS to find HO individuals. F_2-F_4 : Modified SSD breeding program. F_5-F_8: Pedigree selection. O/L= 32.4	-	201300199	9.30.2033	Florida Foundation Seed Producers, Inc.
AT 9899	-	S	Maturity similar to Flavorunner 458 in West Texas. Not resistant to TSWV	-	-	-	-
AT 215	-	R	Maturity: 120 - 125 days in Southeast USA, 130 -135 days in West Texas	-	-	-	-

Source: http://www.ars-grin.gov/cgi-bin/npgs/html/pvp.pl?Peanut and http://apps.ams.usda.gov/CMS/CropSearch.aspx.
Note: V=Virginia type, R=runner type, S=Spanish type. PVP=Plant Variety Protection.

Zhang et al. (2009b) crossed Silihong (a Valencia type peanut cultivar) with *A. pusilla* and obtained 3 hybrid derivatives with O/L ratio of 1.8, 1.8 and 1.7, respectively. The female parent Silihong only had an O/L of lower than 1.0. It is therefore believed that remote hybridization may result in peanut progenies with elevated O/L. Jiang et al. (2009) found the variation in fatty acids from the offspring of remote crosses exceeded the parental difference. Six peanut germplasm accessions were identified as with elevated oleate content (no less than 64%), among which yz8913-8, a hybrid derivative of Lvdasilihong/*A. stenosperma*, contained 67.85% oleate. Some of the materials showed good productivity or had larger seeds or higher shelling outturn.

Wang et al. (2013b) evaluated several lines derived from the cross between CTWE (a high oleate donor) and 06-I8B4 (a normal oleate interspecific hybrid derivative of the cultivated peanut and *A. rigonii*). Some of the lines exhibited variable response to chilling stress, demonstrating the possibility of breeding high oleate peanut cultivars with both high productivity and chilling tolerance (Wang et al., 2013b).

Table 2. Oleate content in wild relatives of the cultivated peanut

Identity	C16:0	C18:0	C18:1	C18:2	C20:0	C20:1	C22:0	C24:0	O/L
A14-1	7.97	1.89	53.26	28.15	0.99	2.02	3.54	2.17	1.89
A14-2	8.22	1.19	49.95	32.02	0.73	2.17	3.50	2.20	1.56
A14-3	7.28	1.91	67.91	13.82	0.92	2.14	3.72	2.30	4.91
A18-1	8.06	3.27	49.46	31.95	1.62	1.20	3.01	1.43	1.55
A24-2	9.55	4.15	48.73	30.55	1.87	0.86	3.16	1.13	1.59
A54-2 s	8.64	4.46	53.08	27.09	2.01	0.81	2.84	1.08	1.96

Source: Tang et al. (2013). Note: A14= *A.correntina* PI331192, A18=*A.rigonii* PI331190, A24= *A.paraguariensis* PI338297, A54= *A.duranensis* PI 262133.

Table 3. Fatty acid composition in a transformant and untransformed control (Huayu 22) (as percentage of total fatty acids, %)

Identity	C16:0	C18:0	C18:1	C18:2	C20:0	C20:1	C22:0	C24:0	O/L
Control 1	11.00	4.60	46.19	30.64	1.90	0.90	3.29	1.48	1.51
Control 2	10.24	3.80	49.32	28.58	1.85	1.10	3.46	1.63	1.73
Positive sample	9.18	4.25	53.27	25.53	1.88	1.03	3.25	1.61	2.09

Gene Engineering

There are several reports on transfer of antisense/RNAi (RNA interference) constructs to the cultivated peanut. Yin et al. (2007) analyzed 4 peanut transformants for seed fatty acids. Oleat content in these transformants ranged from 59.62%-70.01%, whereas in the untransformed control oleate content was only 37.87%. According to our unpublished data, transferring *FAD2B* antisense construct into Huayu 22 resulted in T_0 seeds with an O/L ratio of 2.09, higher than in the control (1.51-1.73) (Table 3). Li et al. (2005) reported increase in oleate content from 38% in untransformed control seeds to 77% in T_1 seeds, and decrease in linoleate content from 36% to 9% accordingly.

Chromatography methods were used for fatty acid analysis in the above-mentioned studies. Huang et al. (2008) used a NIRS machine to predict oleate and linoleate content in Yuhua 7 and Yuanza 9102 transformants, and found 20 single seeds with O/L ratio of over 2.0, higher than in the untransformed control (less than 1.5).

Marker-Assisted Selection (MAS) in Hybridization and Backcrossing

Hybridization

Chen et al. (2009) isolated DNA from leaflets of plants grown from seeds set on Huayu 22 pollinated with SunOleic 95R, and used SSR markers to identify true hybrids. Based on the fact that true F_1 hybrids have both wild type and mutant type *ahFAD2B* (441_442insA) alleles, Wang et al. (2010) used DNA extracted from 3-5 mg cotyledonary tissues of single "F_1" seeds as template (Yu et al., 2010), and *ahFAD2B*-specific PCR primers to amplify the *ahFAD2B* alleles. PCR products were directly sequenced. On the trace file, true hybrids have a series of overlapping peaks, while selfs do not have such peaks. The pitfall of this method is its high cost.

Use of HO peanut materials with the 441_442insA in its *ahFAD2B* in hybridization with high-yielding adapted peanut cultivars to breed peanut with both high yield and high oleate, is undoubtedly the world hot spot for peanut quality breeding research. Using NIRS calibration equations, HO peanut segregants may be identified in F_2 and subsequent generations with ease. Owing to the low frequency of HO segregants in F_2 population (for a digenic trait, it is 1/4; for a monogenic trait, it is only 1/16) and the even lower frequency for segregants with both high yield and high oleate, there is a need to identify segregants with both mutant type *ahFAD2A* and mutant type *ahFAD2B* alleles but at least one of the genes are not homozygous recessive, as in next generation appearance of HO offspring can be expected. Furthermore, to study HO-related genetic factors, it is necessary to genotype each individuals. The genotyping technique, once available, can be used to identify true hybrids and HO segregants as well. Realtime PCR (Barkley et al., 2010; Barkley et al., 2011) and CAPS (Cleaved Amplified Polymorphic Sequences) marker (Chu et al., 2007; Chu et al., 2009) technologies have been used for *ahFAD2A*/*ahFAD2B* genotyping, and achieved satisfactory results. However, realtime PCR needs a realtime PCR machine, and CAPS analysis needs a tedious enzyme digestion step. AS-PCR provides a good option. But the method reported by Chen et al. (2010) was unable to differentiate $Ol_1ol_1Ol_2Ol_2$ and $ol_1ol_1Ol_2Ol_2$, or $Ol_1Ol_1Ol_2ol_2$ and $Ol_1Ol_1ol_2ol_2$. Yu et al. (2013) reported an AS-PCR protocol for accurate genotyping of *ahFAD2A* and *ahFAD2B* in peanut, and this method has been used in hybrid identification (Wang et al., 2011b). Results from the AS-PCR genotyping protocol reported by Yu et al. (2013) are in accordance with the output of direct sequencing of PCR products. This protocol has been used to breed HO peanut in our research group. In Japan, Koilkonda et al. (2013) reported a similar method for *ahFAD2A* genotyping.

Marker-Assisted Backcrossing (MABC)

To breed peanut cultivars with both nematode resistance and high oleate content, in the USA, Chu et al. (2011) crossed nematode resistant cultivar Tifguard with high oleic cultivars Georgia-02C and Florida-07 in April 2008. Tifguard was used as recurrent parent in backcrossing. Only true hybrids heterozygous for both nematode resistance and high oleate were selected as male parent for the first backcrossing in September 2008. Marker analysis was performed on BC_nF_1, and only these individuals heterozygous for HO marker and homozygous for nematode resistance were selected as male parents (In conventional breeding process, both traits have to get homozygous; therefore 2-3 more years are needed). All the 53 BC_3F_1 individuals genotyped with markers for both traits carried only the GM565 allele associated with nematode resistance, and 37 were heterozygous for HO marker. 54 of the 238 BC_3F_2 individuals were homozygous for both traits. Since the coefficient of coancestory between Tifguard and Florida 07 and between Tifguard and Georgia 02C was 0.323 and 0.183, respectively, 3 backcrosses are considered adequate to breed Tifguard High O/L. It only took only 28 months to pyramid high O/L onto nematode resistance in Tifguard by MAS (Chu et al., 2011).

In Japan, efforts have been made, with the help of molecular markers, to transfer the HO trait from YI-0311 (O/L=48.2) into Nakateyutaka, a leading variety of Virginia type in Japan that has a normal O/L ratio (O/L=1.16) (Koilkonda et al., 2013). Nine of the 205 BC_2F_2 plants showed homozygous for the mutational *ahFAD2A* and *ahFAD2B* loci. In January 2012, BC Cycle 3 was in progress (Koilkonda et al., 2013).

ACKNOWLEDGMENT

The study was supported in part by Research Fund from China Agricultural Research System (CARS-14), Ministry of Agriculture, China.

REFERENCES

Anderson, PC; Goebet, DW. Influence of year and planting date on fatty acid chemistry of high oleic acid and normal peanut genotypes. *Journal of Agricultural and Food Chemistry*, 2002, 50, 1298-1305.

Aruna, R; Nigam, SN. Inheritance of fatty acid content and related quality traits in groundnut, *Arachis hypogaea* L. *Journal of Oilseeds Research*, 2009, 26 (1), 10-17.

Barkley, NA; Chenault Chamberli, KD; Wang, ML; Pittman, RN. Development of a real-time PCR genotyping assay to identify high oleic acid peanuts (*Arachis hypogaea* L.). *Molecular Breeding*, 2010, 25(3), 541-548.

Barkley, NA; Chenault Chamberlin, KD; Wang, ML; Pittman, RN. Genotyping and fatty acid composition analysis in segregating peanut (*Arachis hypogaea* L.) populations. *Peanut Science*, 2011, 38, 11-19.

Barkley, NA; Isleib, TG; Wang, ML; Pittman, RN. Genotypic effect of *ahFAD2* on fatty acid profiles in six segregating peanut (*Arachis hypogaea* L) populations. *BMC Genetics*, 2013, 14, 62. DOI: 10.1186/1471-2156-14-62

Braddock, JC; Sims, CA; O'Keefe SF. Flavor and oxidative stability of roasted high-oleic peanuts. *Journal of Food Science*, 1995, 60(3), 489-493.

Brown, DF; Cater, CM; Mattil, KF; Dardanelli, JG. Effect of variety, growing location and their intercation on the fatty acid composition of peanuts. *Journal of Food Science*, 1975, 40, 1055-1060.

Bruner, AC; Jung, S; Abbott, AG; Powellm, GL. The naturally occurring high oleate oil character in some peanut varieties results from reduced oleoyl-PC desaturase activity from mutation of aspartate 150 to asparagine. Crop *Science*, 2001, 41, 522-526.

Butzen, S; Schnebly, S. High oleic soybeans. *Crop Insights*, 2007,17(7), 1-3.

Chamberlin, KD; Melouk, HA; Madden, R; Dillwith, JW; Bannore, Y; Rassi, ZE; Payton, M. Determining the oleic/linoleic acid ratio in a single peanut seed: a comparison of two methods. *Peanut Science*, 2011, 38(2), 78-84.

Chen, CY; Wang, ML; Barkley, NA; Tonnis, B. Effects of G x E interaction on oil content and fatty acid composition of cultivated peanuts. 2013 Proceedings of the American Peanut Research and Education Society, Inc. Meeting, 8-11 July 2013, Young Harris, Georgia, 2013, 45, 29.

Chen, J; Hu, XH; Shi, YQ; Miao, HR, Yu, SL. Identification of peanut hybrids (*Arachis hypogaea* L.) using SSR markers. *Acta Agriculturae Nucleatae Sinica*, 2009, 23(4), 617-620.

Chen, Z; Wang, M; Barkley, NA; Pittman, RN. A simple allele-specific PCR assay for detecting *FAD2* alleles in both A and B genomes of the cultivated peanut for high-oleate trait selection. *Plant Molecular Biology Reporter*, 2010, 28, 542–548.

Chen, SL; Li, YR; Cheng, ZS; Wang, J; Song, YH; Zhang, JN; Zhang, Q; Wang, LY; Kong, HY; Zhang PJ. Breeding of high oleate Jihua 1 and its high yield cultivation techniques. *Chinese Journal of Oil Crops Sciences*, 2013, 35(Supplement), 266-270.

Chiou, RYY; Liu, C-P; Hou, C-J; Liu, C-D. Comparison of fatty acid composition and oxidative stability of peanut oils prepared from spring and fall crops of peanuts. *Journal of Agricultural and Food Chemistry*, 1995, 43,676-679.

Chong, EW; Sinclair, AJ; Guymer, RH. Facts on fats. *Clinical & Experimental Ophthalmology*, 2006, 34(5), 464-471.

Chu, Y; Ramos, ML; Holbrook, CC; Ozias-Akins, P. Genetic mutation of oleoyl-PC desaturase (*ahFAD2A*) in the mini core collection of the U.S. peanut germplasm collection. *Crop Science*, 2007, 47, 2372-2378.

Chu, Y; Holbrook, CC; Ozias-Akins, P. Two alleles of *ahFAD2B* control the high oleic acid trait in cultivated peanut. *Crop Science*, 2009, 49, 2029-2036.

Chu, Y; Wu, CL; Holbrook, CC; Tillman, BL; Person, G; Ozias-Akins, P. Marker-assisted selection to pyramid nematode resistance and the high oleic trait in peanut. *The Plant Genome*, 2011, 4(2), 110-117.

Davis, JP; Sweigart, DS; Price, KM; Dean, LL; Sanders, TH. Refractive index and density measurements of peanut oil for determining oleic and linoleic acid contents. *Journal of American Oil Chemistry Society*, 2013, 90, 199-206.

Ding, JP; Han, ZQ; Zhou, RY; Gao, GQ; Yang, YP. Genetic analysis of oleic/linoleic ratio in peanut. *Chinese Journal of Oil Crop Sciences*, 2007, 29(3), 233-237.

Dwivedi, SL; Nigam, SN; Rao, RCN; Singh, U; Rao, KVS. Effect of drought on oil, fatty acids and protein contents of groundnut (*Arachis hypogaea* L.) seeds. *Field Crops Research*, 1996, 48 (2-3), 125-133.

Fan H. Study on methods for rapid determination of fatty acid in peanut. *Journal of Shandong Agricultural University*, 1991, 22(4), 413-416.

Fang, CQ; Wang, CT; Wang, PW; Tang, YY; Wang, XZ; Cui, FG; Yu, SL. Identification of a novel mutation in *FAD2B* from a peanut EMS mutant with elevated oleate content. *Journal of Oleo Science*, 2012, 61(3), 143-148.

Fox, GP; Cruickshank, A. Near infrared reflectance as a rapid and inexpensive surrogate measure for fatty acid composition and oil content in peanuts (*Arachis hypogaea* L.). *Journal of Near Infrared Spectroscopy*, 2005, 13 (5), 287-291.

Gai, JY; Zhang, YM; Wang, JK. Genetic system for plant quantitative traits. Beijing: Science Press; 2003; 380pp.

Gao, HM; Zhang, YJ. Fast microanalysis of fatty acids of peanut seed by gas chromatography. *Chinese Agricultural Science Bulletin*, 2010, 26(13), 98-103.

Golombek, SD; Sridhar, R; Singh, U. Effect of soil temperature on the seed composition of three Spanish cultivars of groundnut (*Arachis hypogaea* L.). *Journal of Agricultural and Food Chemistry*, 1995, 43, 2067-2070.

Grosso, NR; Lamarque, AL; Zygadlo, JA; Maestri, DM; Guzmán, CA; Giandana, EH. Oleic/linoleic ratio improvement in peanut oil from Cordoba, Argentina. In: Fenwick GR, Hedley C, Richards RL, Khokhar S editors. Agri-Food Quality: An interdisciplinary Approach, Cambridge: The Royal Society of Chemistry; 1996; 171-172.

Gu, JZ; Ren, L; Jin, JM; Li, JH; Deng, L. Rapid evaluation of segregation in F_2 generations involving a high oleic parent in peanut. *Abstract of Wheat: Seed Industry Herald*, 2006, (7), 44.

Gu, JZ; Ren, L; Jin, JM; Li, JH; Deng, L; Fan, JL; Miao, JL; Yin, JH. Development of Kainong 61, a high oleate and high oil peanut cultivar. *Chinese Journal of Oil Crops Sciences*, 2013, 35 (supplement), 279-280.

Han, ZQ; Gao, GQ; Zhou, RY; Tang, RH; Zhou, CQ; Zhong, RC. Major gene plus polygene inheritance of oleic and linoleic acid contents in a cross involving high oleic peanut line. *Chinese Journal of Oil Crop Sciences*, 2010, 32(2), 196-201.

Han, ZQ; Gao, GQ; Zhou, RY; Tang, RH; Zhong, RC; Zhou, CQ; He, LQ. Inheritance of oleic, linoleic acid content and O/L ratio in high oleic acid *Arachis hypogaea* L. var. *hirsuta*. *Journal of Plant Genetic Resources*, 2011, 11(1):17-22.

Hashim, IB; Koehler, PE; Eitenmiller, RR; Kvien, CK. Fatty acid composition and tocopherol content of drought stressed Florunner peanuts. *Peanut Science*, 1993, 20:21-24.

Hinds, MJ. Fatty acid composition of Caribbean-grown peanuts (*Arachis hypogaea* L.) at three maturity stages. *Food Chemistry*, 1995, 53:7-14.

Holladay, CE; Pearson, JL. Effects of genotype and production area on the fatty acid composition, total oil and total protein in peanuts. *Journal of Food Science*, 1974, 39, 1206-1209.

Holley, KT; Hammons, RO. Strains and seasonal effects on peanut characteristics. *Georgia Agricultural Experiment Station Research Bulletin*, 1968, 32:1-27.

Huang, BY; Zhang, XY; Miao, LJ; Yan, M; Hai, Y; Yi, ML; Xu, J; Chen, ZK. RNAi transformation of *ahFAD2* gene and fatty acid analysis of transgenic seeds. *Chinese Journal of Oil Crop Sciences*, 2008, 30(3), 290-293.

Huang, BY; Zhang, XY; Miao, LJ; Liu, H; Qin, L; Xu, J; Zhang, ZX; Tang, FH; Dong, WZ; Han, SY; Liu, ZY. Inheritance of oleic acid and linoleic acid content of *Arachis hypogaea* L. *Scientia Agricultrura Sinica*, 2012, 45(4), 617-624.

Isleib, TG; Young, CT; Knauft, DA. Fatty acid genotypes of five Virginia-type peanut cultivars. *Crop Science*, 1996, 36(3), 556-558.

Isleib, TG; Wilson, RF; Novitzky, WP. Partial dominance, pleiotropism, and epistasis in the inheritance of the high-oleate trait in peanut. *Crop Science*, 2006, 46(3), 1331-1335.

Jiang, HF; Ren, XP; Huang, JQ; Lei, Y; Liao, BS. Genetic variation of fatty acid components in *Arachis* species and development of interspecific hybrids with high oleic and low palmitic acids. *Acta Agronomica Sinica*, 2009, 35(1), 25-32.

Jung, S; Swift, D; Sengoku, E; Patel, M; Teule, F; Powell, G; Moore, K; Abbott. The high oleate trait in the cultivated peanut (*Arachis hypogaea* L.). I. Isolation and characterization of two genes encoding microsomal oleoyl-PC desaturases. *Molecular Genomics and Genetics*, 2000a, 263, 796-805.

Jung, S; Powell, G; Moore K; Abbott, A. The high oleate trait in the cultivated peanut (*Arachis hypogaea* L.). II. Molecular basis and genetics of the trait. *Molecular Genomics and Genetics*, 2000b, 263, 806-811.

Kaveri, SB; Nadaf, HL; Salimath, PM. Comparison of two methods for fatty acid analysis in peanut (*Arachis hypogaea* L.). *Indian Journal of Agricultural Research*, 2009, 43(3), 215-218.

Khan, AR; Emery, DA; Singleton, JA. Refractive index as a basis for assessing fatty acid composition in segregating populations derived from infraspecific crosses of cultivated peanuts (*Arachis Hypogea* L.). *Crop Science*, 1974, 14(3), 464-468.

Kiage, JN; Merrill, PD; Robinson, CJ; Cao, Y; Malik, TA; Hundley, BC; Lao, P; Judd, SE; Cushman, M; Howard, VJ; Kabagambe, EK. Intake of *trans* fat and all-cause mortality in the Reasons for Geographical and Racial Differences in Stroke (REGARDS) cohort. *The American Journal of Clinical Nutrition*, 2013, 97(5), 1121-1128.

Knauft, DA; Moore, KM; Gorbet DW. Further Studies on the inheritance of fatty acid composition in peanut. *Peanut Science*, 1993, 20(2), 74-76.

Koilkonda, P; Kuwata, C; Fukami, M; Shirasawa, K; Aoki, K; Tabata,S; Hasegawa, M; Kiyoshima, H; Suzuki, S; Sasamoto, S; Kurabayashi, A; Tsuruoka, H; Wada, T; Isobe, S. Marker-assisted backcrossing selection for high O/L Ratio in cultivated peanut. In: Varshney RK, Tuberosa R. Editors. Translational Genomics for Crop Breeding: Abiotic Stress, Yield and Quality, Volume 2. John Wiley & Sons, Inc.; 2013;177-191.

Lei, Y; Liao, BS; Jiang, HF; Wang, SY; Huang, JQ; Yan, LY. Rapid method for the identification of high oleic peanut materials. China Patented Invention. Application date: Dec 14, 2009.

Lei, Y. Molecular Mechanism and Genetic Enhancement Technology for High Oleic Acid in Peanut (*Arachis hypogaea* L.). Ph.D Thesis. Chinese Academy of Agricultural Sciences. 2010. Wuhan, China. 84pp.

Lei, Y; Jiang, HF; Wen, QZ; Huang, JQ; Yan, LY; Liao, BS. Frequency of *ahFAD2A* alleles and its association with oleic acid content in the peanut mini core collection from China. *Acta Agronomica Sinica*, 2010, 36(1), 1864-1869.

Li, GM. Genetic Breeding of High Oleic Peanut by dsRNA Gene Silencing. Master's Thesis. Northeast Normal University. 2005. Harbin, China. 38pp.

Li, XH; Guo, HH; Yang, LP. The Effect of climatic factors on peanut quality. *Chinese Agricultural Science Bulletin*, 2010, 26(16), 90-94.

López, Y; Nadaf, HL; Smith, OD; Simpson, CE; Friz, AK. Expressed variants of Δ^{12}-fatty acid desaturase for the high oleate trait in Spanish market-type peanut lines. *Molecular Breeding*, 2002, 9, 183-190.

López, Y; Smith, OD; Senseman, SA; Rooney, WL. Genetic factors influencing high oleic acid content in Spanish market-type peanut cultivars. *Crop Science*, 2001, 41, 51-56.

Mercer, LC; Wynne, JC; Young CT. Inheritance of fatty acid content in peanut oil. *Peanut Science*, 1990, 17(1), 17-21.

Mondal, S; Badigannavar, AM. 2010. Induction of gentic variability for fatty acid composition in a large-seeded groundnut variety through induced mutagenesis. *Journal of SAT Agricultural Research*, 2010, 8.

Mondal, S; Badigannavar, AM; D'souza, SF. Induced variability for fatty acid profile and molecular characterization of high oleate mutant in cultivated groundnut (*Arachis hypogaea* L.). *Plant Breeding*, 2011, 130, 242-247.

Moore, KM; Knauft, DA. The inheritance of high oleic acid in peanut. *The Journal of Heredity*, 1989, 80(3), 252-253.

Mozingo, RW; Coffelt, TA; Wynne, JC. Market grade effects on fatty acid composition of five peanut cultivars. *Agronomy Journal*, 1988, 80, 73-75.

Mozingo, RW; O'Keefe, SF; Sanders, TH; Hendrix, KW. Improving shelf life of roasted and salted inshell peanuts using high oleic fatty acid chemistry. *Peanut Science*, 2004, 31(1), 40-45.

Mugendi, JB; Sims, CA; Gorbet, DW; O'Keefe, SF. Flavor stability of high-oleic peanuts stored at low humidity. *Journal of the American Oil Chemists' Society*, 1998, 75(1), 21-25.

Muitia, A; López, Y; Starr, JL; Schubert, AM; Burow, MD. Introduction of resistance to root-knot nematode [*Meloidogyne arenaria* Neal (Chitwood)] into high-oleic peanut. *Peanut Science*, 2006, 33(2), 97-103.

Mukri, G; Nadaf, HL; Bhat, RS; Gowda, MVC; Upadhyaya, HD; Sujay, V. Phenotypic and molecular dissection of ICRISAT mini core collection of peanut (*Arachis hypogaea* L.) for high oleic acid. *Plant Breeding*, 2012, 131(3), 418-422.

Myer, RO; Johnson, DD; Knauft, DA; Gorbet, DW; Brendemuhl, JH and Walker, WR. Effect of feeding high-oleic-acid peanuts to growing-finishing swine on resulting carcass fatty acid profile and on carcass and meat quality characteristics. *Journal of Animal Science*, 1992, 70, 3734-3741.

Nepote,V; Mestrallet, MG; Grosso, NR. Oxidative stability in fried-salted peanuts elaborated with high-oleic and regular peanuts from Argentina. *International Journal of Food Science & Technology*, 2006, 41(8), 900-909.

Norden, AJ; Gorbet, DW; Knauft, DA; Young, CT. Variability in oil quality among peanut genotypes in the Florida breeding program. *Peanut Science,* 1987, 14,7-11.

O'Byrne, DJ; Knauft, DA; Shireman, RB. Low fat-monounsaturated rich diets containing high-oleic peanuts improve serum lipoprotein profiles. *Lipids*, 1997, 32(7), 687-95.

O'Keefe, SF; Wiley, VA.; Knauft, DA. Comparison of oxidative stability of high- and normal- oleic peanut oils. *Journal of the American Oil Chemists' Society*, 1993, 70(5), 489-492.

Pandey, M; Wang, ML; Qiao, L; Wang, H; Feng, S; Barkley, NA; Wang, J; Culbreath, A; Holbrook, C; Varshney, R; Guo, B. Mapping *FAD2* genes on peanut (*Arachis hypogaea* L.) genome and contribution to oil quality. Plant & Animal Genome, XXII. Jan 11-15, 2014, San Diego, CA. Available from: https://pag.confex.com/pag/xxii/webprogram/Paper11835.html (accessed March 1, 2014)

Patel, M; Jung, S; Moore, K; Powell, G; Ainsworth, C; Abbott, A. High-oleate peanut mutants result from a MITE insertion into the *FAD2* gene. *Theoretical and Applied Genetics*, 2004,108(8),1492-502.

Pretorius, AE; Dreyer, J; Salomon, L. Release of SA Juweel -- a new South African groundnut cultivar with high oleic acid. *Journal of SAT Agricultural Research*, 2010, 8.

Rathnakumar, AL. Chapter 16. Groundnut (*Arachis hypogaea* L.). In: Bharadwaj, DN. editor. Breeding of field crops. Jodhpur, India: Agrobiosis; 2012; 340-383.

Ray, TK; Holly, SP; Knauft, DA; Abbott, AG; Powell, GL. The primary defect in developing seed from the high oleate variety of peanut (*Arachis hypogaea* L.) is the absence of Δ^{12}-desaturase activity. *Plant Science*, 1993, 91, 15-21.

Sanders, T. H. Maturity distribution in commercially sized Florunner peanuts. *Peanut Science*, 1989, 16, 91-95.

Sanders, TH; Landsden, JA; Greene, RL; Drexler, JS; Williams, EJ. Oil characteristics of peanut fruit separated by a nondestructive maturity classification method. *Peanut Science*, 1982, 9, 20-23.

Sarvamangala, C; Gowda, MVC; Varshney, RK. Identification of quantitative trait loci for protein content, oil content and oil quality for groundnut (*Arachis hypogaea* L.). *Field Crops Research*, 2011, 122 (1). 49-59.

Shin, E-C; Pegg, RB; Phillips, RD; Eitenmiller, RR. Commercial runner peanut cultivars in the USA: fatty acid composition. *European Journal of Lipid Science and Technology*, 2010, 112, 195-207.

Shirasawa, K; Koilkonda, P; Aoki, K; Hirakawa, H; Tabata, S; Watanabe, M; Hasegawa, M; Kiyoshima, H; Suzuki, S; Kuwata, C; Naito, Y; Kuboyama, T; Nakaya, A; Sasamoto, S; Watanabe, A; Kato, M; Kawashima, K; Kishida, Y; Kohara, M; Kurabayashi, A; Takahashi, C; Tsuruoka, H; Wada, T; Isobe S. *In silico* polymorphism analysis for the development of simple sequence repeat and transposon markers and construction of linkage map in cultivated peanut. *BMC Plant Bioogy*, 2012, 12, 80. DOI : 10.1186/1471-2229-12-80.

Singkham, N; Jogloy, S; Kesmala, T; Swatsitang, P; Jaisil, P; Puppala, N; Patanothai, A. Estimation of hereditability by parent-offspring regression for high-oleic acid in peanut. *Asian Journal of Plant Sciences*, 2010a, 9(6), 358-363.

Singkham, N; Jogloy, S; Kesmala, T; Swatsitang, P; Jaisil, P; Puppala, N. Genotypic variability and genotype by environment interactions in oil and fatty acids in high, intermediate, and low oleic acid peanut genotypes. *Journal of Agricultural and Food Chemistry*, 2010b, 58(10),6257-6263.

Singkham, N; Jogloy, S; Kesmala, T; Swatsitang, P; Jaisil, P; Puppala, N; Patanothai, A. Combining ability for oleic acid in peanut (*Arachis hypogaea* L.). *SABRAO Journal of Breeding and Genetics*, 2011, 43(1), 59-72.

Singkham, N; Jogloy, S; Suriharn, B; Kesmala, T; Swatsitang, P; Jaisil, P; Puppala, N; Patanothai, A. Types of gene effects governing the inheritance of oleic and linoleic acids in peanut (*Arachis hypogaea* L.). *African Journal of Biotechnology*, 2012, 11(67), 13147-13152.

Sundaram, J; Kandala, CV; Holser, RA; Butts, CL; Windham, WR. Determination of In-Shell Peanut Oil and Fatty Acid Composition Using Near-Infrared Reflectance Spectroscopy. *Journal of the American Oil Chemists' Society*, 2010, 87(10), 1103-1114.

Sundaram, J; Kandala, CV; Butts, CL; Chen, CY; Sobolev, V. Nondestructive NIR reflectance spectroscopic method for rapid fatty acid analysis of peanut seeds. *Peanut Science*, 2011, 38(2), 85-92.

Sweigart, DS; Homich, CA; Stuart, DA. Rapid single kernel refractive index test that differentiates regular from high oleic peanuts. Proceedings of American Peanut Research and Education Society, Inc., 2011, 43, 27-28.

Sykes, EE; Michaels, TE. Combining Ability of Ontario-grown peanuts (*Arachis hypogaea* L.) for oil, fatty acids, and taxonomic characters. *Peanut Science*, 1986, 13, (2), 93-97.

Tang, YY; Wang, XZ; Wu, Q; Sun, QX; Tang, RH; Gao, HY; Wang, CT. Evaluation of wild peanut species for fatty acid composition. *Journal of Today's Biological Sciences: Research & Review*, 2013, 2(2).

Tillman, B; Gorbet, D; Person, G. Predicting oleic and linoleic acid content of single peanut seeds using near-infrared reflectance spectroscopy, *Crop Science*, 2006, 46, 2121-2126.

Upadhyaya, HD; Nigam SN. Detection of epistasis for protein and oil contents and oil quality parameters in peanut. *Crop Science*, 1999, 39, 115-118.

USDA/FAS. PSD online. Table 13. Peanut area, yield, and production. Date Created 1/10/2014 11:12:59 AM. Available from: http://apps.fas.usda.gov/psdonline/psdReport.aspx?hidReportRetrievalName=Table+13+Peanut+Area%2c+Yield%2c+and+Production++++++++++++++++++++++++++&hidReportRetrievalID=918&hidReportRetrievalTemplateID=1 (accessed Jan 29, 2014).

Vassiliou, EK; Gonzalez, A; Garcia, C; Tadros, JH; Chakraborty, G; Toney, GH. Oleic acid and peanut oil high in oleic acid reverse the inhibitory effect of insulin production of the inflammatory cytokine TNF-α both *in vitro* and *in vivo* systems. *Lipids in Health and Disease*, 2009, 8, 25. DOI:10.1186/1476-511X-8-25

Wan, YS; Li, XD; Fan, H. Effect of sowing date and temperature on O/L ratio of peanut. *Shandong Agricultural Sciences*, 1995, (2):6-8.

Wan, YS; Tan, Z. Combinability analysis of O/L and main traits of economic importance in peanut. *Shandong Agricultural Science*, 1995, (1), 8-11.

Wan, YS; Tan, Z; Fan, H; Li, XD; Zhang, GY; Liu, FZ; Wang, S. Genetic effect of major fatty acid com[position in groundnut. *Chinese Journal of Oil Crop Sciences*, 2002, 24(1), 26-28.

Wang, CT. Application of Biotechniques and NIRs in Peanut Breeding. PhD Thesis. Ocean University of China. 2010. Qingdao, China. 136pp.

Wang, CT; Yu, SL; Zhang, SW; Wang, XZ; Tang, YY; Zhang, JC; Chen, DX. 2010. Novel protocol to identify true hybrids in normal oleate x high oleate crosses in peanut. *Electronic Journal of Biotechnology*, 2010, 13(5). DOI: 10.2225/vol13-issue5-fulltext-18

Wang, CT; Tang, YY; Wang, XZ; Zhang, SW; Li, GJ; Zhang, JC; Yu, SL. Sodium azide mutagenesis resulted in a peanut plant with elevated oleate content. *Electronic Journal of Biotechnolog*, 2011a, 14(2). DOI: 10.2225/vol14-issue2-fulltext-4

Wang, CT; Hu, DQ; Ding, YF; Yu, HT; Tang, YY; Wang, XZ; Zhang, JC; Chen, DX. A new set of allele-specific PCR primers for identification of true hybrids in normal oleate x high oleate crosses in groundnut. *Journal of SAT Agricultural Research*, 2011b, vol.9.

Wang, CT; Tang, YY; Wang, XZ; Qi, W; Gao, HY; Feng, T; Su, JW; Yu, ST; Fang, XL; Ni, WL; Jiang, YS; Qian, L; Hu, DQ. Mutagenesis: a useful tool for the genetic improvement of the cultivated peanut (*Arachis hypogaea* L.). In: Mishra R, editor. Mutagenesis. Crotia: InTech; 2012; 1-12.

Wang, CT; Tang, YY; Wang, XZ; Wu, Q; Yang, Z; Jiao, K; Song, GS; Xu, JZ. Effect of *FAD2A/FAD2B* genes on fatty acid profiles in peanut seeds. *Research on Crops*, 2013a, 14 (4), 1110-1113.

Wang, CT; Tang, YY; Wang, XZ; Wu, Q; Guan, SY; Yang, WQ; Wang, PW. Development and characterization of four new high oleate peanut lines. *Research on Crops*, 2013b, 14 (3), 845-849.

Wang, CT; Wang, XZ; Tang, YY; Wu, Q; Xu, JZ; Hu, DQ; Qu, B. Predicting main fatty acids, oil and protein content in intact single seeds of groundnut by near infrared reflectance spectroscopy. *Advanced Materials Research*, 2014, 860-863, 490-496.

Wang, ML; Barkley, NA; Chen, Z; Pittman, RN. *FAD2* gene mutations significantly alter fatty acid profiles in cultivated peanuts (*Arachis hypogaea*). *Biochemical Genetics*, 2011c, 49(11-12), 748-759.

Wang, ML; Sukumaran, S; Barkley, NA; Chen, Z; Chen, CY; Guo, B; Pittman, RN; Stalker, HT; Holbrook, CC; Pederson GA; Yu J. Population structure and marker-trait association analysis of the US peanut (*Arachis hypogaea* L.) mini-core collection. *Theoretical and Applied Genetics*, 2011d, 123(8), 1307-1317.

Wheeler, RA; Smith, RL; Knauft, DA. Microsomal polypeptide comparisons between high and normal oleic acid isogenic peanut lines using two-dimensional gel electrophoresis. *Peanut Science*, 1994, 21(1), 75-78.

Wilkin, JD; Ashton, IP; Fielding, LM.; Tatham, AS. Storage stability of whole and nibbed, conventional and high oleic peanuts (*Arachis hypogeae* L.). *Food and Bioprocess Technology*, 2014, 7(1), 105-113.

Wilson, JN; Baring, MR; Burow, MD; Rooney, WL; Chagoya, JC; Simpson, CE. Generation means analysis of fatty acid composition in peanut. *Journal of Crop Improvement*, 2013, 27(4), 430-443.

Xu, Y; Gan, X; Cao, Y; Gu, S; Liu, F. Studies on combining ability of major nutritional quality characters and agronomic characters in peanut. *Scientia Agricutura Sinica*, 1995, 28(2), 15-23.

Yamaki, T; Nagamine, I; Fukumoto, K; Yano, T; Miyahara, M; Sakurai, H. High oleic peanut oil modulates promotion stage in lung tumorigenesis of mice treated with methyl nitrosourea. *Food Science and Technology Research*, 2005, 11(2), 231-235.

Yang, CD; Guan, SY; Tang, YY; Wang, XZ; Qi, W; Gong, QX; Wang, CT. Rapid non-destructive determination of fatty acids in single groundnut seeds by gas chromatography. *Journal of Peanut Science*, 2012, 41(3), 21-26.

Yin, D; Deng, S; Zhan, K; Cui, D. 2007. High-oleic peanut oils produced by hpRNA-mediated gene silencing of oleate desaturase. *Plant Molecular Biology Reporter*, 2007, 25, 154-163.

Yu, HT; Yang, WQ; Tang, YY; Wang, XZ; Wu, Q; Hu, DQ; Wang, CT; Yu, SL. An AS-PCR assay for accurate genotyping of *FAD2A/FAD2B* genes in peanuts (*Arachis hypogaea* L.). *Grasas y Aceites*, 2013, 64 (4), 395-399.

Yu, S; Min, P. Studies on two improved groundnut varieties and their O/L ratios. In: Seed Industry and Agricultural Development. Beijing: China Agricultural Press; 1997; 464.

Yu, S; Pan, L; Yang, Q; Min, P; Ren, Z; Zhang, H. Comparison of the Δ^{12} fatty acid desaturase gene between high-oleic and normal-oleic peanut genotypes. *Journal of Genetics and Genomics*, 2008, 35, 679-685.

Yu, SL; Zhu, YJ; Min, P; Yang, QL; Cao, YL; Wang, CT; Liu, X; Zhou, XQ. Non-destructive measurement of main fatty acid composition in peanut seeds with Near Infrared Reflectance Spectroscopy. In: Wang SB, editor. Principles and Techniques for Cost-Effective Production of Quality Peanut. Beijing: China Agricultural Science & Technology Press; 2003; 344-349.

Yu, SL; Wang, CT; Yang, QL; Zhang, DX; Zhang, XY; Cao, YL; Liang, XQ; Liao, BS. Peanut Genetics and Breeding in China, Shanghai: Shanghai Science and Technology Press; 2011; 378.

Yu, ST; Wang, CT; Yu, SL;, Wang, XZ; Tang, YY; Chen, DX; Zhang, JC. Simple method to prepare DNA templates from a slice of peanut cotyledonary tissue for polymerase chain reaction. *Electronic Journal of Biotechnology*, 2010, 13(3). DOI: 10.2225/vol13-issue4-fulltext-9

Zeile, WL; Knauft, DA; Kelly, CB. A rapid and non-destructive technique for fatty acid determination in individual peanut seed. *Peanut Science*, 1993, 20, 9-11.

Zhang, J ; Wang, C ; Tang, Y ; Wang, X. Effects of grading on the main quality attributes of peanut kernels. *Frontiers of Agriculture in China*, 2009a, 3(3), 291–293.

Zhang, JC; Wang, CT; Wang, XZ. Quality analysis of 27 peanut breeding lines. Abstracts of 2009 Annual Meeting of China Crops Society. 2009b, 159.

Zhang, XY; Zhu, SJ; Han, SY; Xu, J; Liu, H; Tang, FS; Dong, WZ; Zang, XW; Zhang, ZX. 2011. Inheritance of fat and fatty acid compositions in peanut (*Arachis hypogaea* L.). *Agricultural Science & Technology*, 2011, 12(7), 943-946, 974.

Zhou, LX; Tang, GY; Chen, G; Bi, YP; Shan, L. Correlation between *ahFAD2* polymorphism and oleic acid/linoleic acid ratio in peanut seeds. *Acta Agronomica Sinica*, 2011, 37(3), 415-423.

Reviewed by Prof. Yue Huang, Qingdao Academy of Agricultural Sciences.

In: Peanuts
Editor: Richard W. Cook
ISBN: 978-1-63321-013-4

Chapter 7

PEANUT PRODUCTION, TRADE AND COMPETITIVENESS

*Chen Di**
College of Economics and Management, Shenyang Agricultural University Shenyang, Liaoning, China

ABSTRACT

In this chapter, we mainly do the statistical and econometric analysis on peanut production, trade situation and competitiveness, through data from the FAO database.

Firstly, the statistical analysis of world's peanut production and trade situation was done.

In which, we statistically analyzed the gross production, gross exports, and their changes of the world, and the production, unit area yield, export volume and their changes of the main peanut production and export countries, and especially classified the export objects of the main peanut export countries, during the year 1991-2012.

Then, the competitiveness of the world's primary peanut export countries was measured through the general competitiveness indexes.

According to the results of the statistical analysis above, respectively choose the four countries of China, the United States, India and Argentina as the world's primary peanut export countries.

* Chen Di: College of Economics and Management, Shenyang Agricultural University, Dong Ling Road No.120, Shenyang, Liaoning Province, China.

The indexes that we put to use respectively are the International Market Price (IMS), the International Market Share (IMS), the Trade Competitiveness Index (TC) and the Revealed Comparative Advantage Index (RCA). And especially, we analyzed the competitiveness situation of the four primary peanut export countries comprehensively with the indexes that measured.

1. Overview of the World's Peanut Production and Exports

1.1. Total Peanut Production Trend of the World

The world's total peanut production has been raised from 24 million tons to 41 million tons, with an average annual growth of 2.63%, during the year 1991-2012[1]. The upward trend was more obvious relatively in the year 1991-2000, with an average annual growth of 3.89%. Then, it slightly fluctuated from 33 million tons to 38 million tons and basically stable with only 0.62% growth rate from the year 2001, and reached a high level of over 38 million tons in the year 2005. The rising trend suspended in 2006 with only 33 million tons, then recovered stably and recorded to the highest of 41 million tons in the year 2012. (See figure 1-1)

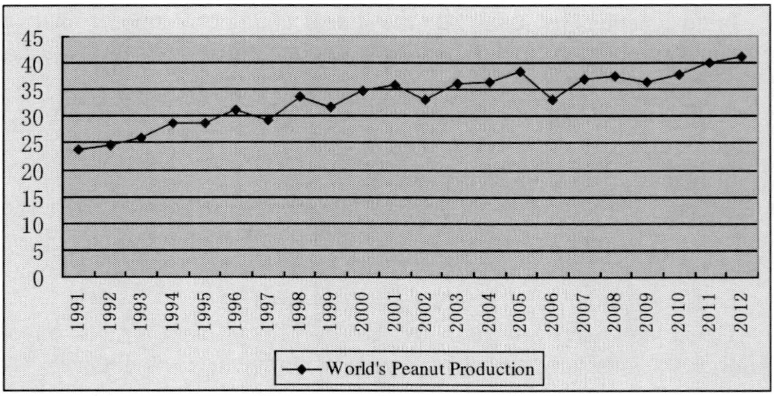

Source: Statistical Database [MT].

Figure 1-1. The peanut production trend of the world in 1991-2012.

[1] Considering the characteristics of world economic development and data available, we take the period in 1991-2011.

1.2. Total Peanut Export Trend of the World

The world's total peanut export volume appeared a slight fluctuation growth trend, with an average annual growth of 1.83% during the year 1991-2011.

The total export volume raised rapidly in the year 1991-1995, reached the highest historical of 1.38 million tons in 1995, then continued declining to the lowest 1.12 million tons in 1998. It came to slightly fluctuated increasing from 1999 and break a high level of 1.38 million in 2009. Just after one year, it increased sharply to 1.79 million tons in the year 2011.

In regional view, Asia, America and Africa are the main world's main peanut export areas. The total peanut export quantity of the three continents accounted for more than 90% of the world total during the year 1991-2011. In the three continents, Asia ranked first in most years, which accounted for 40%-50% of the world total, America ranked the second, which accounted for 30%-40% of the world total; Africa ranked the third, which accounted for less than 10% of the world total in most of the years. The peanut export quantity of Asia appeared a significant turning point in the year 1998 which affected by the Asian financial crisis, declined to a historical lowest 0.375 million tons. Then, it turned to increase stably soon by the economic form recovery, upward to a high level of 0.75 million tons in the year 2003 and 2005. After a slight decline during 2006 to 2010, the peanut export quantity of Asia reached historical highest of 0.95 million tons in the year 2011. The peanut export quantity of America presented a certain complementary form with that of Asia, but it continued to rise and was very close to that of Asia in recent years. Meanwhile, the peanut export quantity of Africa remained relatively stable of 0.1 million tons during the statistical year. As a result, it can be seen that the soar of peanut export in the year 2011 was mainly due to Asia. (see figure1-2)

2. Overview of Peanut Production in Primary Peanut Producing Countries

2.1. Peanut Production of Primary Peanut Producing Countries

It is found that, Asia, America and Africa are the major peanut producing areas all over the world, through the world peanut production statistics in nearly 20 years.

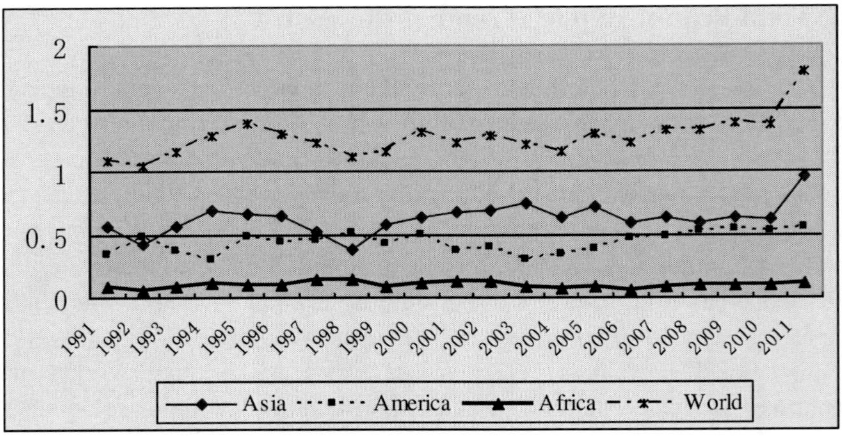

Source: Statistical Database [MT].

Figure 1-2. Total peanut export trend in main peanut export areas in 1991-2011.

In those continents, Asia ranked the first which was represented by China, India, Myanmar and Vietnam, Africa ranked the second which was representted by Nigeria, Senegal, Sudan and Ghana, America ranked the third which was represented by American and Argentina.

The summation peanut production of the 10 countries accounted for more than 80% of the world total during the year 1991-2012, which can represent overall level of the world's peanut production. (see table 2-1)

In those 10 countries, the percentage of peanut production in China and India remained in top two, but with different changing trends. Previously, India was the first place with the percentage of 30% and 35% in the year 1991 and 1992, which was higher than 27% and 25% of China. But since the year 1993, China replaced India, jumped to the first place, and kept relatively stable rising.

Meanwhile, Indian peanut production continued to decline with high volatility. The percentage of peanut production in Nigeria and the United States were ranked the third and the fourth, both of that stably accounted for 5%-10% to the world's.

Peanut production in the other countries is relatively lower to the four countries above, with only 1%-4% of the world's total production.

Among which, Myanmar had a rising trend, and the rest of the countries remained relatively stable.

Table 2-1. Peanut production of Major peanut producing countries in 1991-2012

Year	World	CH	IN	NG	US	MM	SD	SN	GH	VN	AR	Account (%)
1991	23.74	6.39	7.09	1.36	2.24	0.47	0.18	0.72	0.07	0.24	0.31	80
1992	24.46	6.03	8.57	1.30	1.94	0.38	0.38	0.58	0.10	0.23	0.22	81
1993	26.07	8.50	7.83	1.32	1.54	0.43	0.43	0.63	0.14	0.26	0.23	82
1994	28.65	9.76	8.06	1.45	1.93	0.43	0.71	0.68	0.18	0.29	0.21	83
1995	28.61	10.33	7.58	1.58	1.57	0.50	0.74	0.79	0.17	0.33	0.24	83
1996	31.15	10.22	8.64	2.28	1.66	0.59	0.82	0.65	0.16	0.36	0.46	83
1997	29.40	9.73	7.37	2.53	1.61	0.56	1.10	0.54	0.15	0.35	0.28	82
1998	33.82	11.95	8.98	2.53	1.80	0.54	0.78	0.58	0.21	0.39	0.63	84
1999	31.89	12.71	5.26	2.89	1.74	0.56	1.05	1.01	0.19	0.32	0.34	82
2000	34.73	14.52	6.48	2.90	1.48	0.63	0.95	1.06	0.21	0.36	0.42	84
2001	35.88	14.47	7.03	2.68	1.94	0.73	0.99	0.89	0.26	0.36	0.39	83
2002	33.13	14.90	4.12	2.86	1.51	0.76	1.27	0.26	0.52	0.40	0.36	81
2003	36.08	13.49	8.13	3.04	1.88	0.88	0.79	0.44	0.44	0.41	0.22	82
2004	36.44	14.41	6.77	3.25	1.95	0.95	0.79	0.60	0.39	0.47	0.29	82
2005	38.44	14.40	7.99	3.48	2.21	1.04	0.52	0.70	0.42	0.49	0.44	82
2006	33.19	12.81	4.86	3.83	1.58	1.11	0.56	0.46	0.52	0.46	0.35	80
2007	36.98	13.08	9.18	2.85	1.70	1.22	0.56	0.33	0.30	0.51	0.60	82
2008	37.65	14.34	7.17	2.87	2.34	1.30	0.72	0.73	0.47	0.53	0.63	83
2009	36.46	14.76	5.51	2.97	1.67	1.36	0.94	1.03	0.49	0.53	0.61	82
2010	37.95	15.71	5.64	2.64	1.89	1.34	0.76	1.29	0.53	0.49	0.61	81
2011	40.02	16.11	6.96	2.96	1.66	1.40	1.19	0.53	0.47	0.47	0.70	81
2012	41.27	16.88	5.78	3.07	3.06	1.37	1.03	0.67	0.48	0.47	0.82	81

Source: Statistical Database [MT].

2.2. Peanut Yield of Primary Peanut Producing Countries

With the progress of production technology and the improvement of the production environment, the world peanut yield level overall showed a gently rising trend in 20 the past years. It rose from 11509 kg/ha in the year 1991 to 16759 kg/ha in the year 2012, with the average growth rate of 1.93%.

In the 10 major peanut producing countries, there were 4 countries peanut yield higher than the world average level in most of the years, which are China, the United States, Vietnam, and Argentina.

China and the United States alternately kept the first and the second with an obvious high advantage, much higher than the other countries. But since 2007, the United States surpassed China and kept up with the gap gradually increasing. It is worth noting that the peanut yield of the United States increased significantly in 2012, from 37948 kg/ha in 2011 to 46990 kg/ha in 2012, with the growth rate as high as 23.83% in that single year, and the average annual growth rage of 3.49%in the statistical 20 years. At the same term, the average annual growth rate of the world was only 1.93%. The peanut yield of Vietnam was much close to that of the world, and growth steadily. It surpassed the world's level in the year 2002, met the historical high of 21343 kg/ha in the year 2012. The peanut yield of Argentina was fluctuated greatly in the statistical years. It surged over 21000 kg/ha since the year 2005 and remained in the relative high level of 21000 kg/ha to 27900 kg/ha.

The yield of the other major producers were relatively low to the above 4 countries, but India and Myanmar are deserved to concern. India was the second largest peanut producing country, as mentioned above, but it's yield was much lower than the other main peanut producing countries, with the average annual of only 10683 kg/ha, and instability. It was relatively weak in Myanmar's peanut production basis, so the yield was low in the early years, but it showed a stably rising trend and met the world average level in the year 2008. The yield of Ghana, Nigeria, Sudan, Senegal and Nigeria were all low. Their production of the international leading level mainly depended on the large sown area. (see table 2-2 and figure 2-1)

From the above, it can be seen that, the peanut yield of America which presented by the United States, and Argentina, and Asia which presented by China and Vietnam ranked among the top of the world in the 3 major peanut producing continents.

Besides, although Africa was one of the major continent, the yield level is generally low.

Table 2-2. Peanut Yield of Major peanut producing countries in 1991-2012

Year	World	CH	IN	NG	US	MM	SD	SN	GH	VN	AR
1991	11509	21873	8185	12076	27400	8920	7848	8311	6700	11181	17369
1992	11870	20009	10489	12400	28764	8081	6969	6046	7692	10428	14461
1993	12390	24909	9409	11802	22505	8929	5485	8493	8750	11938	21218
1994	13038	25618	10271	9249	29415	9251	8045	7601	9368	11861	15565
1995	12977	26837	10073	8936	25576	10082	6811	9397	9324	12874	15332

Year	World	CH	IN	NG	US	MM	SD	SN	GH	VN	AR
1996	13912	28001	11378	10053	29737	11459	8621	7027	8982	13611	19361
1997	13096	25916	10395	11241	28066	11694	7207	6913	8741	13858	9422
1998	14564	29373	12144	9729	30282	12106	5595	10425	10928	14328	16360
1999	13969	29587	7657	15003	29890	11453	6911	11062	10432	12847	10318
2000	14939	29715	9881	15000	27396	11320	6474	9691	9587	14508	19137
2001	15548	28849	11265	15500	33951	12473	6465		10157	14845	15725
2002	14423	30115	6943	15202	28702	13340	9384	3204	13542	16230	16275
2003	15639	26551	13574	15300	35404	13412	7488	8397	9447	16661	14122
2004	15370	30231	10202	15498	34479	14469	7399	8064	9027	17785	17492
2005	16069	30729	11867	15903	33507	15195	5409	9107	9333	18149	21099
2006	15442	32182	8661	17199	32211	15143	9334	7749	10833	18747	21220
2007	16431	32962	14594	12927	35085	16168	9433	5455	8833	20039	27901
2008	15629	33599	11636	12296	38396	16010	7507	8738	13406	20768	27501
2009	15245	33568	10073	11263	38348	16215	9964	9750	14416	21071	23521
2010	15807	34541	11440	13621	37124	15477	6621	10764	15023	21004	27923
2011	16242	34998	13115	12646	37948	15779	6977	6093	13036	20935	22851
2012	16759	35670	11794	12686	46990	15585	6372	9490	13762	21343	25625

Source: Statistical Database [Kg/Ha].

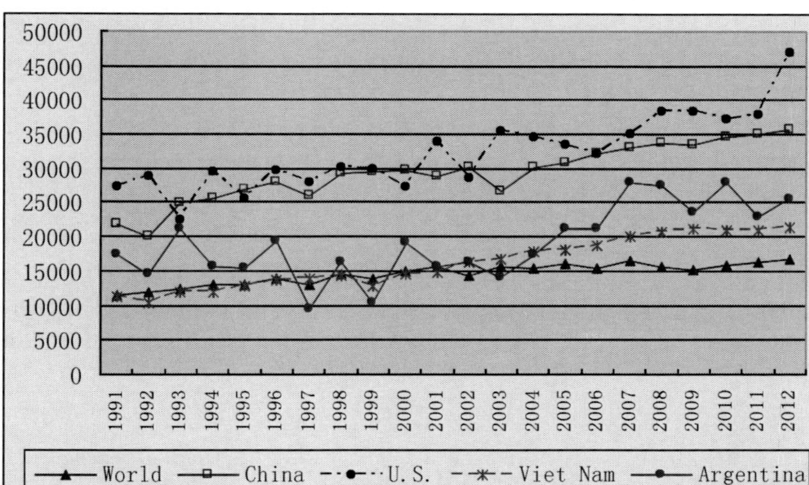

Source: Statistical Database [Kg/Ha].

Figure 2-1. The peanut yield trend of major peanut producing countries in 1991-2011.

3. Overview of Peanut Export in Primary Peanut Export Countries and Classification of Their Export Objects

3.1. Overview of Peanut Export in Primary Peanut Export Countries

There are several major peanut export countries in the world wide, which are China, India, Vietnam, Myanmar, and Indonesia in Asia, the United States Brazil and Argentina in America, Egypt and Nigeria in Africa. The total annual export quantity of the above 10 countries accounted for about 80% of the world in the year 1991-2011.

Among them, the annual export quantity of China, the United States, India, Argentina, peanut exports are all up to 100 thousand tons, the total export quantities of the 4 countries accounted for 70% of the world. In Vietnam, the export quantity was over 100 thousand tons annually before the year 2002, but it fell rapidly to a low level since 2003. Peanut exports of the rest of the 10 countries are relatively low, but still in the top 10 countries.

Among the statistical year 1991-2011, annual peanut export quantity of China had the greatest change, which presented the trend of down - up - down: It fell from 0.41 million tons in 1991 down to 0.16 million tons in 1997, then rose to the historical high level of 0.49 million tons in 2002, and finally fell wandering down to the lowest level of 0.15 million tons. The export quantity in the United States kept around 0.2 million tons steadily. In India, the annual export quantity has grown substantially during the statistical years; it reached over 0.26 million tons in the year 2007, which ranked first, exceeding China and the United State. Moreover, it surged to the world's highest level of 0.75 million tons. In Argentina, the peanut exports showed a certain complementary situation with China, with a trend of up - down – up. (see figure 3-1 and table 3-1)

3.2. Export Objects Classification in the Major Peanut Export Countries

From the above, there are 4 leading peanut export countries which are China, the United State, India and Argentina. But with the formation of the world peanut export pattern, they all had different export objects.

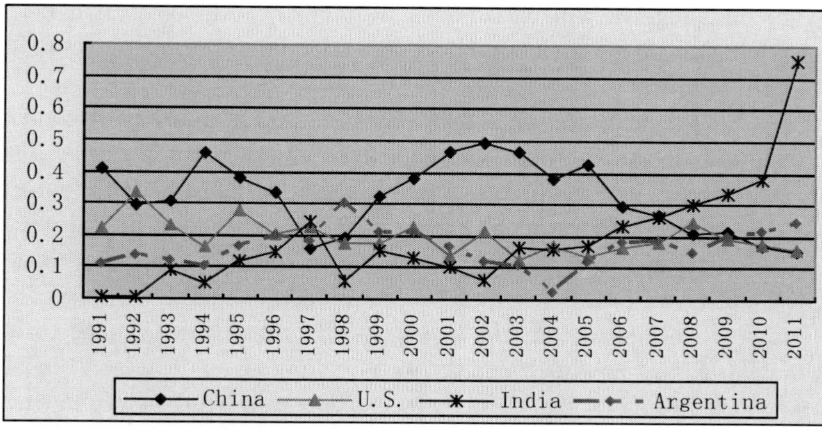

Source: Statistical Database [MT].

Figure 3-1. The trend of peanut exports in main peanut exporting area in 1991-2010.

Table 3-1. Peanut exports in main peanut exporting area in 1991-2010

Year	CN	US	IN	AR	VN	EG	MM	BR	NG	ID	Account (%)
1991	0.4107	0.2208	0.0036	0.1064	0.0789	0.0014	0.0009	0.0019	0.0004	0.0002	0.7631
1992	0.2936	0.3361	0.0043	0.1349	0.0628	0.0033	0.0002	0.0037	0.0001	0.0005	0.8022
1993	0.3043	0.2312	0.0914	0.1193	0.1050	0.0108	0.0002	0.0029	0.0001	0.0009	0.7537
1994	0.4606	0.1633	0.0505	0.1044	0.1192	0.0064	0.0001	0.0042	0.0003	0.0018	0.7118
1995	0.3779	0.2780	0.1180	0.1651	0.1150	0.0087	0.0001	0.0021	0.0002	0.0019	0.7721
1996	0.3359	0.2017	0.1474	0.1980	0.1270	0.0048	0.0036	0.0012	0.0004	0.0024	0.7930
1997	0.1576	0.2271	0.2425	0.1793	0.0864	0.0099	0.0110	0.0003	0.0011	0.0020	0.7515
1998	0.1950	0.1752	0.0563	0.3001	0.0870	0.0131	0.0015	0.0009	0.0052	0.0037	0.7487
1999	0.3247	0.1768	0.1538	0.2089	0.0555	0.0040	0.0012	0.0006	0.0001	0.0023	0.8080
2000	0.3792	0.2286	0.1310	0.2124	0.0762	0.0027	0.0052	0.0008	0.0000	0.0019	0.7890
2001	0.4678	0.1355	0.0994	0.1626	0.0782	0.0032	0.0005	0.0066	0.0006	0.0014	0.7788
2002	0.4932	0.2140	0.0608	0.1185	0.1066	0.0096	0.0000	0.0061	0.0007	0.0025	0.7878
2003	0.4631	0.1260	0.1642	0.1072	0.0850	0.0078	0.0004	0.0133	0.0001	0.0037	0.8016
2004	0.3797	0.1676	0.1577	0.0205	0.0478	0.0136	0.0008	0.0378	0.0000	0.0057	0.7164
2005	0.4269	0.1362	0.1725	0.1173	0.0581	0.0153	0.0006	0.0581	0.0003	0.0036	0.7649
2006	0.2973	0.1660	0.2331	0.1816	0.0150	0.0083	0.0020	0.0475	0.0002	0.0013	0.7804
2007	0.2655	0.1818	0.2606	0.1860	0.0409	0.0071	0.0015	0.0321	0.0003	0.0040	0.7400
2008	0.2122	0.2418	0.3008	0.1490	0.0160	0.0158	0.0012	0.0445	0.0001	0.0059	0.7465
2009	0.2183	0.1913	0.3369	0.2007	0.0234	0.0338	0.0013	0.0530	0.0001	0.0033	0.7703
2010	0.1721	0.1753	0.3802	0.2178	0.0142	0.0096	0.0001	0.0511	0.0000	0.0029	0.7461
2011	0.1509	0.1588	0.7572	0.2431	0.0030	0.0270	0.0006	0.0531	0.0002	0.0031	0.7801

Source: Statistical Database [MT].

The following we will classify the different export object, and list the objects with annual export quantity over 5 thousand tons during the year 1991-2011 (see table 3-2).

It can be seen that, the objects of the 4 leading peanut export countries were mainly their neighboring countries and some European countries. There were competitive relationship between the major peanut exporters, but each had its own competitive advantages. Take China for example, the main export object to European countries was Russia, which did not compete with other major peanut exporters obviously. Some developed countries such as Canada and Germany were also main export objects of China, which competed with the United States, meanwhile, Japan ranked first among all the export object of China in Asia, which was also the main export object of the Unite States. There was competitive relationship between China and India in most export objects. China did not compete with Argentina in most objects due to the geographical position, but had a few exceptions in the objects of Canada and Netherland. Specific analysis of national export object is as follows:

There were a lot of peanut export objects of China, but the quantities were focused on 5-10 thousand tons. They were mainly countries in Asia and some of the European countries. The export quantities were relatively stable in the objects of Japan, Canada, Germany, Greece, Italy, Lebanon, Malaysia, Russia and Spain, fluctuated in the other main export objects. The average export quantity to Netherland was 74.3 thousand tons, highest of the all objects. It met 100 thousand tons in the 1990's. But recently it went done significantly to lower than 10 thousand tons in the year 2009. The similar situation of down trend in recent years appeared in several countries, such as Philippines, Poland, Ukraine, Singapore and Hong Kong.

The main export objects of the United States were the neighboring countries of America continent and parts of European countries. It was relatively stable that the export quantities of the United States to Canada, Japan and Spain, among which, the average highest was 66 thousand tons of Canada. To Germany, it presented a down-up trend. Meanwhile, in Netherland and the UK, it kept the down trend. The export quantities of the United States to Mexico showed rising trend, it met the historical high of 46 thousand tons in the year 2010, and a little reduce to 39 thousand tons in the last statistical year 2011.

The main export objects of India were less, mostly Asian countries, and the quantities of almost all objects presented growth trend year by year, which caused the total peanut export rising. Indonesia was the largest export object of India, and it had a huge increase in recent years.

To Indonesia, the average annual export was 72.3 thousand tons before 2009, rose to 170 thousand tons in 2010, and then surged greatly to 270 thousand tons in 2011. To Malaysia, the average annual export was 30 thousand tons before 2008, which went up to 60 thousand tons in 2009, and then high up to 90 thousand tons in 2011.

To Philippine, it also showed a rising trend with 50-60 thousand tons in recent years in 2009-2011. It is worthy concern that, China became one of the major export objects of India, the export quantity went up to over 10 thousand tons in 2010, and then surged to 40 thousand tons in 2011.

The main export objects of Argentina were even more limited, mainly countries in America, Africa and parts of European countries. Argentina's peanut export quantities all over the world were fluctuant significantly, the same as to the major export objects. To Canada, it was as high as 71 thousand tons in 2007, but then descended rapidly. Although a little rise in 2009, it was still lower than 10 thousand tons until 2011. The export quantities of Argentina to Netherland kept an average of 70 thousand tons with an up trend, and went up to over 100 thousand tons in the year 2010 and 2011. It was the highest standard in all export objects.

Table 3-1. Export object of main peanut exporting area in the world

Exporter	Export Object		
	Annual Average over 20 Thousand tons	Annual Average in 10-20 thousand tons	Annual Average in 5-10 thousand tons
China	Japan, Netherland, Philippine, Russia	German, Indonesia, Spain	Canada, Hong Kong, Greece, Italy, Lebanon, Malaysia, Poland, Singapore, Ukraine
the US	Canada, Mexico, Netherlands, UK	——	Germany, Japan, Spain
India	Indonesia, Malaysia	Philippine, UK	Singapore
Argentina	Netherland	Canada, UK, Algeria	Mexico

Source: Statistical Database.

4. Measurements of Competitiveness Indexes in Primary Peanut Producing Countries

4.1. Introduction

The World Economy Forum (WEF, 1990) and the Swiss International Management Development (IMD, 1990) institute early gave the definition international competitiveness from the national level. Later, Competitiveness and Evaluation Research Center of Renmin University of China innovatively developed by combing the actual situation of China, that national competitiveness factors should be divided into three levels, including the core competitive ability, the basic competitiveness and environmental competitiveness.

In addition, Michael Porter put forward the famous "diamond theory" to research competitiveness from the industry level. However the above research methods show limitations in agricultural industry research.

This part of the artical general evaluated the production and trade of 4 major peanut export countries with comparative analysis.

Based on the above, calculated several international competitiveness indexes of the world four major peanut producers in the year 1991-2011 with statistical analysis.

Summarized the international status and trend of current Chinese peanut industry, and further discussed countermeasures.

4.2. Indexes and Data Sources

Indexes of international competitive analysis generally divide into two kinds, namely revealed indexes and analytical indexes. We will choose three revealed indexes----the international market share, trade competitiveness index, revealed comparative advantage index, and one absolute index----export price, to measure the international competitiveness of peanut industry in the 4 major peanut export countries.

In this part, we chooses 1991-2011 annual world statistical data from The United Nations food and agriculture organization online database (http://www.fao.org/), and calculates peanut production and trade.

The data consist of peanut with shell and shelled peanut, without proceeded peanut, and may include official and semi-official estimated result.

4.3. Empirical Analysis

4.3.1. International Market Price

Table 4-1 show the Export Prices based on the United Nations Food and Agriculture Organization (FAO) database statistics calculation in the year 1991-2011, in the 4 major countries. Generally speaking, the 4 major peanut exporters' prices all represented decending to increasing trend, especially high in recent years.

Overall, the United States ranked first, China ranked second, India and Argentina are relatively low. A faster growth characteristic reflected in Chinese peanuts export prices,surpassed the United States in the year 2007 and 2008, leaped into the front ranks of the world, and then had a little drop in the year 2009-2011. The export price of the United States showed a relatively stable trend with an average of about 800 USD/ton, but it surged in the recent several years of 2007-2011 with over 1000 USD/ton. In India, it also presented an up trend in recent 10 years, and it also exceeded 1000 USD/ton since the year 2010. The avrage export price in Argentina was about 700 USD/ton before the year 2007, the lowest in the 4 major countries. It then fluctuated greatly since 2008, especially got the highest of the 4 countries with over 1400 USD/ton in the year 2011.

4.3.2. International Market Share

International Market share (IMS) is one of the main measures of the international competitiveness. It refers to export product in a country account for the world market share. The higher the IMS, the stronger international competitiveness is, otherwise, the weak.

Table 4-1. Export Price Comparison of World Major Peanut Exporters during 1991-2011

	1991	1992	1993	1994	1995	1996	1997	1998	1999	2000	2001
China	877.41	648.21	645.38	683.97	679.76	757.29	879.16	797.55	597.83	611.08	562.12
the US	678.21	613.60	743.15	906.81	795.92	831.34	904.51	913.46	899.05	860.22	890.55
India	844.99	688.00	599.45	811.71	606.10	619.15	630.57	594.89	561.59	537.98	562.08
Argentina	747.77	465.16	780.72	811.71	746.92	768.43	782.33	721.69	691.42	721.89	702.40

	2002	2003	2004	2005	2006	2007	2008	2009	2010	2011	
China	534.76	686.41	813.01	748.66	820.38	1058.70	1444.22	1000.06	1113.11	1073.24	
the US	807.84	924.18	968.44	961.04	873.32	969.45	981.69	1086.87	1254.20	1401.40	
India	602.63	712.14	704.02	675.32	756.49	979.94	952.86	874.81	1051.26	1245.19	
Argentina	564.51	679.76	2627.19	618.61	656.98	922.55	1214.45	813.43	933.82	1428.66	

Source: Statistical database [USD/Tonnes].

Its computation formula is:

$$IMS_{ij}=X_{ij}/X_{wj}\times 100\%$$

X_{ij} means the export quantity of product j from the exporter i; similarly, X_{wj} means that from all over the world. It can be seen from table 4-2, Chinese international market share of peanut export kept in the first position in the world before the year 2006, even above 30% in most of the years, far higher than other exporters. But it showed a rapid decline later, fell to just 15.5% in 2009, even plunged to 10% in 2011, ranked the third of the 4 exporters.

Meanwhile, the United States remained relatively smooth in recent years, only fell in 2011. What worth to concern is, the IMS of India increased year by year, especially high in 2011. It even surpassed that of China in 2011-2005 when entering WTO. The IMS of Argentina were strong fluctuated, but stable at around 12% in recent years. It can be seen that, from the index of IMS, India and Argentina have exceeded China and the United States.

4.3.3. Trade Competitiveness Index

Trade Competitiveness index (TC) measures the net exports account for the total volume of imports and exports of an exporter, formula is:

$$TC_{ij}=(X_{ij}-M_{ij})/(X_{ij}+M_{ij})$$

X_{ij} and M_{ij} means the export and import number of product j from the exporter i. TC value scope for [-1, 1], when positive means exports are higher than imports, namely the production efficiency is higher than international average, and it more close to 1 shows that more competitive.

It can be seen from table 4-3 that, trade competitiveness indexes are all very close to 1. China peanuts TC reached the higher in the year 2005, decreased from 2006, even became the lowest of the 4 exporters in the year 2010 and 2011. In 2011, it was even down to 0.5562. The TC of United States was quiet low before 2001, it then jumped to high level and showed small-scope fluctuation after rising since 2002, but always lower than that of India and Argentina. India always maintained a high position, which means the exports are far higher than imports. It showed 1 in 1991-1996 and 2004-2005 means there were almost no imports. Argentina keeped a high stable state after rising.

Table 4-2. IMS Comparison of World Mainly Peanut Exporters during 1991-2011

	1991	1992	1993	1994	1995	1996	1997	1998	1999	2000	2001
China	41.30	28.74	24.80	32.28	24.80	25.48	14.67	18.59	24.58	25.92	33.52
the US	17.16	31.14	21.70	15.17	21.36	16.80	21.76	19.13	20.14	22.00	15.39
India	0.34	0.44	6.91	3.32	6.90	9.14	16.19	4.01	10.94	7.88	7.12
Argentina	9.12	9.48	11.76	8.69	11.91	15.24	14.85	25.89	18.29	17.15	14.56
	2002	2003	2004	2005	2006	2007	2008	2009	2010	2011	
China	33.68	35.51	32.70	32.76	25.31	21.80	20.06	15.47	15.27	10.29	
the US	22.08	13.01	17.19	13.41	15.05	13.67	15.54	14.73	13.85	8.78	
India	4.68	13.06	11.76	11.94	18.30	19.81	18.76	20.88	25.18	37.20	
Argentina	8.54	8.14	5.71	7.44	12.38	13.31	11.85	11.57	12.81	13.70	

Source: Statistical Database [%].

Table 4-3. TC Comparison of World Mainly Peanut Exporters during 1991-2011

	1991	1992	1993	1994	1995	1996	1997	1998	1999	2000	2001
China	0.9976	0.9974	0.9960	0.9853	0.9939	0.9981	0.9644	0.9744	0.9965	0.9985	0.9990
the US	0.9079	0.9976	0.9997	0.9806	0.7585	0.5409	0.6425	0.5925	0.5729	0.4325	0.4016
India	1.0000	1.0000	1.0000	1.0000	1.0000	1.0000	0.9993	0.9909	0.9996	0.9997	0.9997
Argentina	0.9995	0.9974	0.9964	0.9904	0.9983	0.9984	0.9964	0.9948	0.9991	0.9890	0.9935
	2002	2003	2004	2005	2006	2007	2008	2009	2010	2011	
China	0.9895	0.9920	0.9839	0.9857	0.9509	0.9610	0.9212	0.9328	0.8290	0.5562	
the US	0.8104	0.9503	0.9831	0.9976	0.9851	0.8892	0.9311	0.9306	0.9308	0.8373	
India	0.9993	0.9998	1.0000	1.0000	0.9997	0.9998	0.9999	0.9976	0.9989	0.9990	
Argentina	0.9966	0.9901	0.9963	0.9994	0.9996	0.9992	0.9995	0.9996	0.9979	0.9996	

Source: Statistical Database.

4.3.4. Revealed Comparative Advantage Index

Revealed Comparative Advantage index (RCA), refers to the rate of the number of export of one product account for the total export of one country, to the product export number account for the world's total exports, formula is:

$$RCA_i=(X_i/X_{it})/(X_w/X_{wt})$$

X_i and X_w respectively for the export number of the product in one exporter and all over the world; X_{it} and X_{wt} respectively for all export commodities' number of the exporter i and all over the world. $RCA_i>1$ reveals comparative advantage, conversely, no comparative advantage.

This index is a relatively good measure for relative advantage of an export product in a country so as to reflect the competitiveness of an industry in the international market, for it eliminate the influence of national and world exports fluctuation to the outcome. Table 4-4 shows the RCA of 4 main peanut exporters.

Almost all of them are larger than 1, means they all have comparative advantage throughout the world. Among them, China's RCA continued declining from relatively high index of 9.76 in 1991 to 1.03 in 2010 year by year, with comparative advantage position diminishing. It was even lower than 1 in 2011, comperatative advantage lost. The United States' RCA remained stable, keeping between 1-2, relatively weak; India maintained in more than 10, surged to 17.54 in 2006, even higher to 22.48 in 2011.

Argentina outclassed the other exporters with the highest comparative advantage, which means peanut is the main export products in Argentina.

CONCLUSION

The pitfall of single index analysis is that it is one-sided; hence it cannot explain the issue very well. For example, in the above TC calculation, we found the reason for Indian peanut trade competitiveness index high is that India almost has no peanut imports.

Therefore, this paper will make the comparison using the above 4 indexes that measures peanut international competitiveness.

Table 4-4. RCA Comparison of World Mainly Peanut Exporters during 1991-2011

	1991	1992	1993	1994	1995	1996	1997	1998	1999	2000	2001
China	9.76	6.48	5.26	6.45	4.87	5.10	2.67	3.45	4.40	4.14	5.23
the US	1.42	2.61	1.75	1.27	1.87	1.44	1.75	1.53	1.63	1.80	1.29
India	0.67	0.82	11.61	5.37	10.71	14.56	25.04	6.47	16.73	11.14	9.85
Argentina	26.63	29.06	33.61	23.45	29.05	34.18	31.13	53.55	44.43	41.70	33.59
	2002	2003	2004	2005	2006	2007	2008	2009	2010	2011	
China	4.71	4.53	3.84	3.54	2.53	2.08	1.56	1.12	1.03	0.71	
the US	2.05	1.35	1.91	1.54	1.73	1.64	1.92	1.74	1.65	1.09	
India	5.63	15.58	13.41	11.97	17.54	18.84	15.45	15.85	16.99	22.48	
Argentina	21.46	20.43	15.03	19.23	31.81	33.36	27.14	26.00	28.71	29.87	

Source: Statistical Database.

China's peanut export price has had comparative advantage in the early years especially when entering into WTO, but was gradually losing since 2005.

It can be seen that, the price advantage of Chinese peanuts relying on traditional resources was hard to maintain in recent years, even losing.

Meanwhile, the other three indexes were successively lower. Therefore, in recent years, under the high absolute number of Chinese peanut output and export, China was losing its world's leading position in terms of competitiveness in peanut industry.

Although the United States peanuts kept high export prices and low RCA, but it can still sustain a stable international market share, given government subsidies and other policies in the hope of protect agricultural sector implemented. Comprehensive index analysis showed that, the international competitiveness of the US was relatively low compared with the other three main peanut exporters, but still kept a high status in recent years and ensure the US edible oil safety.

Due to low quality, geographic attributes and cheap domestic input prices, the output price of Indian peanut was relatively low. Thus it has had comparative advantage over its international competitors. Better still, for Indian domestic producers, some importers do not care much about quality. That might be the reason why it kept a high export rate that even exceeded that of China who kept a leading position before. Its TC and RCA indexes were also higher than that of China and the United States, and kept stable. The result of comprehensive index analysis showed that Indian peanuts international market competitiveness was higher, and is also rising slowly.

Argentina's peanut production share of the world total output was relatively low. The fluctuation of international market share index might be related to its domestic industry policies; the high TC indexes were caused by small import volume. What worth noting is, the export prices were gradually reduced in recent years, even below that of China in 2005, and the RCA indexes were continuously ranked first. Thus it is clear that, Argentine peanut production takes an important position in its domestic export products and growing fast and that may be a great threat to the further development of the other peanut exporters.

INDEX

B

C

D

E

F

G

H

I

J

K

L

M

N

O

P

T

U

V

W

Y

ENVIRONMENTAL HEALTH -
PHYSICAL, CHEMICAL AND BIOLOGICAL FACTORS

U.S. WATERS PROTECTED UNDER THE CLEAN WATER ACT

ANALYSES OF A PROPOSAL

CAROLINE M. EDNIE
EDITOR

nova publishers
New York

For permission to use material from this book please contact us:
Telephone 631-231-7269; Fax 631-231-8175
Web Site: http://www.novapublishers.com

Additional color graphics may be available in the e-book version of this book.

Library of Congress Cataloging-in-Publication Data

ISBN: 978-1-63321-275-6

Published by Nova Science Publishers, Inc. † New York

CONTENTS

PREFACE

On March 25, 2014, the Environmental Protection Agency (EPA) and the U.S. Army Corps of Engineers (Corps) jointly proposed a rule defining the scope of waters protected under the Clean Water Act (CWA). The proposal would revise regulations that have been in place for more than 25 years. This book describes the proposed rule and includes a table comparing the existing regulatory language that defines "waters of the United States" with the proposal. In 2006, the Supreme Court decided Rapanos v. United States, the most recent and well-known of three Supreme Court decisions wrestling with the question of which wetlands are covered by the wetlands permitting program in the Clean Water Act. This book also provides background including the pre-Rapanos Supreme Court opinions, then moves on to Rapanos itself and the Corps/EPA guidance documents.

Chapter 1 - On March 25, 2014, the Environmental Protection Agency (EPA) and the U.S. Army Corps of Engineers (Corps) jointly proposed a rule defining the scope of waters protected under the Clean Water Act (CWA). The proposal would revise regulations that have been in place for more than 25 years. Revisions are proposed in light of 2001 and 2006 Supreme Court rulings that interpreted the regulatory scope of the CWA more narrowly than previously, but created uncertainty about the precise effect of the Court's decisions.

In 2011, EPA and the Corps proposed guidance on policies for determining CWA jurisdiction to replace guidance issued in 2003 and 2008; all were intended to lessen confusion over the Court's rulings. The 2011 proposed guidance was extremely controversial, with some contending that it represented an overreach beyond the agencies' statutory authority. Most environmental groups welcomed the proposed guidance, although some would have preferred a stronger document. The 2014 proposed rule would replace the existing 2003 and 2008 guidance, which remains in effect because the 2011 proposed guidance was not finalized.

According to the agencies, the proposed rule would revise the existing administrative definition of "waters of the United States" consistent with legal rulings and science concerning the interconnectedness of tributaries, wetlands, and other waters and effects of these connections on the chemical, physical, and biological integrity of downstream waters. Waters that are "jurisdictional" are subject to the multiple regulatory requirements of the CWA. Non-jurisdictional waters do not have the federal legal protection of those requirements.

This report describes the proposed rule and includes a table comparing the existing regulatory language that defines "waters of the United States" with the proposal. The proposed rule is particularly focused on clarifying the regulatory status of waters located in isolated places in a landscape. It does not modify some categories of waters that currently are jurisdictional by rule (traditional navigable waters, interstate waters and wetlands, the territorial seas, and impoundments). Proposed changes would increase the asserted scope of CWA jurisdiction, in part as a result of expressly declaring some types of waters categorically jurisdictional (such as all waters adjacent to a jurisdictional water), and also by application of new definitions, which give larger regulatory context to some types of waters, such as tributaries.

Beyond the categories of waters that would be categorically jurisdictional under the proposal is a category sometimes referred to as "other waters." The regulatory term "other waters" applies to wetlands and non-wetland waters such as prairie potholes that are not considered traditionally navigable or meet other of the proposed rule's jurisdictional definitions. Much of the controversy since the Supreme Court rulings has focused on the degree to which "other waters" are jurisdictional. According to the agencies' analyses, 17% of these "other waters" would be categorically jurisdictional under changes in the proposal. It also lists waters and features that would not be jurisdictional, such as prior converted cropland and certain ditches. It makes no change to existing statutory and regulatory permit exclusions, such as exemptions for normal farming and ranching activities.

The agencies believe that the proposal does not exceed the CWA's coverage or protect new types of waters that have not been protected historically. While it would enlarge jurisdiction beyond that under the existing EPA-Corps guidance, they believe that it would not enlarge jurisdiction beyond what is consistent with the Supreme Court's narrow reading of jurisdiction. Others may disagree. Overall, the agencies estimate that approximately 3% of U.S. waters will additionally be subject to CWA jurisdiction as a result of the proposed rule (including additional "other waters"), compared with current field practice. EPA and the Corps estimate that costs of the proposal, from additional permit application expenses, for example, range from $162 million to $279 million annually. Benefits, including the value of ecosystem services such as flood protection, are estimated to range from $318 million to $514 million per year. They acknowledge uncertainties and limitations in these estimates.

Chapter 2 - The U.S. Army Corps of Engineers (Corps) and the Environmental Protection Agency (EPA), collectively "the agencies", proposed a rule for public comment that that defines the scope of waters protected under the Clean Water Act (CWA), in light of the U.S. Supreme Court cases in *U.S. v. Riverside Bayview, Rapanos v. United States,* and *Solid Waste Agency v. U.S. Army Corps of `Engineers (SWANCC).* The effect of the *SWANCC* decision is primarily on so-called "isolated" (other) waters. These waters do not meet the agencies' definition of "adjacent" and often include vernal pools, prairie potholes and playa lakes that lie entirely within a single state and lack a direct, surface water connection to the river network. In practice, the effect of the *Rapanos* decision has been primarily on some small streams, rivers that flow for part of the year, and nearby wetlands. The agencies believe this proposal would enhance protection for the nation's public health and aquatic resources, and increase CWA program predictability and consistency by increasing clarity on the scope of "waters of the United States" protected under the Act.

Specifically, the agencies propose to define the waters of the United States for all sections of the Clean Water Act to mean: traditional navigable waters (TNWs); interstate waters, including interstate wetlands; the territorial seas; impoundments of waters otherwise defined as waters of the United States; tributaries, as defined, to traditional navigable waters, interstate waters, or the territorial seas; adjacent waters, including wetlands; and, on a case-specific basis, other waters that have a significant nexus to a traditional navigable water, interstate water, or the territorial seas.

The agencies also propose to exclude specified waters from the definition of "waters of the United States." The agencies are not proposing changes to the existing exclusions for waste treatment systems designed consistent with the requirements of the Clean Water Act, nor are the agencies are proposing any changes for prior converted cropland. The agencies are, for the first time, proposing to exclude by regulation certain waters and features over which the agencies have as a policy matter generally not asserted CWA jurisdiction.

The agencies propose for the first time to define the term "neighboring" as it is used as a component of the existing term “adjacent”, and in turn define the terms "riparian area" and "floodplain" that appear in the new definition of “neighboring”. The agencies also define the terms "tributary" and "significant nexus." The goal is to ensure the regulatory definition is consistent with the CWA, as interpreted by the Supreme Court, to protect water quality, public health, and the environment.

Chapter 3 - In 1985 and 2001, the Supreme Court grappled with issues as to the geographic scope of the wetlands permitting program in the federal Clean Water Act (CWA). In 2006, the Supreme Court rendered a third decision, *Rapanos v. United State*s, on appeal from two Sixth Circuit rulings. The Sixth Circuit rulings offered the Court a chance to clarify the reach of CWA jurisdiction over wetlands adjacent only to *non*navigable tributaries of traditional navigable waters—including tributaries such as drainage ditches and canals that may flow intermittently. (Jurisdiction over wetlands adjacent to traditional navigable waters was established in the 1985 decision.)

The Court’s decision provided little clarification, however, splitting 4-1-4. The four-Justice plurality decision, by Justice Scalia, said that the CWA covers only wetlands connected to relatively permanent bodies of water (streams, rivers, lakes) by a continuous surface connection. Justice Kennedy, writing alone, demanded a substantial nexus between the wetland and a traditional navigable water, using an ambiguous ecological test. Justice Stevens, for the four dissenters, would have upheld the existing broad reach of Corps of Engineers/EPA regulations.

Because no rationale commanded the support of a majority of the Justices, lower courts are extracting different rules of decision from *Rapanos* for resolving future cases. Corps/EPA guidance issued in December 2008 says that a wetland generally is jurisdictional if it satisfies either the plurality or Kennedy tests. In April 2011, the agencies proposed revised guidance intended to clarify whether waters are protected by the CWA, but this proposal was controversial. The ambiguity of the *Rapanos* decision and questions about the agencies’ guidance have increased pressure on EPA and the Corps to initiate a rulemaking to promulgate new regulations. In September 2013, EPA and the Corps withdrew the controversial proposed guidance and submitted a draft rule to the Office of Management and Budget for review. The substance of the draft rule, and when it might be proposed, are unknown for now. There also has been pressure on Congress to provide legislative clarification. In the 111th

Congress, legislation intended to do so was approved by a Senate committee, but no further legislative action occurred. Similar legislation was not introduced in the 112th Congress or so far in the 113th Congress. Instead, proposals to bar issuance of the Corps/EPA revised guidance and to narrow the regulatory scope of the CWA have been introduced.

The legal and policy questions associated with *Rapanos*—regarding the outer geographic limit of CWA jurisdiction and the consequences of restricting that scope—have challenged regulators, landowners and developers, and policymakers for 40 years. The answer may determine the reach of CWA regulatory authority not only for the wetlands permitting program but also for other CWA programs, since the CWA uses but one jurisdiction-defining phrase ("navigable waters") throughout the statute.

While regulators and the regulated community debate the legal dimensions of federal jurisdiction under the CWA, scientists contend that there are no discrete, scientifically supportable boundaries or criteria along the continuum of wetlands to separate them into meaningful ecological or hydrological compartments. Wetland scientists believe that all such waters are critical for protecting the integrity of waters, habitat, and wildlife downstream. Changes in the limits of federal jurisdiction highlight the role of states in protecting waters not addressed by federal law. From the states' perspective, federal programs provide a baseline for consistent, minimum standards to regulate wetlands and other waters. Most states are either reluctant or unable to take steps to protect non-jurisdictional waters through legislative or administrative action.

In: U.S. Waters Protected …
Editor: Caroline M. Ednie

ISBN: 978-1-63321-275-6

Chapter 1

EPA AND THE ARMY CORPS' PROPOSED RULE TO DEFINE "WATERS OF THE UNITED STATES"*

Claudia Copeland

SUMMARY

On March 25, 2014, the Environmental Protection Agency (EPA) and the U.S. Army Corps of Engineers (Corps) jointly proposed a rule defining the scope of waters protected under the Clean Water Act (CWA). The proposal would revise regulations that have been in place for more than 25 years. Revisions are proposed in light of 2001 and 2006 Supreme Court rulings that interpreted the regulatory scope of the CWA more narrowly than previously, but created uncertainty about the precise effect of the Court's decisions.

In 2011, EPA and the Corps proposed guidance on policies for determining CWA jurisdiction to replace guidance issued in 2003 and 2008; all were intended to lessen confusion over the Court's rulings. The 2011 proposed guidance was extremely controversial, with some contending that it represented an overreach beyond the agencies' statutory authority. Most environmental groups welcomed the proposed guidance, although some would

* This is an edited, reformatted and augmented version of a Congressional Research Service publication R43455, prepared for Members and Committees of Congress dated April 21, 2014.

have preferred a stronger document. The 2014 proposed rule would replace the existing 2003 and 2008 guidance, which remains in effect because the 2011 proposed guidance was not finalized.

According to the agencies, the proposed rule would revise the existing administrative definition of "waters of the United States" consistent with legal rulings and science concerning the interconnectedness of tributaries, wetlands, and other waters and effects of these connections on the chemical, physical, and biological integrity of downstream waters. Waters that are "jurisdictional" are subject to the multiple regulatory requirements of the CWA. Non-jurisdictional waters do not have the federal legal protection of those requirements.

This report describes the proposed rule and includes a table comparing the existing regulatory language that defines "waters of the United States" with the proposal. The proposed rule is particularly focused on clarifying the regulatory status of waters located in isolated places in a landscape. It does not modify some categories of waters that currently are jurisdictional by rule (traditional navigable waters, interstate waters and wetlands, the territorial seas, and impoundments). Proposed changes would increase the asserted scope of CWAjurisdiction, in part as a result of expressly declaring some types of waters categorically jurisdictional (such as all waters adjacent to a jurisdictional water), and also by application of new definitions, which give larger regulatory context to some types of waters, such as tributaries.

Beyond the categories of waters that would be categorically jurisdictional under the proposal is a category sometimes referred to as "other waters." The regulatory term "other waters" applies to wetlands and non-wetland waters such as prairie potholes that are not considered traditionally navigable or meet other of the proposed rule's jurisdictional definitions. Much of the controversy since the Supreme Court rulings has focused on the degree to which "other waters" are jurisdictional. According to the agencies' analyses, 17% of these "other waters" would be categorically jurisdictional under changes in the proposal. It also lists waters and features that would not be jurisdictional, such as prior converted cropland and certain ditches. It makes no change to existing statutory and regulatory permit exclusions, such as exemptions for normal farming and ranching activities.

The agencies believe that the proposal does not exceed the CWA's coverage or protect new types of waters that have not been protected historically. While it would enlarge jurisdiction beyond that under the existing EPA-Corps guidance, they believe that it would not enlarge jurisdiction beyond what is consistent with the Supreme Court's narrow reading of jurisdiction. Others may disagree. Overall, the agencies estimate that approximately 3% of U.S. waters will additionally be subject to CWA jurisdiction as a result of the proposed rule (including additional "other waters"), compared with current field practice. EPA and the Corps estimate that costs of the proposal, from additional permit application expenses, for example, range from $162 million to $279 million annually. Benefits, including the value of ecosystem services such as flood protection, are estimated to range from $318 million to $514 million per year. They acknowledge uncertainties and limitations in these estimates.

INTRODUCTION

On March 25, 2014, the Environmental Protection Agency (EPA) and the U.S. Army Corps of Engineers (Corps) jointly proposed a rule defining the scope of waters protected under the Clean Water Act (CWA). The proposed rule would revise regulations that have been in place for more than 25 years.[1] Revisions are proposed in light of Supreme Court rulings in 2001 and 2006 that interpreted the regulatory scope of the CWA more narrowly than previously, but created uncertainty about the precise effect of the Court's decisions.[2]

In April 2011, EPA and the Corps proposed guidance on policies for determining CWA jurisdiction to replace guidance previously issued in 2003 and 2008; all were intended to lessen confusion over the Court's rulings for the regulated community, regulators, and the general public. The guidance documents sought to identify, in light of the Court's rulings, categories of waters that remain jurisdictional, categories not jurisdictional, and categories that require a case-specific analysis to determine if CWA jurisdiction applies. The 2011 proposed guidance identified similar categories as in the 2003 and 2008 documents, but it would have narrowed categories that require case-specific analysis in favor of asserting jurisdiction categorically for some types of waters. The 2014 proposed rule would replace the existing 2003 and 2008 guidance, which remains in effect because the 2011 proposed guidance was not finalized.[3]

The 2011 proposed guidance was extremely controversial, especially with groups representing property owners, land developers, and the agriculture sector, who contended that it represented a massive federal overreach beyond the agencies' statutory authority. Most state and local officials were supportive of clarifying the extent of CWA-regulated waters, but some were concerned that expanding the CWA's scope could impose costs on states and localities as their own actions (e.g., transportation projects) become subject to new requirements. Most environmental advocacy groups welcomed the proposed guidance, which would more clearly define U.S. waters that are subject to CWA protections, but some in these groups favored even a stronger document. Still, both supporters and critics of the 2011 proposed guidance urged the agencies to replace guidance with revised regulations that define "waters of the United States." Three opinions in the 2006 Supreme Court *Rapanos* ruling similarly urged the agencies to initiate a rulemaking, as they now have done.

In Congress, a number of legislative proposals were introduced to bar EPA and the Corps from implementing the 2011 proposed guidance or developing regulations based on it; none of these proposals was enacted. Similar criticism followed almost immediately after release of the proposed rule on March 25, 2014, with some Members asserting that the proposed rule would result in job losses and would damage economic growth. Supporters of the Administration, on the other hand, defended the agencies' efforts to protect U.S. waters and reduce frustration that has resulted from the unclear jurisdiction of the act.[4] Support was expressed by environmental and conservation organizations, among others.[5]

THE CWA AND THE PROPOSED RULE

The proposed rule was published in the *Federal Register* on April 21, 2014. The deadline for public comments is July 21, 2014.[6] **Table 1** in this report provides a comparison of the current regulatory language that defines "waters of the United States" with language in the proposed rule.

The CWA protects "navigable waters," a term defined in the act to mean "the waters of the United States, including the territorial seas."[7] Waters that are jurisdictional are subject to the multiple regulatory requirements of the CWA: standards, discharge limitations, permits, and enforcement. Non-jurisdictional waters, in contrast, do not have the federal legal protection of those requirements. The act's single definition of "navigable waters" applies to the entire law. In particular, it applies to federal prohibition on discharges of pollutants except in compliance with the act's requirements (§301), requirements for point sources to obtain a permit prior to discharge (§§402 and 404), water quality standards and measures to attain them (§303), oil spill liability and oil spill prevention and control measures (§311), certification that federally permitted activities comply with state water quality standards (§401), and enforcement (§309). It impacts the Oil Pollution Act and other environmental laws, as well.[8] The CWA leaves it to the agencies to define the term "waters of the United States," which EPA and the Corps have done several times, most recently in 1986.

According to the agencies, the proposed rule would revise the existing administrative definition of "waters of the United States" in regulations consistent with legal rulings—especially the recent Supreme Court cases—and science concerning the interconnectedness of tributaries, wetlands, and other waters to downstream waters and effects of these connections on the chemical, physical, and biological integrity of downstream waters. It is particularly focused on clarifying the regulatory status of waters located in isolated places in a landscape, the types of waters with ambiguous jurisdictional status following the Supreme Court's 2001 ruling in *SWANCC,* and small streams, rivers that flow for part of the year, and nearby wetlands, the types of waters affected by the Court's 2006 ruling in *Rapanos*. In developing the proposed rule, EPA and the Corps relied on a draft synthesis of more than 1,000 published and peer-reviewed scientific reports; the synthesis discusses the current scientific understanding of the connections or isolation of streams and wetlands relative to large water bodies such as river, lakes, estuaries, and oceans. The purpose of the report is to summarize current understanding of these connections, the factors that influence them, and the mechanisms by which connected waters affect the function or condition of downstream waters.[9] This draft assessment document is under review by EPA's Science Advisory Board (SAB), which provides independent engineering and scientific advice to the agency. A number of EPA's critics have suggested that the agencies should have deferred developing or proposing a revised rule until a final scientific review document is complete. In the preamble to the proposed rule, the agencies state that the rule will not be finalized until the SAB's review and a final report are complete. However, some have expressed concern that the final report will not be available during the public comment period on the rule.

Under the first section of the March 25 proposal, the following waters would be jurisdictional by rule:

- Waters susceptible to interstate commerce, known as traditional navigable waters (no change from current rules);
- All interstate waters, including interstate wetlands (no change from current rules);
- The territorial seas (no change from current rules);

- Impoundments of the above waters or a tributary, as defined in the rule (no change from current rules);
- Tributaries of the above waters (more inclusive than current rules because "tributary" is newly and broadly defined); and
- All waters, including wetlands, that are adjacent to a water identified in the above categories (by including all adjacent waters—not simply adjacent wetlands—the proposal is more inclusive than current rules; these waters are considered jurisdictional under the proposed rule because they have a significant nexus to a traditional navigable water, interstate water, or the territorial seas).

The concept of significant nexus is critical because courts have ruled that, to establish CWA jurisdiction between waters, there needs to be "some measure of the significance of the connection for downstream water quality," as Justice Kennedy found in the 2006 *Rapanos* case. He said, "Mere hydrologic connection should not suffice in all cases; the connection may be too insubstantial for the hydrologic linkage to establish the required nexus with navigable waters as traditionally understood."[10] However, as EPA and the Corps observe in the March 25 proposed rule, significant nexus is not itself a scientific term, but rather a determination of the agencies in light of the law and science. Functions that might demonstrate significant nexus include sediment trapping and retention of flood waters. In the proposed rule, the agencies note that a hydrologic connection is not necessary to demonstrate significant nexus, because the function may be demonstrated even in the absence of a connection (e.g., pollutant trapping is another such function).

"Other Waters"

Beyond the categories of waters that would be categorically jurisdictional under the proposed rule is a category sometimes referred to as "other waters." The regulatory term "other waters" applies to wetlands and non-wetland waters that do not fall into the category of waters susceptible to interstate commerce (traditional navigable waters), interstate waters, the territorial seas, tributaries, or waters adjacent to waters in one of these four categories. Current rules contain a non-exclusive list of "other waters," such as intrastate lakes, mudflats, prairie potholes, and playa lakes (see **Table 1**). Headwaters, which constitute most "other waters," supply most of the water to downstream traditional navigable waters, interstate waters, and the territorial seas.

EPA and the Corps recognize that the Supreme Court decisions in *SWANCC* and *Rapanos* put limitations on the scope of "other waters" that may be determined to be jurisdictional under the CWA. Much of the controversy since the Court's rulings has focused on uncertainty as to what degree "other waters" are jurisdictional, either by definition/rule, or as determined on a case-by-case basis to evaluate significant nexus to a jurisdictional water. Under the 2008 guidance, which remains in effect today, all "other waters" require a case-by-case evaluation to determine if a significant nexus exists, thus providing a finding of CWA jurisdiction. There likewise has been uncertainty as to what degree "other waters" that are similarly situated may be aggregated or combined for a significant nexus determination.[11] In the proposed rule, "other waters," including wetlands, that are adjacent to a jurisdictional water are categorically jurisdictional. Non-adjacent "other waters" and wetlands will continue to require a case-by-case determination of significant nexus. Also, the proposed rule allows broader aggregation of "other waters" that are similarly situated than under the 2008 guidance, which could result in more "other waters" being found to be jurisdictional following a significant nexus evaluation.

Some in the regulated community have urged EPA and the Corps to provide metrics, such as quantifiable flow rates or minimum number of functions for "other waters," to establish a significant nexus to jurisdictional waters. The agencies declined to do so in the proposed rule, saying that absolute standards would not allow sufficient flexibility to account for variability of conditions and the varied functions that different waters provide.

The agencies acknowledge that there may be more than one way to determine which waters are jurisdictional as "other waters," and they are requesting comment on alternate approaches, combination of approaches, scientific and technical data, case law, and other information that would clarify which "other waters" should be considered categorically jurisdictional or following a case-specific significant nexus determination.

In addition, EPA and the Corps are asking for public comment on whether to conclude by rule that certain types of "other waters"—prairie potholes, western vernal pools, Carolina and Delmarva bays, pocosins, Texas coastal prairie wetlands, and perhaps other categories of waters—have a significant nexus and are *per se* jurisdictional. These waters would not require a case-by-case analysis. At the same time, the agencies are asking for comment on whether to determine by rule that playa lakes and perhaps other categories of waters do not have a significant nexus and are not jurisdictional. If so determined, these waters would not be subject to a case-by-case analysis of significant nexus.

Exclusions and Definitions

The second section of the proposed rule excludes specified waters from the definition of "waters of the United States." The listed waters and features would not be jurisdictional even if they would otherwise be included within categories that are jurisdictional. The exclusions are:

- Waste treatment systems, including treatment ponds or lagoons, that are designed to meet CWA requirements;
- Prior converted cropland;
- A list of features that have been excluded by long-standing practice and guidance and would now be excluded by rule, such as artificially irrigated areas that would revert to upland should application of irrigation water to the area cease (see **Table 1** for the full list); and
- Two types of ditches: ditches that are excavated wholly in uplands, drain only uplands or non-jurisdictional waters, and have less than perennial (i.e., permanent) flow; and ditches that do not contribute flow, either directly or through another water, to a traditional navigable water, interstate water, impoundment, or the territorial seas. Other ditches, if they meet the rule's definition of "tributary," would continue to be "waters of the United States"—a point of much controversy with some stakeholders.

The proposed rule makes no change to and does not affect existing statutory and regulatory exclusions, such as exemptions for normal farming, ranching, and silviculture activities (CWA §404(f)); exemptions for permitting of agricultural stormwater discharges and return flows from irrigated agriculture; or exemptions for water transfers that do not introduce pollutants into a waterbody. Nor would it change permitting processes.

In the third section of the proposed rule, the agencies define terms, including "floodplain," "riparian area," "tributary," "significant nexus," and "neighboring" as a component of the existing term "adjacent." The terms "adjacent" and "wetland" are not redefined. (See **Table 1**.)

Finally, the proposed rule includes two appendixes. One is an abbreviated, but lengthy, version of the scientific assessment document currently being reviewed by EPA's Science Advisory Board, plus additional detail of the agencies' reasoning concerning science in support of the proposed rule; the other is an analysis of relevant case law.

IMPACTS OF THE PROPOSED RULE

The agencies acknowledge that the proposed rule would increase the asserted geographic scope of CWA jurisdiction, when compared to a baseline of current practices under the existing regulations and the 2003-2008 EPA-Corps guidance. This results in part from the agencies' expressly declaring some types of waters categorically jurisdictional (such as all waters adjacent to a jurisdictional water), and also by application of definitions, which give larger regulatory context to some types of waters, such as tributaries.

The agencies believe, however, that the proposed rule does not protect any new types of waters that have not been protected historically (i.e., prior to the *SWANCC* and *Rapanos* rulings) or exceed the CWA's coverage. That is, while it would enlarge jurisdiction beyond that under the 2003 and 2008 EPA-Corps guidance, which the agencies believe was narrower than is justified by science and the law, they believe that it would not enlarge jurisdiction beyond what is consistent with the Supreme Court's narrow reading of jurisdiction. Others may disagree. Many stakeholders are concerned with what changes the proposed rule will make, how much additional waters will be considered jurisdictional, and what additional costs will result.

The agencies' broader assertion of jurisdiction, compared to existing regulation and current practice, does not identify specific waters that will be found to be jurisdictional—that is, this or that particular stream or pond—but the proposed rule attempts to draw more of a bright line of CWA jurisdiction than in the past.

In an Economic Analysis document accompanying the proposed rule, EPA and the Corps estimate that approximately 3% of U.S. waters would additionally be subject to CWA jurisdiction as a result of the proposed rule, compared with current field practice, and thus subject to CWA requirements. The estimated increase includes about 17% of "other waters" (discussed above) that were not jurisdictional under the 2003/2008 guidance.[12]

Table 1. Comparison of "Definition of Waters of the United States" Regulatory Language Current Regulatory Language and Proposed Rule Announced by EPA and the Army Corps of Engineers March 25, 2014

Current Regulatory Language[a]	Proposed Regulatory Language (3/25/2014)	Comments[b]
(a) The term *waters of the United States* means	(a) For purposes of all sections of the Clean Water Act, 33 U.S.C. 1251 *et seq*. and its implementing regulations, subject to the exclusions in subsection (b) of this section, the term "waters of the United States" means:	
(1) All waters which are currently used, or were used in the past, or may be susceptible to use in interstate or foreign commerce, including all waters which are subject to the ebb and flow of the tide;	(1) All waters which are currently used, were used in the past, or may be susceptible to use in interstate or foreign commerce, including all waters which are subject to the ebb and flow of the tide;	These waters are often referred to as "traditional navigable waters" (TNWs), which include but are not limited to the "navigable waters of the United States" within the meaning of Section 10 of the Rivers and Harbors Act of 1899. No change from the existing rule.
(2) All interstate waters including interstate wetlands;	(2) All interstate waters, including interstate wetlands;	These waters include tributaries to interstate waters, waters adjacent to interstate waters, waters adjacent to tributaries of interstate waters, and "other waters" that have a significant nexus to interstate waters. No change from the existing rule. Interstate waters would continue to be "waters of the United States" even if they are not navigable in fact and do not connect to such waters.

Current Regulatory Language[a]	Proposed Regulatory Language (3/25/2014)	Comments[b]
(3) All other waters such as intrastate lakes, rivers, streams (including intermittent streams), mudflats, sandflats, wetlands, sloughs, prairie potholes, wet meadows, playa lakes, or natural ponds, the use, degradation or destruction of which could affect interstate or foreign commerce includeing any such waters:	(7) On a case-specific basis, other waters, including wetlands, provided that those waters alone, or in combination with other similarly situated waters, including wetlands, located in the same region, have a significant nexus to a water identified in paragraphs (a)(1) through (3) of this section.	In the existing rule, there is a non-exclusive list of the types of "other waters" which may be found to be "waters of the U.S." The existing description is omitted under the proposal as unnecessary and confusing because it includes some waters that would be jurisdictional under one of the categories of waters that are jurisdictional by rule under the proposal (for example, an intermittent stream that meets the definition of tributary). Under the proposed rule, "other waters" are not jurisdictional as a single category but require a case-specific analysis of a significant nexus to a traditional navigable water, an interstate water, or the territorial seas. They may be evaluated either individually, or as a group of waters where they are determined to be similarly situated in a region. "In the region" means the watershed that drains to the nearest water, or the territorial seas through a single point of entry. How other waters are aggregated for a case-specific significant nexus analysis depends on the functions they perform and their spatial arrangement

Table 1. (Continued)

Current Regulatory Language[a]	Proposed Regulatory Language (3/25/2014)	Comments[b]
		traditional navigable water, interstate within the region or watershed. It is the landscape position within the watershed that is the determinative factor for the analysis, which will focus on the degree to which the functions provided by the other waters affect the chemical, physical, or biological integrity of (a)(1) through (a)(3) waters.
		Current rule asserts jurisdiction more broadly than what is proposed; the proposal deletes language requiring that an "other water" be one "the use, degradation or destruction of which could affect interstate commerce" and replaces it with requirement that the "other water" meet the significant nexus standard. The agencies consider this a substantial change from the current rule.
(i) Which are or could be used by interstate or foreign travelers for recreational or other purposes; or		Specific examples are omitted in the proposed rule as unnecessary. The agencies say that the listing has led to confusion where it has been incorrectly read as an exclusive list.

Current Regulatory Language[a]	Proposed Regulatory Language (3/25/2014)	Comments[b]
(ii) From which fish or shellfish are or could be taken and sold in interstate or foreign commerce; or		
(iii) Which are used or could be used for industrial purpose by industries in interstate commerce;		
(4) All impoundments of waters otherwise defined as waters of the United States under the definition;	(4) All impoundments of waters identified in paragraphs (a)(1) through (3) and (5) of this section;	Impoundments of a traditional navigable water, interstate water, the territorial seas, or a tributary are jurisdictional by rule. As a matter of policy and law, impoundments do not de-federalize a water, even where there is no longer flow below the impoundment. That is, damming or impounding a water of the United States does not make the water non-jurisdictional.
(5) Tributaries of waters identified in paragraphs (a)(1) through (4) of this section;	(5) All tributaries of waters identified in paragraphs (a)(1) through (4) of this section;	Tributaries, as defined in the proposed rule, of a traditional navigable water, interstate water, the territorial seas, or an impoundment would be jurisdictional by rule. Unless excluded under subsection (b) of the proposed rule, any water that meets the proposed definition of tributary is a water of the United States, whether it is perennial, intermittent, or ephemeral. The water may contribute flow directly or may contribute

Table 1. (Continued)

Current Regulatory Language[a]	Proposed Regulatory Language (3/25/2014)	Comments[b]
		flow to another water or waters that eventually flow into a jurisdictional water. The tributary must drain, or be part of a network of tributaries that drain, into an (a)(1) through (a)(4) water. "Tributary" is defined below.
(6) The territorial seas;	(3) The territorial seas;	Jurisdictional by rule; no change from the existing rule.
(7) Wetlands adjacent to waters (other than waters that are themselves wet-lands) identified in paragraphs (a)(1) through (6) of this section.	(6) All waters, including wetlands, adjacent to a water identified in paragraphs (a)(1) through (5) of this section; and (b) The following are not "waters of the United States"	All waters, including wetlands, adjacent to a traditional navigable water, interstate water, the territorial seas, impoundment, or tributary would be jurisdictional by rule. Under the proposed rule, wetlands, ponds, lakes, and similar waterbodies that are adjacent to traditional navigable waters, interstate waters, and the territorial seas, as well as waters and wetlands adjacent to other jurisdictional waters such as tributaries and impoundments, would be jurisdictional by rule.
(8) Waters of the United States do not include prior converted cropland.[c] Notwithstanding the determination of an area's status as prior converted	(2) Prior converted cropland. Notwith-standing the determination of an area's status as prior converted cropland by any other federal agency, for the purposes of	No change proposed.

Current Regulatory Language[a]	Proposed Regulatory Language (3/25/2014)	Comments[b]
cropland by any other Federal agency, for the purposes of the Clean Water Act, the final authority regarding Clean Water Act jurisdiction remains with EPA.	the Clean Water Act, the final authority regarding Clean Water Act jurisdiction remains with EPA.	
Waste treatment systems, including treatment ponds or lagoons designed to meet the requirements of CWA (other than cooling ponds as defined in 40 CFR 423.11(m) which also meet the criteria of this definition) are not waters of the United States.[d]	(1) Waste treatment systems, including treatment ponds or lagoons, designed to meet the requirements of the Clean Water Act. (3) Ditches that are excavated wholly in uplands, drain only uplands or non-jurisdictional waters, and have less than perennial flow.	The agencies do not believe that omitting the parenthetical reference to 40 CFR 423.11(m) is a change in substance to the waste treatment exclusion or how it is applied. Proposed rule would codify long-standing practice and guidance (including 1986 and 1988 preamble language), which has been to exclude these waters from jurisdiction. Excluded ditches must be dug only in uplands, drain only uplands, and have ephemeral or intermittent flow. Water that only stands or pools in a ditch is not considered perennial flow and, therefore, any such upland ditch would not be subject to regulation. Other ditches, if they meet the new proposed definition of "tributary," would continue to be waters of the U.S. Ditches may function as point sources that discharge pollutants, thus subject to CWA Section 402.

Table 1. (Continued)

Current Regulatory Language[a]	Proposed Regulatory Language (3/25/2014)	Comments[b]
	(4) Ditches that do not contribute flow, either directly or through another water, to a water identified in paragraphs (a)(1) through (4) of this section.	Proposed rule would codify long-standing practice and guidance (includ-ing 1986 and 1988 preamble language), which has been to exclude these waters from jurisdiction. These waters would not be jurisdictional by rule.
		Ditches that do not contribute flow to the tributary system of a traditional navigable water, interstate water, impoundment, or the territorial seas are not "waters of the United States," even if the ditch has a perennial flow. Other ditches, if they meet the new proposed definition of "tributary," would continue to be waters of the U.S. Ditches may function as point sources that discharge pollutants, thus subject to CWA Section 402.
	(5) The following features: (i) Artificially irrigated areas that would revert to upland should application of irrigation water to that area cease; (ii) artificial lakes or ponds created by excavating and/or diking dry land and used exclusively for such purposes as	Proposed rule would codify long-standing practice and guidance (including 1986 and 1988 preamble language), which has been to exclude these waters from jurisdiction. These waters would not be jurisdictional by rule.

Current Regulatory Language[a]	Proposed Regulatory Language (3/25/2014)	Comments[b]
	stock watering, irrigation, settling basins, or rice growing; (iii) artificial reflecting pools or swimming pools created by excavating and/or diking dry land; (iv) small ornamental waters created by excavating and/or diking dry land for primarily aesthetic reasons; (v) water-filled depressions created incidental to construction activity; (vi) groundwater drained through subsurface drainage systems; and (vii) gullies and rills and non-wetland swales.	
	(c) Definitions—	
(b) The term *wetlands* means those areas that are inundated or saturated by surface or ground water at a frequency and duration sufficient to support, and that under normal circumstances do support, a prevalence of vegetation typically adapted for life in saturated soil conditions. Wetlands generally include swamps, marshes, bogs, and similar areas.	(6) **Wetlands:** The term *wetlands* means those areas that are inundated or saturated by surface or ground water at a frequency and duration sufficient to support, and that under normal circumstances do support, a prevalence of vegetation typically adapted for life in saturated soil conditions. Wetlands generally include swamps, marshes, bogs, and similar areas.	No change proposed. Wetlands are ecosystems that often occur at the edge of aquatic (water, fresh or salty) or terrestrial (upland) systems. Wetlands typically represent transitional zones between aquatic and upland systems.
(c) The term *adjacent* means bordering, contiguous, or neighboring. Wetlands separated from other waters of the United	(1) **Adjacent:** The term *adjacent* means bordering, contiguous or neighboring. Waters, including wetlands, separated	Current rule limits consideration of adjacency to wetlands. Proposed rule would change "adjacent wetlands" to "adjacent

Table 1. (Continued)

Current Regulatory Language[a]	Proposed Regulatory Language (3/25/2014)	Comments[b]
States by man-made dikes or barriers, natural river berms, beach dunes and the like are ''adjacent wetlands.''	from other waters of the United States by man-made dikes or barriers, natural river berms, beach dunes and the like are "adjacent waters."	waters" so that waterbodies such as ponds and oxbow lakes [a U-shaped body of water formed when a wide meander from a river is cut off to form a lake] as well as wetlands that are adjacent to jurisdictional waters are "waters of the U.S." by regulation. The rule would include wetlands and other waterbodies that meet the proposed definition of adjacent, including "neighboring," which is defined separately. Adjacent waters are those that provide similar functions which, *together with functions provided by tributaries to which they are adjacent*, have a significant nexus to traditional navigable waters (TNWs), interstate waters, and the territorial seas. "In the aggregate, all adjacent waters have a significant nexus with their downstream TNWs or interstate waters." The lateral limits of an adjacent water, other than wetlands or tributaries, are determined by the presence of an ordinary high water mark (OHWM) without the need for a bed and banks. Deletion of parenthetical

Current Regulatory Language[a]	Proposed Regulatory Language (3/25/2014)	Comments[b]
		phrase in the existing rule is intended to ensure that all waters that meet the proposed definitions of “adjacent”are “waters of the U.S.” regardless of whether or not another adjacent water is located between those waters and the tributary.
(d) The term *high tide line* means the line of intersection of the land with the water’s surface at the maximum height reached by a rising tide. The high tide line may be determined, in the absence of actual data, by a line of oil or scum along shore objects, a more or less continuous deposit of fine shell or debris on the foreshore or berm, other physical markings or characteristics, vegetation lines, tidal gages, or other suitable means that delineate the general height reached by a rising tide. The line encompasses spring high tides and other high tides that occur with periodic frequency but does not include storm surges in which there is a departure from the normal or predicted reach of the tide due to the piling up of water against a coast by strong winds such as	No change proposed	

Table 1. (Continued)

Current Regulatory Language[a]	Proposed Regulatory Language (3/25/2014)	Comments[b]
those accompanying a hurricane or other intense storm.		
(e) The term *ordinary high water mark* means that line on the shore established by the fluctuations of water and indicated by physical characteristics such as clear, natural line impressed on the bank, shelving, changes in the character of soil, destruction of terrestrial vegetation, the presence of litter and debris, or other appropriate means that consider the characteristics of the surrounding area.	No change proposed	
(f) The term *tidal waters* means those waters that rise and fall in a predictable and measurable rhythm or cycle due to the gravitational pulls of the moon and sun. Tidal waters end where the rise and fall of the water surface can no longer be practically measured in a predictable rhythm due to masking by hydrologic, wind, or other effects.	No change proposed	
	(2) **Neighboring:** The term *neighboring*, for purposes of the term "adjacent" in this section, includes waters located within the riparian area	Waters, including wetlands, that are located within the riparian area or floodplain of an (a)(1) through (a)(5) water would be jurisdictional without a

Current Regulatory Language[a]	Proposed Regulatory Language (3/25/2014)	Comments[b]
	or floodplain of a water identified in paragraphs (a)(1) through (a)(5) of this section, or waters with a surface or shallow subsurface hydrologic connection to such a jurisdictional water.	case-specific significant nexus analysis. Even if separated from such a water by natural or man-made features (e.g., a berm), the water would be adjacent and thus jurisdictional.
	(3) **Riparian area:** The term *riparian area* means an area bordering a water where surface or subsurface hydrology influence the ecological processes and plant and animal community structure in that area. Riparian areas are transitional areas between aquatic and terrestrial ecosystems that influence the exchange of energy and materials between those ecosystems.	The term "riparian area" is used to help identify waters, including wetlands, that may be "adjacent" and would, therefore, be "waters of the United States" under the proposed rule. No uplands located in "riparian areas" can ever be "waters of the United States."
	(4) **Floodplain:** The term *floodplain* means an area bordering inland or coastal waters that was formed by sediment deposition from such water under present climatic conditions and is inundated during periods of moderate to high water flows. (5) **Tributary:** The term *tributary* means a waterbody physically characterized by the presence of a bed and banks and ordinary high water mark, as defined at 33 CFR § 328.3(e), which	The term "floodplain" is used to help identify waters, including wetlands, that may be "adjacent" and would, therefore, be "waters of the United States" under the proposed rule. No uplands located in "floodplains" can ever be "waters of the United States." This term has not previously been defined in any regulation or preamble. Bed and banks and ordinary high water mark (OHWM) are features that generally

Table 1. (Continued)

Current Regulatory Language[a]	Proposed Regulatory Language (3/25/2014)	Comments[b]
	contributes flow, either directly or through another water, to a water identified in paragraphs (a)(1) through (4) of this section. In addition, wetlands, lakes, and ponds are tributaries (even if they lack a bed and banks or ordinary high water mark) if they contribute flow, either directly or through another water to a water identified in paragraphs (a)(1) through (3) of this section. A water that otherwise qualifies as a tributary under this definition does not lose its status as a tributary if, for any length, there are one or more man-made breaks (such as bridges, culverts, pipes, or dams) or one or more natural breaks (such as wetlands at the head of or along the run of a stream, debris piles, boulder fields, or a stream that flows underground) so long as a bed and banks and an ordinary high water mark can be identified upstream of the break. A tributary, including wetlands, can be a natural, man-altered, or man-made waterbody and includes waters such as	are physical indicators of flow. OHWM generally defines the lateral limits of a water. In many tributaries, the bed is that part of the channel below the OHWM, and the banks often extend above the OHWM. Wetland tributaries are wetlands that are located within the stream channel itself or that form the start of the stream channel. Man-altered and man-made tributaries perform many of the same functions as natural tributaries and provide connectivity between streams and downstream rivers.

Current Regulatory Language[a]	Proposed Regulatory Language (3/25/2014)	Comments[b]
	rivers, streams, lakes, ponds, impoundments, canals, and ditches not excluded in paragraph (b)(3) or (4) of this section.	
	(7) **Significant nexus:** The term *significant nexus* means that a water, including wetlands, either alone or in combination with other similarly situated waters in the region (i.e., the watershed that drains to a water identified in paragraphs (a)(1) through (3) of this section), significantly affects the chemical, physical or biological integrity of a water identified in paragraphs (a)(1) through (3) of this section. For an effect to be significant, it must be more than speculative or insubstantial. Other waters, including wetlands, are similarly situated when they perform similar functions and are located sufficiently close together or close to a "water of the U.S." so that they can be evaluated as a single landscape unit with regard to their effect on the chemical, physical, or biological integrity of a water identified in	A significant nexus analysis may be based on a particular water alone or on the effect that the water has in combination with other similarly situated waters in the region. "Region" means the watershed that drains to a water identified in (a)(1) through (a)(3) through a single point of entry. Proposed rule adopts the concept of aggregating certain waters to determine whether they meet the "alone or in combination with similarly situated waters" test of Justice Kennedy. Waters must perform similar functions and be located sufficiently close together or close to a traditional navigable water, interstate water, or the territorial seas so that they can be evaluated as a single landscape unit with regard to their effects. Examining both functionality and proximity limits the "other waters" that can be aggregated for purposes of determining jurisdiction.

Table 1. (Continued)

Current Regulatory Language[a]	Proposed Regulatory Language (3/25/2014)	Comments[b]
	paragraphs (a)(1) through (3) of this section.	Functions that might demonstrate significant nexus include sediment trapping and retention of flood waters. A hydrologic connection is not necessary, because the function may be demonstrated even in the absence of a connection (e.g., pollutant trapping).

Source: Prepared by CRS.

Notes:

a. 33 C.F.R. 328.3, 40 C.F.R. 122.2, 40 C.F.R. 230.3, and 40 C.F.R. 232.2 (definition of "waters of the United States"). The term "navigable waters" is defined at 40 C.F.R. 110.1 (Discharge of Oil); 40 C.F.R. 112.2 (Oil Pollution Prevention); 40 C.F.R. 116.3 (Designation of Hazardous Substance); 40 C.F.R. 117.1(i) (Determination of Reportable Quantities for Hazardous Substances); 40 C.F.R. 300.5 and Appendix E 1.5 to Part 300 (National Oil and Hazardous Substances Pollution Contingency Plan); and 40 C.F.R. 302.3 (Designation, Reportable Quantities, and Notification).

b. Comments in this table are drawn in large part from the preamble to the proposed rule.

c. The term "prior converted cropland" is included in the U.S. Department of Agriculture's administrative definition of the term "wetland" (see 7 C.F.R. 12.2).

d. A definition of "waste treatment system is found in EPA regulations (35 C.F.R. 35.905): "Complete waste treatment system. A complete waste treatment system consists of all of the treatment works necessary to meet the requirements of title III of the Act, involved in (a) The transport of waste waters from individual homes or buildings to a plant or facility where treatment of the waste water is accomplished; (b) the treatment of the waste waters to remove pollutants; and (c) the ultimate disposal, including recycling or reuse, of the treated waste waters and residues which result from the treatment process. One complete waste treatment system would, normally, include one treatment plant or facility, but also includes two or more connected or integrated treatment plants or facilities."

According to the analysis, costs to regulated entities and governments (federal, state, and local) are likely to increase. Direct and indirect costs would result from additional permit application expenses (for CWA Section 404 permitting, stormwater permitting for construction and development activities, and permitting of pesticide discharges and confined animal feeding operations [CAFOs] for discharges to waters that would now be determined jurisdictional) and additional requirements for oil storage and production facilities needing to develop and implement spill prevention, control and countermeasure (SPCC) plans. Federal and state governments would likely experience costs to administer and process additional permits. Other costs would likely include compensatory mitigation requirements for permit impacts (if applicable), affecting land developers and state and local governments. In all, the agencies estimate that incremental costs associated with the rule range from $162 million to $279 million per year.

The agencies believe that benefits accruing from the proposed rule include the value of ecosystem services provided by the waters and wetlands protected as a result of CWA requirements, such as habitat for aquatic and other species, support for recreational fishing and hunting, and flood protection. Other benefits would include government savings on enforcement expenses, because the rule is intended to provide greater regulatory certainty, thus reducing the need for government enforcement. Business and government may also achieve savings from reduced uncertainty concerning where CWA jurisdiction applies, they believe. In all, the agencies estimate that benefits of the proposed rule range from $318 million to $514 million per year. However, they note that "there is uncertainty and limitations associated with the results," due to data and information gaps, as well as analytic challenges. The analysis does not quantify all possible costs and benefits.[13] Overall, they conclude that benefits would exceed costs.

Unclear for now is a question of the extent to which case law construing the existing administrative definition of "waters of the United States" will continue to apply. Some of that case law has been in place for more than 35 years. The preamble to the proposed rule does not address this issue.

The agriculture sector has been vigorous in criticizing and challenging EPA regulatory actions that may affect the sector's operations, making potential impacts of the proposed rule on agriculture a likely focus of controversy. One of the sector's concerns about a new "waters of the United States" rule has been whether it would modify existing statutory and regulatory exemptions that exclude certain discharges from agricultural activities from CWA permitting. As described above, the proposed rule makes no change and does not affect these exemptions, which are self-implementing. An EPA fact sheet discusses the continued exclusions and exemptions.[14]

In addition, simultaneous with proposing the rule, EPA and the Corps issued an interpretive rule that identifies 53 conservation practices approved by the U.S. Department of Agriculture's Natural Resources Conservation Service (NRCS) that additionally qualify for exemption under the CWA Section 404(f)(1)(A) exclusion of "normal farming" activities from Section 404 permit requirements and do not require determination whether the discharge involves a "water of the United States." Through this interpretive rule, the agencies intend to resolve uncertainties about "normal farming" activities that are exempt from permitting when these conservation practices are used. In other words, effective immediately, producers who utilize any of the 53 identified practices according to NRCS technical standards need not seek a determination of CWA jurisdiction and need not seek a CWA permit. The three agencies also have signed a Memorandum of Understanding detailing implementation of the interpretive rule and identifying a process for reviewing and updating the list of qualifying NRCS conservation practices. Although the interpretive rule is already in effect, the agencies are accepting public comment until June 5, 2014.[15]

CONCLUSION

The Corps and EPA will accept public comment on the proposed rule for 90 days, until July 21, 2014. If past experience regarding controversial proposals is a guide, however, it is likely that the public comment period will be extended. Further, as noted above, the agencies pledge that a final rule will not be promulgated before completion of EPA's scientific assessment report; so, when that may occur is likely to be some months in the future.

The EPA Administrator recently stated at a congressional hearing that it generally takes about one year to finalize a rule. Complex and controversial rules can take much longer from proposal to promulgation. Once a rule is finalized, legal challenges are likely, possibly delaying implementation of any rule for years. New regulations may clarify many current questions, but they are unlikely to please all of the competing interests, as one environmental advocate observed.

However, a rulemaking would only benefit wetlands if it did not reduce the jurisdiction offered by current regulations and if the Administration remained faithful to sound science. If politics were to trump science in the rulemaking process, the likelihood of such a protective rule would not be promising. Also, rules are subject to legal challenge and can be tied up in court for years before they are implemented.[16]

End Notes

[1] Definition of "waters of the United States" is found at 33 C.F.R. § 328.3 (Corps) and 40 C.F.R. § 122.2 (EPA). The term is similarly defined in other EPA regulations, as is the term "navigable waters." See **Table 1**.

[2] Solid Waste Agency of Northern Cook County v. U.S. Army Corps of Engineers (SWANCC), 531 U.S. 159 (2001), and Rapanos v. United States, 547 U.S. 715 (2006).

[3] For background on the Supreme Court rulings, subsequent guidance, and other developments, see CRS Report RL33263, *The Wetlands Coverage of the Clean Water Act (CWA):* Rapanos *and Beyond*, by Robert Meltz and Claudia Copeland.

[4] Anthony Adragna and Amena Saiyid, "Republicans Contend EPA Overreached on Clean Water Act Jurisdiction Proposal," *Daily Environment Report*, vol. 58 (March 26, 2014), pp. A-7.

[5] U.S. Environmental Protection Agency, "Here's What They're Saying About the Clean Water Act Proposed Rule," press release, March 26, 2014, http://yosemite.epa.gov/opa/admpress.nsf/3881d73f4d4aaa0b85257359003f5348/3f954c179cf0720985257ca7004920fa!OpenDocument.

[6] Department of Defense, Department of the Army, Corps of Engineers, and Environmental Protection Agency, "Definition of 'Waters of the United States' Under the Clean Water Act, Proposed Rule," 79 *Federal Register* 22188-22274, April 21, 2014.

[7] CWA §502(7); 33 U.S.C. § 1362(7).

[8] For example, the reach of the Endangered Species Act (ESA) is affected, because that act's requirement for consultation by federal agencies over impacts on threatened or endangered species is triggered through the issuance of federal permits.

[9] U.S. Environmental Protection Agency, Office of Research and Development, Connectivity of Streams and Wetlands to Downstream Waters: A Review and Synthesis of the Scientific Evidence, External Review Draft, EPA/600/R-11-098B, September 2013, http://yosemite.epa.gov/sab/sabproduct.nsf/0/7724357376745F48852579E60043E88C/$File/WOUS_ERD2_Sep2013.pdf.

[10] 547 U.S. at 784-785.

[11] In the *Rapanos* ruling, Justice Kennedy stated that wetlands possess the requisite significant nexus if the wetlands, "either alone or in combination with similarly situated [wet]lands in the region, significantly affect the chemical, physical, and biological integrity of other covered waters more readily understood as 'navigable.'" 547 U.S. at 780.

[12] U.S. Environmental Protection Agency and U.S. Army Corps of Engineers, *Economic Analysis of Proposed Revised Definition of Waters of the United States*, March 2014, http://www2.epa.gov/uswaters/economic-analysis-proposed-revised-definition-waters-united-states, p. 12.

[13] Ibid., pp. 21-22, 32.

[14] See http://www2.epa.gov/sites/production/files/2014-03/documents/cwa_ag_exclusions_exemptions.pdf.

[15] Department of Defense, Department of the Army, Corps of Engineers, and Environmental Protection Agency, "Notice of Availability Regarding the Exemption From Permitting Under Section 404(f)(1)(A) of the Clean Water Act to Certain Agricultural Conservation Practices," 79 *Federal Register* 22276, April 21, 2014.The list of practices, the Memorandum of Understanding, and the interpretive rule are available at http://water.epa.gov/lawsregs/guidance/ wetlands/agriculture.cfm. USDA had no formal role in developing the Corps-EPA proposed rule, but it was among the federal agencies commenting on it during interagency review.

[16] James Murphy, "*Rapanos v. United States*: Wading Through Murky Waters," *National Wetlands Newsletter*, vol. 28, no. 5, September-October 2006, p. 19.

In: U.S. Waters Protected …
Editor: Caroline M. Ednie

ISBN: 978-1-63321-275-6

Chapter 2

ECONOMIC ANALYSIS OF PROPOSED REVISED DEFINITION OF WATERS OF THE UNITED STATES*

U.S. Environmental Protection Agency; U.S. Army Corps of Engineers

SECTION 1: OVERVIEW OF PROPOSED RULE

The U.S. Army Corps of Engineers (Corps) and the Environmental Protection Agency (EPA), collectively "the agencies", proposed a rule for public comment that that defines the scope of waters protected under the Clean Water Act (CWA), in light of the U.S. Supreme Court cases in *U.S. v. Riverside Bayview, Rapanos v. United States,* and *Solid Waste Agency v. U.S. Army Corps of `Engineers (SWANCC).* The effect of the *SWANCC* decision is primarily on so-called "isolated" (other) waters. These waters do not meet the agencies' definition of "adjacent" and often include vernal pools, prairie potholes and playa lakes that lie entirely within a single state and lack a direct, surface water connection to the river network. In practice, the effect of the *Rapanos* decision has been primarily on some small streams, rivers that flow for part of the year, and nearby wetlands. The agencies believe this proposal would enhance protection for the nation's public health and aquatic resources,

* This is an edited, reformatted and augmented version of a document issued by the U.S. Environmental Protection Agency, dated March 2014.

and increase CWA program predictability and consistency by increasing clarity on the scope of "waters of the United States" protected under the Act.

Specifically, the agencies propose to define the waters of the United States for all sections of the Clean Water Act to mean: traditional navigable waters (TNWs); interstate waters, including interstate wetlands; the territorial seas; impoundments of waters otherwise defined as waters of the United States; tributaries, as defined, to traditional navigable waters, interstate waters, or the territorial seas; adjacent waters, including wetlands; and, on a case-specific basis, other waters that have a significant nexus to a traditional navigable water, interstate water, or the territorial seas.

The agencies also propose to exclude specified waters from the definition of "waters of the United States." The agencies are not proposing changes to the existing exclusions for waste treatment systems designed consistent with the requirements of the Clean Water Act, nor are the agencies are proposing any changes for prior converted cropland. The agencies are, for the first time, proposing to exclude by regulation certain waters and features over which the agencies have as a policy matter generally not asserted CWA jurisdiction.

The agencies propose for the first time to define the term "neighboring" as it is used as a component of the existing term "adjacent", and in turn define the terms "riparian area" and "floodplain" that appear in the new definition of "neighboring". The agencies also define the terms "tributary" and "significant nexus." The goal is to ensure the regulatory definition is consistent with the CWA, as interpreted by the Supreme Court, to protect water quality, public health, and the environment.

SECTION 2: GENERAL APPROACH FOR THE ECONOMIC ANALYSIS

The definition of "waters of the U.S.," by itself, imposes no direct costs. The potential costs and benefits incurred as a result of this proposed action are considered indirect because the action involves a definitional change to a term that is used in the implementation of a variety of CWA programs. Each of these programs may subsequently impose direct or indirect costs as a result of implementation of their specific regulations.

Estimates of the economic costs and benefits that may indirectly be imposed on governments and regulated entities can help inform the public and policymakers of some of the implications associated with this proposal. Just over 10 years ago, almost all waters were considered "waters of the U.S." Following the *SWANCC* (2001) and *Rapanos* (2006) decisions, field practice changed to limit assertion of CWA jurisdiction for some types of waters. For purposes of identifying a set of potential costs and benefits associated with this action, this analysis compares the projected outcome of implementing the proposed rule to the best approximation of field practices during the 2009-2010 time period (post *SWANCC* and *Rapanos*), following issuance of program guidance in 2008. The agencies expect that the outcome of the proposed rule will be an approximate 3 percent increase in assertion of jurisdiction when compared to 2009-2010 field practices, but not as extensive as when the existing regulation went into effect.[1]

In April 2011, the agencies published revised draft guidance on policies for determining CWA jurisdiction to replace guidance issued in 2003 and 2008. The agencies expect that the outcome of the proposed rule would be similar to the outcome of fully implementing the April 2011 draft guidance. As such, this analysis builds on an analysis prepared in association with the April 2011 draft guidance, described in the *Potential Indirect Economic Impacts and Benefits Associated with Guidance Clarifying the Scope of Clean Water Act Jurisdiction* document. This document is available in the administrative record for the proposed rule and available at http://water.epa.gov/lawsregs/guidance/wetlands/upload/cwa guidance impacts benefits.pdf.

The economic analysis is necessarily based on readily available information and the resulting cost and benefit estimates are incomplete. Nonetheless, the agencies have considered the effects on a variety of CWA programs and provide quantitative estimates for many potential impacts. Readers should be cautious in examining these results in light of the many data and methodological limitations, as well as the inherent assumptions in each component of the analysis.

SECTION 3: PROGRAMS AFFECTED

Any water found not to be a "water of the U.S." generally is not subject to CWA requirements. Exhibit 1 depicts the CWA programs that are affected by the definition of "waters of the U.S.," along with the government entities that are responsible for administering the programs. Among its many provisions, the CWA establishes oil spill prevention programs (section 311); requires permits for pollutant discharges (section 402); requires permits for the placement of dredged or fill material in waters of the United States, including wetlands (section 404); calls for states to set standards for meeting water quality goals and develop plans to restore polluted waters (section 303); establishes state roles in certifying that federal permits will not violate state water quality standards (section 401); and allows the federal government, states, and communities to enforce the law.

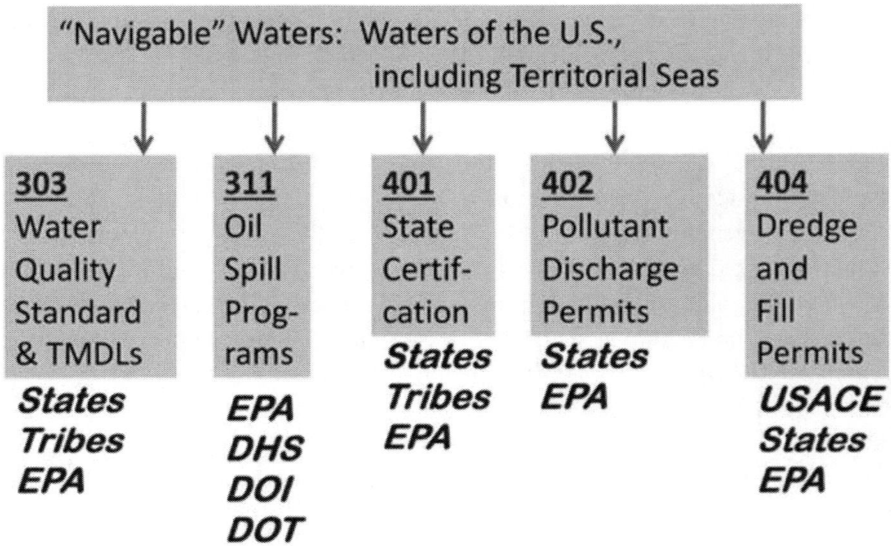

Exhibit 1. Clean Water Act Programs Affected.

As shown in Exhibit 1, states and tribes have a large role in administering many CWA programs. This economic analysis does not account for the possibility that some states may already be considering a broader set of waters to be subject to their implementation of certain CWA programs. Although the extent of their CWA jurisdiction may not be smaller than the definition of waters of the U.S., states and tribes may elect to implement CWA programs more broadly according to a definition of "waters of the state" or "waters of the tribe". To the extent states have elected to do this, the economic impacts may be smaller than presented here (because states may already be asserting jurisdiction over waters for which this analysis presumed jurisdiction was not generally asserted in practice). The particulars of state laws and regulations are often complex and subject to change. At present, it is believed that approximately two-thirds of all states place some legal constraint on the authority of state and local government officials to adopt aquatic resource protections beyond waters of the U.S. These may be straightforward stringency limitations, property-based limitations, or combinations of the two. The provisions may be partial limitations, affecting only some applications. It is further believed that approximately half the states have some provisions that extend protections beyond waters of the U.S. Some of these provisions pre-date stringency limitations and may not be retro-active.

SECTION 4: POTENTIAL AREAS OF NEW INDIRECT COSTS

CWA Section 404 and 401

This proposed rule could result in new indirect costs on regulated entities such as the energy, agricultural, and transportation industries; land developers, municipalities, industrial operations; and on governments administering regulatory programs, at the tribal, state and federal levels. The recent challenges to CWA jurisdiction have arisen from the CWA 404 program, and it is likely that this program has seen the greatest impact from the *SWANCC* and *Rapanos* decision and subsequent joint agency guidance. As such, the CWA 404 program would also see the greatest impact of a regulatory change that would result in broader assertion of CWA jurisdiction. These indirect costs may include application costs, associated environmental compliance costs, wetlands mitigation, stream mitigation, and project re-design and relocation expenses. In addition, there would be program management, training, and associated environmental compliance costs to government associated with administering the CWA. For example, the Corps may process more permit requests, conduct jurisdictional determinations (JDs) if needed, manage data, coordinate with federal and state resource agencies, and determine compensatory mitigation needs. These potential costs are described in detail below. Because most CWA 404 permits are issued by the Corps, states or tribes may incur additional costs of certifying that such permits do not violate their water quality standards under CWA 401. The impact on the CWA 404 program can be measured from data records of jurisdictional determination status of aquatic resources maintained by the Corps. There are no comparable data from other CWA programs. Nevertheless, the regulatory change to the definition of waters of the U.S. applies to all CWA programs and the potential impact to each of these programs should be assessed.

CWA Section 402

EPA does not believe that the *SWANCC* and *Rapanos* decisions have greatly affected traditional CWA 402 permits, such as those issued for municipal wastewater treatment plants or industrial facilities. Neither in its capacity as permitting authority, nor in fulfilling its oversight role of permitting programs delegated to states, has the EPA witnessed a large number of permit holders asserting they no longer required such a permit because of the non-jurisdictional status of a receiving water. While EPA is aware of occasional inquiries on this matter, no such inquiries have resulted in a permitting authority determining that a discharger no longer needed a permit. There are several potential explanations for this. The first is that the nature of a traditional discharge permit where a facility is seeking to have wastewater dispersed and carried away is different than a 404 permit where an entity is, for example, seeking to drain and fill a portion of a natural water for development. As such, it is possible that a CWA 402 permitted discharger may have the effect of creating a permanent water where there once was an intermittent or ephemeral water because of continuous discharge (i.e., an "effluent dependent" or "effluent dominated" water). In these cases, jurisdiction may not come under question. A second explanation is that EPA has authorized most (46) states to operate the CWA 402 permitting program, and states apply jurisdiction to "waters of the state" which must be as inclusive as "waters of the U.S" but may be more inclusive. In contrast, only two states (Michigan and New Jersey) have assumed the 404 program (to the extent it can be assumed for "non-navigable" waters). Additionally, facilities may have invested the capital in treatment and simply be willing to continue operating under their permit and see no need to challenge jurisdiction.

Permitting for construction and development stormwater, concentrated animal feeding operations (CAFOs), and pesticide application are three areas of CWA 402 implementation where there may be potential new costs. This is because these activities relate to collection of runoff rather than disposal of wastewater, and EPA and states typically regulate them through CWA 402 general permits rather than individual permits. In addition, these newer requirements have changed in the last decade. Entities engaged in actions requiring general permit coverage can submit a Notice of Intent (NOI) to the permitting authority to obtain coverage. Under the existing CWA jurisdictional implementation, many of these entities may not believe their discharge affects a jurisdictional water and may not have applied for permit coverage. Under the proposed rule, a portion of these entities may be subject to an assertion of jurisdiction to a similar extent of those seeking 404 permits. Construction-related stormwater discharges, CAFO discharges, and application of pesticides likely occur in similar locations as CWA 404 dredge and fill discharge with respect to proximity to "isolated waters," small streams, and their adjacent wetlands. Indirect costs for these programs include implementing best management practices (BMPs) for regulated entities and administering permitting programs for government.

CWA Section 303 and 305

CWA Section 303 includes development of state water quality standards, monitoring and assessment of water quality, and development of total maximum daily loads (TMDLs) for impaired waters. These programs involve costs to states (standards development, monitoring and assessment, TMDL development). EPA's position on these costs is that an expanded assertion of jurisdiction would not have an effect on annual expenditures.

States typically develop water quality standards for general categories of waters, which have been and are inclusive of the types of waters where jurisdiction comes into question (e.g., for wetlands, the vast majority of which have been and are jurisdictional). Therefore, requirements for state water quality standards to be consistent with the CWA (designated uses, criteria to protect those uses, antidegradation policies) will not change as a result of this proposed action. What could change is whether or not those standards apply. To the extent a state believes there are needs for water quality standards development for specific types of waters, those needs would exist with or without this proposed rule.

CWA 305(b) requires a report from states that includes (among other items) a description of the water quality of all navigable waters in the state and an analysis of the extent to which they meet the 101(a)(2) goals of the Act. In practice, states typically have a set budget for these activities and make plans accordingly. Many states strive to be as comprehensive as possible and balance the needs to identify all impaired waters with probabilistic surveys designed to track general status and trends. To the extent that this proposed rule may increase the coverage where a state would wish to apply its monitoring resources, states are likely to adjust sampling locations or sampling frequency without a net cost increase.

States conduct assessments based on all existing and readily available monitoring data. States are required to list waters that are impaired, but have discretion to prioritize this list for TMDL development, which may proceed over a period of several years under EPA policy. Monitoring, assessment, and TMDL development tend to occur in water segments where the agencies assert jurisdiction under current practices. It is not clear that additional cost burdens for TMDL development would result from this action. In watersheds where there are impaired water segments, waters where the agencies may more clearly assert jurisdiction under the proposed rule are likely to lie upstream of existing impaired segments. Because tribal or state–initiated water quality pollution control strategies are typically applied throughout the watershed of an impaired segment, all upstream waters typically benefit. In addition, clarifying jurisdiction may reduce the cost of returning an impaired water to a condition of meeting water quality standards by allowing better control of upstream sources of pollution.

CWA Section 311

CWA Section 311 covers oil spill prevention and preparedness, reporting obligations, and response planning. These requirements apply to facilities engaged in production or storage of oil products based on total volume. In particular, inland non-transportation oil facilities of a certain size that have potential to discharge to navigable waters must prepare and implement Spill Prevention, Control, and Countermeasure (SPCC) plans. Similar to traditional 402 permits, these requirements have been in place since 1973 and it is not clear how regulated facilities have adjusted their behavior in response to *SWANCC* and *Rapanos*. However, EPA does have some limited anecdotal information from regional offices on facilities that have expressed no discharge potential relevant to jurisdictional water. Based on inferences from this information, EPA can present some potential cost implications, as described in section 9.

Section 5: Potential Areas of New Indirect Benefits

Although costs are a very important component of any economic analysis, the value of benefits received is equally important. Failure to account for the full economic values of ecosystems could result from a lack of recognition of benefits that 1) traditional market valuation techniques may not capture, 2) may be public goods that are not subject to any valuation reporting, or 3) may be intangible by their nature (these categories are not mutually exclusive). A common concern is that government agencies might not effectively manage what they do not measure, and they might undervalue resources that are not identified or quantified.

Ecosystem Services

The term "ecosystem services" refers to the many natural processes by which ecosystems, and the species they include, sustain and fulfill human life. A sufficient quantity and quality of water is important for public health, safety, and quality of life. Polluting or destroying waterways can affect drinking water, places where people recreate, the fish and shellfish people eat, the irrigation water used on food crops, and how floods affect people and property. Waters affected by this proposed rule also provide habitat and biodiversity, support recreational fishing and hunting, filter sediment and contaminants, reduce flooding, stabilize shorelines and prevent erosion, recharge ground water, and maintain biogeochemical cycling. Fishing and hunting expenditure estimates, major flood losses, and the value of wetlands for storm protection services all total in the tens of billions of dollars per year. Any economic valuation exercise would have to account for the incremental portion of these values attributable to the incremental number of waters affected by the proposed rule.

The ecosystem services identified in Exhibit 2 have no market values. Some are closely related to marketed goods, which may facilitate valuation, whereas others are far removed from the end product of market value or contribute to consumer value directly. There are basically two types of effects: 1) direct effects on non-market ecosystem goods and services, and 2) effects on hydrogeology and biochemical processes and on life support services that are valued for themselves as well as for their contribution to other ecosystem goods and services. Exhibit 2 is not an exhaustive list.

One category of benefits includes goods and services that a proposed action or activity generates. Although potentially easier to identify than other categories, these benefits may or may not be easy to measure or ascribe value. In terms of protecting waters, an example benefit might be supporting fish and shellfish populations in downstream waters as well as protecting the waters themselves. Ponds, streams, and wetlands provide habitat for a robust and diverse assemblage of organisms that are necessary to support the whole aquatic community structure and ecological function. Some associated attributes may have market value (such as the fish themselves) and some may have non-market value (such as biodiversity).

Exhibit 2. Examples of Ecosystem Services Relevant to CWA Regulation

Input in Production of Marketed Goods & Services

- Flood storage & conveyance
- Support for commercial fisheries
- Water input and land productivity for agriculture and commercial & industrial production

Direct Use

- Municipal & home water supply
- Recreation & aesthetics (including fishing and hunting)

Hydrogeology and Biochemical Processes

- Sediment and contaminant filtering
- Nutrient cycling
- Groundwater recharge
- Shoreline stabilization and erosion prevention

Life Support (Ecological)

- Biodiversity
- Wildlife habitat (food chain, nursery, etc.)

Benefits also include costs avoided. Costs avoided represent what you don't have to pay because of the action you have taken. For example, floodplain preservation prevents costly damage from frequent flooding. Although dams and levees are built to control potential flooding, altering the natural hydrologic regime contributes to the potential for flooding. Waters affected by this proposed rule store water and slow down its movement across the landscape. When these systems no longer perform this function, the potential losses from flooding may increase.

Government Efficiency

Administration of government programs may also benefit from avoided costs. The federal government and states are currently spending resources on site-by-site evaluations of jurisdiction against a standard that is unclear and somewhat ambiguous. This represents an investment of resources that could be put to other use (and may in fact be needed to process additional CWA 404 permits) if the agencies articulated the decision criteria more clearly. While incurring additional costs to process additional permits, this proposed rule may reduce some permitting costs and speed the permit review process in the long-term by clarifying jurisdictional matters that have been time-consuming and cumbersome for field staff and the regulated community for certain waters. The two Supreme Court cases and subsequent guidance have, in some circumstances, required agency staff to spend resources to understand and apply complex jurisdictional standards. The uncertainty surrounding jurisdictional questions has increased the paperwork, costs, and time associated with jurisdictional determinations. However, any cost savings will be at least partially offset by reviews of additional mitigation plans, associated environmental compliance for larger permit areas, and implementation costs, including additional documentation and data management requirements.

Comprehensive Enforcement

Benefits may also be realized from more comprehensive enforcement efforts that could result from the proposed rule. Because it can be difficult to establish where the CWA applies after the Supreme Court's decisions in *SWANCC* in 2001 and *Rapanos* in 2006, EPA enforcement managers have indicated that enforcement efforts have shifted away from small streams high in the watershed where jurisdiction is a potential issue. In short, EPA is focusing efforts on larger streams and rivers, where there is more certainty of establishing jurisdiction. A rule that more clearly protects small streams may lead to more comprehensive enforcement and therefore greater compliance with CWA program regulations. This, in turn, could ultimately save the costs of additional drinking water filtration, stream restoration, and other costs of repairing damage caused by pollution.

Reduced Uncertainty

Land developers, the energy and transportation sectors, the agricultural community, and other businesses face uncertainty surrounding CWA jurisdiction that may lead to reduced willingness to invest in projects or lost investment when entities must alter or abandon project plans. Businesses operate best in an environment of regulatory certainty. Business professionals are equipped to plan accordingly for known factors. However, uncertainty can lead businesses to sit on capital rather than take unknown risks. The current lack of clarity in where the CWA applies can delay building roads and houses, developing natural resources, and engaging in other activities where CWA 404 permits are needed. A rule that more clearly identifies small streams and wetlands that require protection under the CWA may reduce uncertainty and the costs that go with it. Depending on how significant uncertainty-related costs are, this proposed rule might ultimately reduce net costs for people seeking CWA permits, and increase consistency, predictability, and timeliness of the permitting process.

SECTION 6: SCOPE OF IMPACT

To evaluate the extent to which EPA and the Corps may assert CWA jurisdiction as a result of this proposed rule, the agencies evaluated data records from FY2009-10 in the Corps' ORM2 (Operation and Maintenance Business information Link, Regulatory Module) database that documents Corps jurisdictional status decisions associated with various aquatic resource types. The aquatic resource data records include the following categories: isolated waters, relatively permanent waters, traditional navigable waters, non-relatively permanent waters, and wetlands associated with these categories. The isolated waters category is used in the Corps' ORM2 database to represent intrastate, non-navigable, waters that lack a direct surface connection to other waterways; these waters are hereafter referred to as "other waters."[2]

The data available in ORM2 allows for an evaluation of how decisions on jurisdictional determinations completed in the last two fiscal years (FY2009-10) may change under different jurisdictional policies. This analysis will allow for an estimation of a change in assertion of CWA jurisdiction as viewed through the lens of potential CWA 404 permitting activity during the baseline period of FY2009-10. Landowners and developers may assume that some waters are non-jurisdictional and not request a determination or engage in the permitting process. These waters would not be represented in the ORM2 FY2009-2010 data base. However, these waters are also likely to be the most isolated and the least connected to other waters and therefore the least likely to have their status changed under this proposed rule. To the extent the waters evaluated are representative of waters of the U.S. as a whole, the proportions of each water type that would change their jurisdictional status is more broadly representative.

The ORM2 aquatic resource records may be placed into three groups: streams (ORM2 categories of traditionally navigable waters, relatively permanent waters, and non-relatively permanent waters), wetlands (associated with the various above categories of streams), and other waters. Streams comprise 67 percent of the records and 98 percent were found jurisdictional in the FY2009-2010 baseline period. Wetlands comprise 27 percent of the records and 98.5% were found jurisdictional in the FY2009-2010 baseline period. Other waters comprise 6 percent of the records, none of which are considered to be jurisdictional for the FY2009-2010 baseline period. As was done for the economic analysis for the April 2011 draft guidance, the agencies assume that all streams and wetlands would be found jurisdictional under this proposed rule for purposes of this economic analysis. The agencies presume that all "streams" from the ORM2 grouping are presumed to meet the definition of "tributary" in the proposed rule, and all "wetlands" from the ORM2 grouping meet the definition of "adjacent" in the proposed rule. This represents a scenario that results in the highest estimates of costs for these groups of waters.

To determine how jurisdiction might change for the "other waters" group from ORM2, a team of Corps experts examined a sample of 262 project files previously coordinated with Corps headquarters from June 2008 – January 2011, representing over 1,000 individual waters in 30 states. Of the waters that the Corps examined, 73 percent were wetlands, and the remaining waters were ponds, streams, or other resource types. Based on data available in the record files, the team judged whether or not the Agencies would determine the waters to be jurisdictional under the policies outlined in the April 2011 draft guidance. Overall, the team found that 17 percent of these other waters would be determined to be jurisdictional. An EPA team independently examined a sub-sample of 50 of these files and similarly estimated that 15 percent of these other waters would become jurisdictional.

Exhibit 3 depicts the results of the analysis of ORM2 FY2009-2010 records to estimate scope of impact with respect to CWA 404 permitting. Overall, assuming all tributary streams and adjacent wetlands as well as 17 percent of other waters (based on the ORM2 records grouping) are projected to be jurisdictional under the proposed rule increases overall jurisdiction under the CWA by 2.7 percent (95.2% - 92.5%), or roughly 3 percent, over current field practices.

Exhibit 3. Analysis of FY2009-2010 ORM2 Records Showing Jurisdictional Status of Aquatic Resources

	Number of ORM2 Records	Positive Jurisdiction Records (09-10)	Projected Positive Jurisdiction Records	Percent of Total ORM2 Records	Percent Positive Jurisdiction (09-10)	Projected Percent Positive Jurisdiction
Streams	95,476	93,538	95,476	67%	98.0%	100.0%
Wetlands	38,280	37,709	38,280	27%	98.5%	100.0%
Other Waters	8,209	0	1,396	6%	0.0%	17.0%
Total	141,965	131,247	135,152	100%	92.5%	95.2%

This representation may or may not accurately represent a proportional change for CWA program activity other than CWA 404 permitting. As described above, EPA is more comfortable with these data representing a proportional change for stormwater, CAFO, and pesticide application permitting than for other CWA 402 permitting and CWA 311 SPCC plan imposition, because the locations of these latter activities may not be similar to CWA 404 permitting and the regulatory history of these types of entities is different. For example, a large portion of traditional CWA 402 permit holders are located nearby large water sources to support their operations.

SECTION 7: ESTIMATE OF CWA 404 PROGRAM COSTS

Under CWA Section 404, entities seeking to discharge dredge or fill material to waters of the U.S. must obtain a permit. A change in assertion of CWA jurisdiction could result in indirect costs of implementation of the CWA 404 program: a greater share of development projects would intersect with jurisdictional waters, thus requiring the sponsors of those additional projects to obtain and comply with CWA 404 permits. Exhibit 4 provides a descriptive overview of four types of CWA 404 permitting costs the regulated community would face —permit application costs, compensatory mitigation costs, permitting time costs, and impact avoidance and minimization costs.

Exhibit 4. Conceptual Overview of CWA Section 404 Permit Compliance Costs

Cost Category	Description (costs vary considerably by permit type and by region)
Permit Application Costs	Financial costs to finalize a permit application that the Corps deems to be complete. Includes costs for delineation and survey of jurisdictional waters; preparing project area and impact drawings and maps; alternatives analysis that investigates opportunities to avoid and minimize project impacts (on-site alternatives in the case of general permits, both on- and off-site alternatives in the case of individual permits); developing a Corps-approved compensatory mitigation plan; submitting a completed application that includes all notification and other requirements. In general, permit application costs increase with the size of the project area, size of impacts to jurisdictional waters, the number of separate impact locations, and any actions needed to comply with other Federal laws before a permit can be issued (e.g., Endangered Species Act, National Historic Preservation Act). The cost of the alternatives analysis often dominates application costs for individual permits in the case of projects involving relatively large impacts to jurisdictional waters.
Compensatory Mitigation Costs	Financial and opportunity costs to implement the Corps-approved compensatory mitigation plan that is written into the permit as a special condition. In the case of a mitigation plan that involves third-party mitigation providers (commercial mitigation banks or in-lieu fee programs), cost is driven by credit prices and the number of credits required. In the case of a permittee-responsible mitigation plan, includes opportunity costs of reserving a portion of development project lands for mitigation, and the financial costs of mitigation project implementation as well as mitigation monitoring, maintenance, and reporting until success criteria have been achieved. Could also include financial and opportunity costs of posting any required financial assurances for mitigation project success and/or providing any required endowment for long-term site management after mitigation success has been achieved.

Exhibit 4. (Continued)

Cost Category	Description (costs vary considerably by permit type and by region)
Permitting Time Costs	Potential financial and opportunity costs associated with any delay in project implementation resulting from the time it takes to secure a permit. In the case of private sector, for-profit development projects, time costs could include financial or opportunity costs of carrying development capital for longer periods of time. In the case of public sector projects, time costs could include opportunity costs of foregone public services and benefits from not proceeding with the project sooner rather than later.
Impact Avoidance and Minimization Costs	Potential financial and opportunity costs associated with project redesign that may be required in order to avoid and minimize impacts on jurisdictional waters. Opportunity costs could include foregone net returns to development in the case of private sector, for-profit development projects, or lower levels of public service provision and benefits in the case of public sector projects (e.g., road construction and maintenance, repair of flood control infrastructure, etc.).

The sponsors of all projects subject to CWA 404 regulation incur costs to finalize a permit application (or a pre-construction notification in the case of general permits) that the Corps deems to be complete. Similarly, the sponsors of virtually all permitted projects also incur costs to implement compensatory mitigation actions required by permits to offset permitted impacts to jurisdictional waters. The analysis of incremental costs to the regulated community focused on the estimation of these two categories of compliance costs.

Depending on circumstances, the sponsors of many private sector as well as public sector projects that are subject to 404 permitting can also incur non-trivial permitting time costs and/or impact avoidance and minimization costs. Permitting time costs include potential financial and opportunity costs associated with delays in project implementation resulting from the time it takes to secure a permit. Impact avoidance and minimization costs include potential financial and opportunity costs associated with permit requirements to redesign projects so as to avoid and minimize project impacts on jurisdictional waters to the extent practicable. The agencies recognize that time and impact avoidance and minimization costs can be significant for some share of permit applicants. However, because there is not a defensible, ready basis for estimating these costs, the agencies did not estimate compliance costs for these categories as part of this economic analysis.

Estimate of Permit Application Costs

Estimated permit application costs relied on estimates of the number of additional permit applications, and the average impact per additional application, that would result from the proposed rule coupled with estimates of unit permit application costs. Exhibit 5 shows estimates of additional Individual Permits (IP) and General Permits (GP), and average per permit impact to jurisdictional waters (in acres) for each permit type.

Exhibit 5. Estimated Additional CWA 404 Permits and Impacts to Jurisdictional Waters

Permit Type	Permits Issued in FY2010 (Sec. 404 only)	Added Permits w/Rule (2.7% increase in jurisdiction)	Average Impact Per Added Permit (Acres)	Total Added Impacts (Acres)
IP	2,766	75	12.81	960
GP	49,151	1,327	0.28	372

The Corps derived the total number of permits issued and associated impact totals by permit type (IP vs GP) from FY2010 ORM2 data, using only records from permits issued under CWA 404 authority (excluding data associated with permits issued under Section 9, 10, and 103 authority). The Corps system of tracking impacts has expanded over the past few years to include the ability to distinguish between permanent and temporary impacts, as well as different impact activity types (e.g. discharge of dredged material, discharge of fill material, excavation associated with fill, conversion, ecological restoration, and Section 10 impact types - structures and work). There are also fields to record area and/or linear values and activity specific fields for these impact activity types. To produce the table values for average impact per added permit, the Corps selected only records with permanent impacts associated with the discharge of dredged or fill material in FY2010, excluding ecological restoration and conversion activities, as well as temporary impacts. Non-zero records with values in the authorized area field were included (entries that contained just a linear feet impact value or null values were excluded). Dividing these acreage totals by the number of CWA 404 permits produces estimates of the average impact acreage per permit. Multiplying the number of added permits by the average impact produces estimates of the total added impacts in acres (1,332 acres in total).

The agencies used two sets of estimates for unit permit application costs to calculate a range of incremental permit application costs associated with the estimated proposed rule-induced permitting changes shown in Exhibit 4. These were obtained from two separate 1999 estimates of permit application costs developed to calculate incremental permit application costs associated with the replacement of Nationwide Permit No. 26 (NWP 26) with a suite of new and modified nationwide permits in the year 2000 (hereafter referred to as the "NWP replacement package").

The Corps developed one set of estimates as part of its analysis of the incremental costs of the NWP replacement package.[3] This estimate relied on data and information obtained through informal phone interviews with permitting consulting firms (companies that help the regulated community to navigate the permitting process) and Corps district regulatory staff based around the country. The Corps asked interviewees to identify major components and component and total costs for finalizing a NWP 26 pre-construction notification and an IP application associated with a "typical" project involving up to three acres of impacts to jurisdictional waters.

The Corps analysis of unit permit application for the NWP replacement package explicitly noted that the cost estimates were developed for a "typical" project, and that IP application costs for some projects could be much higher than the estimates produced for the NWP replacement package (e.g., it noted that in the case of controversial projects, the costs for the alternatives analysis alone could be several times the Corps estimates of IP application costs for a typical project). Further, permit application costs can vary considerably by region, so the cost for a typical project in one region can be considerably different than the cost for a typical project in another region. Also, the Corps analysis of permit application costs for the NWP replacement package was limited to projects affecting up to three acres of jurisdictional waters, whereas the proposed rule considered here could involve new permit application costs for projects involving significantly greater impacts to jurisdictional waters (which is relevant since permit application costs generally increase as the impact size increases). For these reasons, the agencies used the highest Corps estimates of unit permit application costs for the NWP replacement package as a lower bound on total added permit application costs associated with the proposed rule.

To calculate an upper bound on incremental permit application costs associated with the proposed rule, the agencies used estimates of permit application costs produced by a study of the costs of the NWP replacement package conducted by two academic economists in 1999 (hereafter referred to as the "SZ study").[4] The SZ study was commissioned by two groups representing public and private segments of the regulated community: the National Association of Counties and the Foundation for Environmental and Economic Progress (whose members include large real estate development companies).

The SZ study relied on a survey of 103 NWP and IP applications for which the project sponsors were asked to report the costs they incurred in preparing and finalizing the applications. Two-thirds of the applications in the survey sample involved projects in western states and the remainder involved applications in eastern or mid-western states. The sample involved a roughly equal mix of public sector and private sector development projects, including school construction, quarry expansion, sediment containment, home building, road improvements, and flood control.[5]

Exhibit 6. Estimated Annual Additional CWA 404 Permit Application Costs

Permit Type	Added Permits w/Rule	Avg. Impact per permit (acres)	Unit Costs from NWP Analysis (2010$)	Unit Costs from Sunding & Zilberman Study (2010$)	Additional Annual Cost (2010$ millions)
IP	75	12.81	$31,400	$57,180 plus $15,441 per acre impact	$2.4 – $19.1
GP	1,327	0.28	$13,100	$22,079 plus $12,153 per acre impact	$17.4 – $33.8
Total	1,402	-	-	-	$19.8 - $52.9

The SZ study analysis of the survey data found a statistically-significant, positive relationship between the amount of permitted impacts on jurisdictional waters and the cost of preparing a NWP and an IP. The authors used the survey data to develop a relationship between impacts to jurisdictional waters (measured in acres) and the cost of preparing a NWP and an IP. For each permit type, the SZ study produced an estimate of a fixed cost component plus another cost component that varied based on the amount of impact acres.[6]

Exhibit 6 shows the unit permit application costs obtained from the two sources outlined above, and the range of total added permit application costs for individual permits and general permits using the permit change data from Exhibit 5. The unit NWP costs are used to represent unit costs for all types of general permits. Costs figures in Exhibit 6 are adjusted from 1999$ to 2010$ using the CPI-U (1999=166.6, 2010=218.056).

Estimate of Compensatory Mitigation Costs

A portion of costs to applicants will result from compensatory mitigation of wetlands and streams. The cost of compensatory mitigation depends upon land prices and varies substantially across and within states. Additionally, the scale of a project will impact costs as the amount of compensatory mitigation required is typically calculated as a multiple of acreage of wetlands or linear feet of streams to be filled.

To estimate state-specific per-acre costs of wetland mitigation and per linear foot estimates of stream mitigation, the Corps examined published studies and survey results, made phone inquiries to Corps Districts and mitigation banks, and researched web sites. A team of Corps experts agreed on a range of values for each state. These costs vary widely, with average costs nationwide ranging from $24,989 to $49,207 per acre of wetlands mitigated and from $177 to $265 per linear foot of stream mitigation. There is wider variation in costs from state to state (see Appendix A).

The Corps also provided an estimate of 43,000 acres of wetland mitigation and 530 miles of stream mitigation to represent activity in the baseline period. This estimate is based on approximately 32,500 acres of permittee-responsible mitigation documented in the ORM2 database in FY2010; approximately 8,200 acres of bank mitigation documented in the Regional Internet Bank Information Tracking System (RIBITS) database in FY2010, and 2,200 acres of in-lieu fee (ILF) mitigation estimated from the ratio of ORM2 entries for banks (26%) and ILF (7%) in FY2010. This total may be incomplete, but the agencies believe it is a close approximation of mitigation for FY2010, and that it is consistent with the level of mitigation the Corps has estimated for the past 10-15 years.

The agencies used the same methodology to estimate mitigation costs as used previously to estimate these costs for policies proposed in draft guidance in April 2011. The methodology assumes that all permits associated with projected additional jurisdictional waters would require mitigation at the same rate as the baseline permitting profile on a state-specific basis. The agencies assumed all non-isolated streams and wetlands in ORM2 classified as non-jurisdictional in the ORM2 data base in FY2009- 10 would be considered jurisdictional under the proposed rule, and that 17 percent[7] of non-jurisdictional "other waters" would likewise be considered jurisdictional under the proposed rule (please see description under section 6 "Scope of Impact" above). The vast majority of these "other waters" among the 17 percent would be classified as "adjacent wetlands" under the proposed rule and thus, most appropriately associated with wetlands mitigation rates and costs on a state-by-state basis.

EPA and the Corps estimate that the proposed rule could result in an additional 2,042 acres of wetland compensatory mitigation annually, and an additional 49,075 linear feet of stream mitigation annually. Using a range of state-specific unit costs of mitigation, this translates to a total estimated cost of annual incremental mitigation ranging from \$59.7 million to \$113.5 million. Of this amount, the majority of costs (\$51.0 – \$100.5 million) are for wetlands. Exhibit 7 summarizes these results.

Exhibit 7. Estimated Annual Additional CWA 404 Compensatory Mitigation Costs

Water Body Type	Units of Mitigation[1]	Unit Cost[2]	Annual Cost (millions)[3]
Streams	49,075 feet	\$200 - \$300	\$8.7 - \$13.0
Wetlands	2,042 acres	\$25,000 - \$49,200	\$51.0 - \$100.5
Total	--	--	\$59.7 - \$113.5

1. Based on method described in EPA (2011).
2. Weighted average of varying unit costs across states.
3. Calculated by multiplying incremental mitigation with unit costs.

Estimate of Corps Administrative Costs

The Corps anticipates that it will incur additional administrative costs under the proposed rule associated with the increased permitting workload. The Corps is typically, but not always, the permitting authority for CWA 404 permits. Sources of administrative costs include: responding to additional requests for jurisdictional determinations; an overall increase in workload-related tasks such as permit actions, consultations, and compliance and enforcement actions; and additional time to conduct significant nexus analyses. The Corps will also likely face additional costs to provide program management, training, and compliance oversight associated with administering the program. Exhibit 8 briefly summarizes the principal cost categories for administering the CWA 404 program.

Exhibit 8. Overview of CWA 404 Permit Administrative Costs

Cost Category	Description (costs vary considerably by permit type and often by region)
Permitting Costs	Costs associated with the time needed to review additional permits (which may be more complex due to a larger scope of review, reduction in the ability to avoid and minimize impacts, requiring more project modifications and additional mitigation) additional compliance and enforcement costs, additional mitigation plan reviews, effort to conduct additional agency consultations and coordination and possible increase in permit appeal requests and litigation costs.
JD Review and Coordination Costs	Additional time needed to review additional JD requests, more coordination with Corps Headquarters for "other" (isolated) waters, additional time for District staff to prepare a significant nexus evaluation for "other" waters. More appeals of approved JDs may occur.
Automation Costs	Additional costs for automating new JD forms, updating the permit tracking system (ORM2) to reflect needed data elements, updating user documentation.
Training Costs	Additional costs for Corps districts to implement the new guidance/rule, includes webinars, field training, and outreach activities for the regulated public.

The increase in waters that the agencies consider jurisdictional from the 2008 guidance may result in an increase in requests for JDs. Some changes contained in the proposed rule, such as providing a definition of tributaries that are categorically jurisdictional, could reduce the administrative costs of establishing jurisdiction. If such changes balance the expected increase in JD requests, there would be no incremental change administrative costs related to jurisdictional determinations.

Because the agencies expect that most non-isolated waters will be jurisdictional under the policies under the proposed rule, applicants may find "preliminary JDs" (PJDs) more appealing. In a PJD a permit applicant elects to set aside the question of jurisdiction and voluntarily "opts in" to the permitting process and avoids a longer "approved JD" (AJD) process. In FY2010, 58 percent of JDs were PJDs (42 percent were AJDs). PJDs are less time-consuming to document than AJDs, but permit application processing may require more information describing jurisdictional waters (e.g., to assess impacts and formulate compensatory mitigation requirements). Alternatively, some applicants may request an AJD as a means to potentially reduce mitigation requirements and associated costs. If more landowners elect to request AJDs, the workload and administrative costs will increase.

Exhibit 9. Categories of Corps CWA 404 Administrative Tasks

Category	Tasks
Wetland Delineation and Jurisdictional Determination (JD)	Preliminary JD
	Office/Desk JD
	Field JD
Permit Related Tasks	Pre-Application Meetings
	Standard Permit (SP) Processing Base
	Letter of Permissions (LOP)
	Nationwide (NWP) Processing without a Pre-Construction Notification (PCN)
	NWP Processing with PCN
	Regional/Programmatic (RGP/PGP) Processing without PCN (issued by Regulatory)
	RGP/PGP Processing with PCN (issued by Regulatory)
Consultation	Endangered Species Act (ESA) Formal Consultation Process
	ESA Informal Consultation Process
	Historic Properties
	Tribal
Environmental Impact Statement (EIS)	EIS as Lead
	EIS as Cooperating Agency
Compliance	Compliance
	Resolution of Non-Compliance
Enforcement	Unauthorized Activity

The agencies expect that permit applications will increase as the agencies determine that more waters are jurisdictional. This increase in permit activity may increase required consultations under the Endangered Species Act (ESA) and Section 106 of the National Historic Preservation Act. This could increase costs for other agencies, such as the Fish and Wildlife Service, National Marine Fisheries Service, Advisory Council on Historic Preservation, and Tribal and State Historic Preservation Officers.

Exhibit 9 depicts the broad categories and specific tasks related to Corps administration of the CWA 404 program. To derive an estimate of the incremental administrative costs, the Corps identified how many hours per year are devoted to each task at the headquarters and district office level and translated this into dollars using average fully loaded salary rates for the needed personnel. Applying the incremental percentage increase in CWA 404 permits of 2.7 percent, the Corps estimates that their additional administrative costs will range from \$7.4 to \$11.2 million annually. An increase in the Corps permitting budget of this amount would be necessary to maintain current levels of permitting efficiency with the rule in place.

SECTION 8: ESTIMATE OF CWA 404 PROGRAM BENEFITS

The CWA establishes requirements for waters of the U.S., and a revised definition of waters of the U.S as proposed would result in additional waters over which the agencies would clearly assert jurisdiction. This in turn could lead to ecosystem service benefits through 1) avoidance and minimization of permit impacts and 2) compensatory mitigation requirements. This analysis focuses on benefits of incremental compensatory mitigation because the agencies lack reliable data and information to estimate benefits of avoidance and minimization. Further, this analysis focuses on the value of wetlands mitigation. Benefits associated with stream mitigation are not quantified.

Potential benefits of the proposed rule may also accrue from cost savings to federal and state agencies. The policies in the proposed rule may lower the level of effort required to complete a jurisdictional determination or pursue an enforcement case. The additional clarity resulting from the proposed rule may also ultimately reduce the workload associated with jurisdictional determinations for streams and adjacent wetlands in the longer term, resulting in a cost-savings to the Corps.

The agencies estimated the potential benefits from CWA 404 compensatory mitigation using a benefits transfer approach. Benefits transfer involves selecting study cases relevant to the policy case under consideration, and transferring values using a unit value or function-based approach. The major issue with benefits transfer is that economic values for ecosystem services are context (resource/region/user) specific. Thus, it is best suited for transferring estimates between comparable contexts. For example, there is uncertainty involved in completing a benefits transfer where waters vary greatly in their functionality and relative value based on the relative scarcity, location within a watershed, and the degree of human impacts in their vicinity, as do the waters under consideration in this analysis. To the extent that the waters valued in studies from the literature are more functional, and thus more highly valued than the additional resources subject to compensatory mitigation under this proposed rule, the contexts of the transfer would diverge. Also, the users of the services in the original valuation studies may not be comparable to users in other areas; that is, the WTP among service users in different areas could differ significantly. However, without knowing specifically where impacts will occur in the future, benefits transfer remains the only feasible option for quantifying potential benefits. Given these challenges, and the uncertainty as to specific sites that may be affected by this proposed regulatory action, the benefits values presented in this analysis should be viewed as only illustrative. This type of analysis would not be appropriate for a site-specific evaluation.

The specific benefits transfer approach used in this analysis also relies on contingent valuation and aggregation of household level estimates of willingness to pay (WTP). Contingent valuation elicits "stated preferences" rather than revealed (or actual) preferences, which is not ideal for quantifying benefits. Stated preference methods rely on surveys that assess respondents stated WTP for goods or services, such as ecosystem services provided by a natural landscape feature.

In using the household-level WTP information, there are no clear rules for aggregation (i.e., determining which households pay). For this analysis, the agencies attempted to make reasonable and credible choices, but it is important to recognize up front that there is uncertainty and limitations associated with the results.

The April 2011 draft guidance on *Identifying Waters Protected by the Clean Water Act* was accompanied by an assessment of potential benefits that may be indirectly realized from adoption of the jurisdictional policies proposed in the *Guidance*. To estimate benefits from additional mitigation, studies of ecosystem services that reported a monetized value on a per acre basis were examined. A few authors have attempted to value the majority of the services provided by a wetland, although the estimates developed are still considered fairly incomplete by their authors. A synthesis study relied upon for the *Guidance* economic assessment presents average wetland function values for fishing, fur trapping, hunting, recreation, water filtration, flood control, scenic value, and habitat values. Summing the values for each category yields a total "unit benefit" ranging from $129,000 to $292,000 per acre (2010$, capitalized using a 6 percent discount rate). Applying this unit benefit estimate to the estimated incremental number of wetland acres impacted for which mitigation is required yields a rough estimate of the potential indirect benefits. While this approach allows for quantification of many of the functions served by wetlands, combining these values leads to some uncertainty. Not all wetlands fully perform all of the functions evaluated in the literature.

For this economic analysis supporting the proposed rule, the agencies pursued an alternative approach to seek studies from the literature that provide value estimates for a suite of ecosystem services provided by a particular wetland or wetland complex as a whole (i.e., total resource values rather than stacked service-specific values). Wetlands under consideration for their value may provide varying degrees of particular services, or may not provide a particular service at all. A strength of this approach is the values elicited implicitly account for the varying degree and interrelationships among of services provided[8], assuming respondents are sufficiently informed. With a set of values representing a variety of wetlands that provide similar services as those likely to be incrementally protected by the proposed rule, the agencies can develop WTP estimates to apply to aggregate national-scale estimates of impacted acres.

In conducting the literature search, the agencies focused on studies that assess waters expected to provide services similar to the waters incrementally protected under the proposed rule. The economic valuation literature includes a large volume of studies that estimate the value of preserving, protecting, restoring, replacing (mitigation), and increasing the size of wetlands, including several meta-analysis studies (e.g., Moeltner and Woodward 2007).[9] Many of these studies provide values for overseas, tidal, or coastal wetlands that may not well represent waters likely be incrementally protected by the proposed rule. For example, tidal wetlands are valued highly for fishery habitat, which is typically not provided to the same degree by wetlands adjacent to small tributaries or more isolated wetlands. However, the agencies identified 10 studies that provide estimates of WTP to preserve wetlands that provide a suite of services expected to be similar to those provided by waters incrementally protected under the proposed rule. These studies represent riverine or floodplain, forested, emergent, and depression or isolated wetlands in 12 states across the country. These studies are summarized in Appendix B of this report.

For this exercise, it is necessary to express values on a "per acre" basis rather than a "per acre per year" basis to be comparable to the cost figures presented in section VII. The cost figures are annual values, but they reflect an annual summation of one-time compensatory mitigation costs. These "unit costs" are established as the one-time cost per acre to maintain the services provided in perpetuity. Thus, a proper comparison would be to derive marginal benefits as the product of the estimated marginal number of acres affected each year and a "unit benefit" dollar value per acre. Dollar values expressed as "per acre per year" can be converted to a present value dollar value "per acre" by dividing by a discount rate (typically between 3 percent and 7 percent).

The agencies standardized WTP estimates across all studies in three ways: 1) household basis, 2) per acre basis, and 3) annual basis. For estimates reported as annual WTP for wetland preservation, the agencies derived the total present value over a period of 50 years using 3 percent and 7 percent discount rates. For estimates originally reported per individual rather than per household, the agencies assumed one individual per household. The agencies calculated WTP on a per household per acre basis by dividing the per household WTP value by the size of valued wetlands reported in a particular study. The agencies took the geometric mean of WTP values from the 10 studies, weighted by number of respondents in each study, to represent an overall WTP. The majority of the original studies modeled WTP using a log-normal distribution and reported geometric means. As shown in Exhibit 10, this methodology results in a WTP per household per acre of $0.016 using a 3% discount rate. The same approach with a 7% discount rate results in $0.012 WTP per household per acre.

Exhibit 10. Weighted-Average WTP per Acre per Household for Wetland Preservation

States Covered in the Sample Studies	WTP per HH per Acre (3% Discount Rate)	WTP per HH per Acre (7% Discount Rate)
CA, IA, MN, NE, SD, WI IL, IN, KY, MO, SC, and TN	$0.016	$0.012

Benefits values for compensatory mitigation were calculated using estimates of impacted acres rather than estimates of mitigation acres required.

This is because the benefits associated with mitigation reflect the value of pre-project wetlands that will be impacted at the site. The Corps typically requires more mitigation acreage than impacted acres because it may take more mitigation acres to replace the functionality of the impacted acres at the site. To facilitate estimating permit application costs, the Corps estimated that there would be an additional 1,332 acres impacted across the nation each year as a result of the proposed rule (see Section VII, Subsection A, Table 4). The agencies apportioned this estimate of acreage by state according to the number of positive wetland aquatic resource jurisdictional status records from ORM2 in FY2009-2010 (just as the agencies did to apportion mitigation acres by state for the cost analysis), assuming that this serves as a proxy for permitting activity in the state.

As stated above, there are no clear rules for aggregating households to determine a total willingness to pay. One option would be to use the total number of households in the nation and the total incremental impact acreage estimate for the nation. Another option would be to use the total number of households in the state and the incremental impact acreage estimate apportioned by state. The agencies selected an intermediate option of grouping states into similar "wetland regions", assuming that per acre benefits values accrue to all citizens in the region. The USDA Economic Research Service has used a set of eight wetland regions in the contiguous U.S.: Central Plains, Delta and Gulf, Mountain, Midwest, Northeast, Pacific, Prairie Potholes, and Southeast (Heimlich et al. 1998).[10] The agencies assumed that the benefits in Alaska and Hawaii accrue only to households residing in those states. Using the incremental impact acreage estimate apportioned by state and the total number of households in each state, the agencies calculated wetland compensatory mitigation benefits for the proposed rule in each wetland region. As shown on Exhibit 11, the illustrative estimate of present value of wetland mitigation ranges from $257.6 million to $345.1 million annually, using a 7 percent and 3 percent discount rate respectively.

In terms of WTP per household, the annual WTP for all regional acres ranges from $0.36 to $3.86 depending on the region, with an overall average of $2.30. On a per acre basis, benefits vary by region, ranging from approximately $26,000 to $287,000 per year with an overall average of $193,000 (7% discount rate). In comparison, the stacked service-specific approach used in the Guidance benefit assessment yielded per acre benefit ranging from $129,000 to $292,000 (6% discount rate).

Exhibit 11. Estimated Annual CWA 404 Wetland Compensatory Mitigation Benefits

Region	Incremental Impact Acreage Estimate	Number of Households	Present Value of Incremental Benefit Per Year (2010$ millions)	
			7% Discount Rate	3% Discount Rate
Central Plains	30	3,201,336	$1.2	$1.5
Delta and Gulf	85	14,521,178	$14.8	$19.8
Mountain	145	7,390,812	$12.9	$17.3
Midwest	322	23,909,088	$92.3	$123.7
Northeast	240	23,839,690	$68.7	$92.1
Pacific	79	16,163,714	$15.3	$20.5
Prairie Potholes	241	2,176,626	$6.3	$8.4
Southeast	187	20,485,107	$46.1	$61.7
Other	3	234,779	$0.0	$0.0
National	1,332	111,922,330	$257.6	$345.1

Another way to evaluate the results is to look at inferences of the relative proportion of total value for "use" and "non-use" values. The WTP studies evaluated ecosystem services that may be categorized as "use" values such as flood protection and recreation and services that may be categorized as "non-use" values such as wildlife habitat or "bequest" or "existence" values. It is reasonable to suggest that one may value wetlands very far from their home for their "non-use" values more than they would for their "use" values. Because of the holistic valuation approach, the agencies cannot discern "use" or "non-use" components of the WTP estimates. However, the agencies can consider a scenario where the full WTP applies to state households, and a discounted WTP applies to out-of-state households for the impact acreage in each state. To achieve the same totals as the regional approach, the discounted rate for out-of-state households would be approximately 12 percent of the full WTP. If this discounted out-of-state WTP is considered to account for "non-use values" only (which is not necessarily the case because many "use" values, notably flood protection value, may accrue more on a watershed basis that cross state lines), then this implies a "non-use" to "use" ratio of 0.14 (12/88) or a "non-use" to total ratio of 0.12. This is considerably on the lower end of the range for "non-use" to total WTP ratios in the literature. Brown (1993) summarizes 31 studies measuring "use" and "non-use" WTP, finding a range of "non-use" to "use" ratio of 0.11 to 10.74 with a median ratio of 1.92 (equivalent to a "non-use" to total ratio of 0.1 to 0.91, median of 0.66).[11] Carson and Mitchell (1993), used in past EPA regulations, report an out-of-state to total WTP ratio of 0.33.[12] The relatively small contribution (0.12) from out-of-state households lends credibility to the selection of the regional approach to household aggregation.

SECTION 9: COSTS AND BENEFITS TO OTHER PROGRAMS

As discussed above in section III, the definition of waters of the U.S. affects several CWA programs. As further discussed above, EPA anticipates that this proposed rule would be cost neutral or minimal with respect to CWA Section 303 program implementation, as well as for traditional CWA Section 402 discharge permits such as those for municipal wastewater treatment facilities or industrial operations. However, there may be additional indirect costs may be incurred for CWA Section 401 state certification, CWA Section 402 stormwater permits for construction and development and municipalities, and CWA Section 311 oil spill prevention plans. Across the board, EPA may incur enforcement program savings.

CWA Section 401 State Certification

Under the CWA, tribes and states have the authority to review the issuance of federal permits and certify if they will meet applicable tribal/state water quality standards. Tribes and states may also condition federal permits to ensure they will not cause or contribute to a violation of tribal/state water quality standards. There is no uniform level of implementation of CWA Section 401 across all states.[13] Different states dedicate various levels of resources to CWA 401 certification. Based on program experience, EPA estimates that a representative distribution of effort would be 25 states dedicating 0.5 FTE (full time employees) equivalent, 20 states dedicating 10 FTE, and 5 states dedicating 20 FTE for CWA 401 implementation. This tallies to 312.5 FTE nationally. Based on Bureau of Labor Statistics occupational employment statistics (OES) categories, an even mix of scientists, engineers, economists, and managers (representing a team involved in prioritizing and reviewing permits) employed by state government would have an average fully-loaded salary rate of $42 per hour. Assuming an eight hour day, five days a week, 52 weeks a year, this would be $87,360 per year per FTE. Multiplying by a total of 312.5 FTE, this yields an annual estimate of approximately $27.3 million. Although this would represent effort for reviews of all federal permits, applying the incremental percentage increase in CWA 404 permits of 2.7 percent results in a projected incremental costs to states of about $737,100 annually. Exhibit 12 summarizes additional cost information.

Exhibit 12. Estimated Annual Additional CWA 401 Administrative Costs to States

FTE Amount for 401	Number of States	Total FTE	Total Costs (2010$)
0.5	25	12.5	$ 1,092,000
10	20	200	$ 17,472,000
20	5	100	$ 8,736,000
TOTAL:		312.5	$ 27,300,000
2.7% INCREMENT:		8.44	$737,100

To the extent that states condition permits, added costs to permittees and environmental benefits associated with compensatory mitigation would be accounted for in the methodology for assessing those incremental impacts: they would accrue to the same extent as represented in the baseline. Any added costs to permittees and environmental benefits associated with avoidance and minimization that result from state certification are not quantified.

CWA Section 402 NPDES Permits

Under the CWA, the term "discharge of a pollutant" and the term "discharge of pollutants" generally each means any addition of any pollutant to navigable waters from any point source. NPDES permits all address discharge of a pollutant, yet may reflect different statutory and regulatory requirements depending on the type of point source.

Polluted stormwater runoff is commonly transported through Municipal Separate Storm Sewer Systems (MS4s), from which it is often discharged untreated into local waters. To prevent harmful pollutants from being washed or dumped into an MS4, operators must obtain a NPDES permit and develop a stormwater management program. Phase I, issued in 1990, requires medium and large cities or certain counties with populations of 100,000 or more to obtain NPDES permit coverage for their stormwater discharges. Phase II, issued in 1999, requires regulated small MS4s in urbanized areas, as well as small MS4s outside the urbanized areas that are designated by the permitting authority, to obtain NPDES permit coverage for their stormwater discharges. Generally, Phase I MS4s are covered by individual permits and Phase II MS4s are covered by a general permit. Each regulated MS4 is required to develop and implement a stormwater management program (SWMP) to reduce pollutant discharge from stormwater to the "maximum extent practicable" (MEP) and eliminate non-stormwater discharges.

It is unclear specifically how a broader assertion of CWA jurisdiction under this proposed rule would affect MS4 permits. An MS4 may have several different outflows within its service area, and some may be to waters where CWA jurisdiction may not apply. However, in implementing a SWMP, operators likely implement BMPs uniformly across their area without regard to the specific location of a specific outfall, and thus the jurisdictional status of a portion of the receiving water would not matter in terms of costs. In addition, MS4 outfalls tend not to be in wetlands, which represent a large portion of the CWA 404 program aquatic resource records and the most incremental waters where increased assertion of CWA jurisdiction is expected under this proposed rule. Thus, the true cost impact is considered to be negligible.

Stormwater runoff from construction activities can have a significant impact on water quality. As stormwater flows over a construction site, it can pick up pollutants like sediment, debris, and chemicals and transport these to a nearby storm sewer system or directly to a river, lake, or coastal water. Polluted stormwater runoff can harm or kill fish and other wildlife. Sedimentation can destroy aquatic habitat, and high volumes of runoff can cause stream bank erosion. Debris can clog waterways and potentially reach the ocean where it can kill marine wildlife and impact habitat.

The NPDES stormwater program requires construction site operators engaged in clearing, grading, and excavating activities that disturb one acre or more, including smaller sites in a larger common plan of development or sale, to obtain coverage under an NPDES permit for their stormwater discharges. EPA has authorized most states to implement the stormwater NPDES permitting program.

EPA used information from the *Economic Analysis of Final Phase II Storm Water Rule* (October 1999, see Exhibit ES-4) to estimate potential incremental indirect costs for construction stormwater permit holders. The process is to 1) take the costs (in 1988 $/yr) for construction, 2) determine the 2.7 percent increment to account for increased jurisdictional assertion from this proposed rule, 3) account for program growth of 30% representing the increase from 130 thousand "construction starts" in 1994 cited in the 1999 Economic Analysis to 169 thousand construction sites with permit coverage in 2011 cited in EPA's GPRA management measures tracking (any *SWANCC* and *Rapanos* effect would be implicit in this calculation step), and 4) convert to 2010 dollars. This results in incremental costs of $25.6 – 31.9 million annually for construction. The same process applied to benefits calculation yields a range of $25.4 - $32.3 million per year.

Exhibit 13 summarizes costs and benefits for construction and development stormwater CWA 402 permitting. The same process for estimating indirect permitting authority administrative costs for both MS4s and construction yields incremental costs of approximately $250 thousand annually. These costs would generally accrue to states as the typical permitting authority. The original analysis did not adjust the universe of affected entities based on CWA jurisdiction so the incremental impacts are components of costs and benefits previously identified for past rules, not new costs and benefits associated with this proposed rule.

Exhibit 13. Estimated Annual Additional CWA 402 Stormwater Permitting Impacts ($ millions)

	Administrative Costs (States)	Implementation Costs (low)	Implementation Costs (high)	Benefits (low)	Benefits (high)
1998 Values	5.3	545.0	678.7	540.5	686.0
(1) 2.7% Increment	0.143	14.7	18.3	14.6	18.5
(2) Program Growth	0.186	19.1	23.8	19.0	24.1
(3) 2010 Dollars	0.249	25.6	31.9	25.4	32.3

Concentrated Animal Feeding Operations (CAFOs) are point sources under the CWA and are regulated under the NPDES permitting program. Most current permit holders are covered under state-issued general permits. EPA promulgated regulations for Concentrated Animal Feeding Operations (CAFOs) in 2003 that expanded the number of operations covered by the CAFO regulations and included requirements to address the land application of manure from CAFOs (develop and implement nutrient management plans). EPA revised this regulation in 2008 to reflect changes requested by the Second Circuit Court in its decision in response to litigation. However, the basic cost and benefit information from the supporting economic analysis (see Table 8.1 and 8.4 in Federal Register volume 68 number 29 from February 12, 2003) is useful for estimating potential indirect impacts in a similar manner as above for stormwater. The process is to 1) take the costs (in 2001 $/yr) for CAFO operators and permit authority administrators (typically states), 2) determine the 2.7 percent increment to account for increased jurisdictional assertion from this proposed rule, 3) adjust for a program size decrease of 50 percent comparing the approximate 15,000 CAFOs considered in the 2003 Economic Analysis to 7,318 CAFO permit holders in 2011 cited in EPA's GPRA management measures tracking (any *SWANCC* and *Rapanos* effect would be implicit in this calculation step), and 4) convert to 2010 dollars. This results in incremental costs of $5.5 million annually for CAFO operators and $150 thousand annually for administrative costs to permitting authorities. The same process applied to benefits calculation yields a range of $3.4 - $5.9 million per year, although the benefits are only calculated for large CAFOs which comprise 85 percent of the operator costs and 66 percent of the administrative costs. Exhibit 14 summarizes costs and benefits for CAFO CWA 402 permitting. The original analysis did not adjust the universe of affected entities based on CWA jurisdiction so the incremental impacts are components of costs and benefits previously identified for past rules, not new costs and benefits associated with this proposed rule.

Exhibit 14. Estimated Annual Additional CWA 402 CAFO Permitting Impacts ($ millions)

	Administrative Costs (States)	Implementation Costs	Benefits (low)	Benefits (high)
2001 Values	9.0	326.0	204.0	355.0
(1) 2.7% Increment	0.243	8.8	5.5	9.6
(2) Program Size Adjustment	0.122	4.4	2.8	4.8
(3) ($) 2010 Dollars	0.151	5.5	3.4	5.9

On October 31, 2011, EPA issued the final NPDES general permit for point source discharges to waters of the United States from the application of (1) biological pesticides, or (2) chemical pesticides that leave a residue. This permit, also known as the Pesticide General Permit (PGP), was developed in response to a decision by the Sixth Circuit Court of Appeals (National Cotton Council, et al. v. EPA). The Agency's final PGP covers operators that apply pesticides that result in discharges from the following use patterns: (1) mosquito and other flying insect pest control; (2) weed and algae control; (3) animal pest control; and (4) forest canopy pest control. The permit requires permittees to minimize pesticide discharges through the use of pest management measures and monitor for and report any adverse incidents. The general permit will provide coverage for discharges in the areas where EPA is the NPDES permitting authority. In the remaining areas (44 states and the Virgin Islands), states are authorized to develop and issue the NPDES pesticide permits.

Exhibit 15. Estimated Annual Additional CWA 402 PGP Impacts ($ millions)

	Costs (low)	Costs (high)	Notes
2010 Costs	10.4	11.4	Table ES-6 of Economic Analysis of the Pesticide General Permit (PGP) for Point Source Discharges from the Application of Pesticides (2009$ adjusted to 2010$ using CPI)
(1) 2.7% Increment	0.3	0.3	Projected increment attributable to proposed rule
(2) Scale Up for States	2.9	3.2	Scale up from 35,376 affected entities under federal permit to potential universe of 365,000

PGP cost information from the supporting economic analysis is useful for estimating potential indirect impacts in a similar manner as above for stormwater and CAFOs. The process is to 1) take the identified PGP costs, 2) determine the 2.7 percent increment to account for increased jurisdictional assertion from this proposed rule, and 3) scale up from 35,376 affected entities where EPA is the permitting authority to the approximate 365,000 potentially affected entities nationwide once states develop their own general permits for these dischargers (assuming costs will be similar). This results in incremental costs of between $2.9 and $3.2 million annually for operators. EPA did not generate estimates for government costs, nor did EPA attempt to quantify benefits. Exhibit 15 summarizes costs and benefits for CWA 402 PGP. The original analysis did not adjust the universe of affected entities based on CWA jurisdiction so the incremental impacts are components of costs previously identified, not new costs associated with this proposed rule.

CWA Section 311 Oil Spill Prevention Plans

CWA Section 311 covers oil spill prevention and preparedness, reporting obligations, and response planning. These requirements apply to facilities that produce or store oil products based on total volume. In particular, inland non-transportation oil facilities of a certain size that have potential to discharge to navigable waters must prepare and implement Spill Prevention, Control, and Countermeasure (SPCC) plans. Potential costs of this proposed rule associated with CWA Section 311 include SPCC plan development and implementation for oil storage and production facilities. In its 2009 *Regulatory Impact Analysis for the Final Amendments to the Oil Pollution Prevention Regulations*, EPA developed compliance unit costs for SPCC-regulated facilities, including plan preparation and maintenance, secondary containment, integrity testing, drainage, monthly inspections, security, and training. There are four categories of production and storage facilities, with the great majority (more than 80 percent) comprising the lowest two categories in terms of capacity, and the lowest unit costs for compliance. The weighted average annual cost is $9,128 for production facilities (about 35% of total facilities) and $13,038 for storage facilities (values adjusted from 2007 $/year to 2010 $/year).

Anecdotal information from EPA Regional Office program managers and enforcement specialists reveal that some potentially regulated facilities believe that they are not covered by the applicable SPCC regulations because they do not have the potential to discharge to a water of the U.S. Although there is not corresponding jurisdictional determination information as available for the CWA 404 permit program, it is reasonable to assume that a broader assertion of CWA jurisdiction may affect some of these facilities. Each EPA Region inspects approximately 100 facilities per year for compliance. Upon closer inspection, some of these facilities conclude they do need to comply. Generally, less arid EPA Regions report that their facilities do not question CWA jurisdiction, whereas EPA regions that include more arid (western) areas more frequently encounter this claim. Some EPA Regions report that a handful (one to five) facilities claim non-jurisdiction and that some of these facilities report there are a dozen others that are similarly situated. One EPA Region reports that at least 20 have asserted non-jurisdiction. Supposing that 100 of these facilities nationally are correct in their claim, and that there are 10 times more facilities that would also be correct in this claim, and that none of these 1,000 facilities has incurred compliance costs (either for the SPCC rule or to meet self-imposed industry standards), this would result in approximately $11.7 million per year in incremental costs.

One of the benefits of compliance is avoiding risk of incurring cleanup costs should there be a spill. The national average spill volume (2000-2005 data from NRC) is 1,290 gallons. The average clean up costs for a spill of this size is $221 per gallon in 2010 dollars, or a total of $285 thousand in clean up costs per average spill. A bigger spill can cost more. Essentially, complying facilities expend about $10 thousand dollars a year to avoid clean up costs of several hundred thousand dollars (plus fines that range from 4, 400 to 230,400 on average). If the incremental risk associated with taking no steps to prevent a spill is 1 in 10 per year, this would represent an annual benefit of $28,509 (not including fines). If the risk is more like 1 in 20, the annual benefit is $14,255. Applying the lower benefit per facility per year value, incremental benefits for 1,000 non-complying facilities would total approximately $14.3 million annually. This does not consider ecological benefits of avoiding oil spills. Although the precise number of affected facilities is highly uncertain, it does appear that reasonable assumptions with respect to costs and benefits suggest that benefits would justify costs.

EPA Enforcement Savings

EPA has experienced increased resource burden associated with enforcement of CWA 402, 404, and 311 as a result of the decisions in *SWANCC* and/or *Rapanos* and the agencies' implementing guidance. The proposed rule should reduce these impacts by providing clarity on federal CWA jurisdiction. Compared to current practices, the proposed rule will establish jurisdiction for more waters, and increase the certainty regarding CWA program applicability. Although some cases may still require site-specific "significant nexus" analyses, the costs associated with proving federal jurisdiction in the majority of cases should decrease.

The costs associated with enforcement efforts include the time of federal and state staff to conduct the needed jurisdictional analyses in prosecuting civil and criminal cases against CWA violators, primarily under CWA 402, 404, and 311. The staff includes environmental scientists, environmental engineers, and attorneys. Under the current system, EPA often needs to hire contractors to provide support in hydrology, wetlands ecology, etc. Appendix A includes the average labor costs for such staff that are expected to be involved in JD enforcement efforts.

EPA identified a number of representative cases to characterize the potential magnitude of costs or cost savings at the case level. These examples illustrate the incremental level of resources needed to assert jurisdiction post *SWANCC* and *Rapanos*. For example, EPA's Region 9 expended thousands of hours to establish jurisdiction in the case of an Arizona rancher who bulldozed 2,000 acres within the floodplain of the lower Santa Cruz River, filling in over 100 acres of the River and its tributaries. The rancher asserted that the area filled was not subject to CWA jurisdiction, since it was not itself navigable.

In another example, the government filed criminal charges against a pipe manufacturer (as well as several managers with knowledge of and control over the discharges) and won convictions. However, the discharger appealed, arguing that the receiving water is not navigable and is thus not jurisdictional pursuant to *Rapanos*. The 11th Circuit Court rejected the convictions because EPA had not sufficiently demonstrated the "significant nexus," despite the fact that the convictions had occurred before the *Rapanos* decision. Although they ultimately obtained convictions in the case, EPA and DOJ expended thousands of hours in preparation for both the appeal and the retrial, including an extensive demonstration of CWA jurisdiction. The DOJ alone reported spending over 2,400 hours after the reversal, and EPA likely spent approximately half that amount working on the appeal.

Similarly, in a case involving a dairy farm in Texas, the operator discharged a large quantity of wastewater (up to about 43,000 gallons) from a waste lagoon through a hose to the ground of the dairy's property where it flowed to a neighboring property and then entered a creek that flows to Lake Fork Reservoir, a large navigable-in-fact waterbody. Although EPA expended over 300 hours on *Rapanos*-related jurisdictional analyses, the Assistant United States Attorney declined to prosecute the case because of concerns about establishing jurisdiction in light of *Rapanos*.

Although they are likely to be only a subset of cases affected by *SWANCC* and/or *Rapanos*, these three cases may be representative of the resource burdens associated with enforcement under the CWA that has been increased as a result of *SWANCC* and/or *Rapanos*. For example, as an estimate for trial cases, federal resource costs would be approximately $79,100 per case for 1,200 hours, based on a weighted average labor cost of federal environmental scientists and engineers (75%) and federal lawyers (25%). An estimate of non-trial cases would be 300 incremental hours,with federal resource cost at approximately $19,780 based on the same labor rates. These estimates may be conservative in some respects because they do not include additional expenses such as travel, per diem, or equipment utilized in the jurisdictional determination.

EPA pursues enforcement actions though the judicial system and through the administrative enforcement process. The labor costs associated with proving jurisdiction in these cases is on the order of thousands of hours of environmental scientist and attorney labor. Many more judicial cases are settled before trial, and because EPA must still prove CWA jurisdiction in those cases, the associated labor costs are only slightly less than for cases going to trial. The majority of EPA's CWA enforcement cases are resolved through the administrative enforcement process. Many administrative cases involve CWA jurisdictional issues. EPA also conducts inspections and investigations to develop CWA jurisdiction in hundreds of other potential enforcement cases that are never formally pursued and the case file is closed.

SECTION 10: SUMMARY OF ESTIMATED COSTS AND BENEFITS

The agencies project that this proposed action to change the definition of waters of the U.S. would increase assertion of CWA jurisdiction when compared to a baseline of current practices under the existing regulation. CWA jurisdiction does not mean that waters must always be preserved in their natural state and never receive discharges of pollutants. Instead, CWA jurisdiction means water quality must be maintained to meet established water quality standards; discharges must meet minimum technology-based controls (or reduced to the maximum extent practicable); impacts must be avoided (if there is a practicable alternative), minimized, or compensated; and facilities must take actions to prevent oil spills.

As a result of this proposed action, costs to regulated entities will likely increase for permit application expenses, compensatory mitigation (if applicable), and installation of best management practices. Costs are also likely to increase to state and federal governments for permit program administration. Most of the projected costs would likely accrue to landowners and development companies, state and local governments investing in infrastructure, and industries involved in resource extraction. These types of entities are affected by additional need for CWA 404 dredge and fill permits and CWA 402 construction stormwater permits. Any incremental costs for routine maintenance of waterways (such as drainage ditches that might newly meet the definition of tributary as proposed in this rule) incurred by local, state, or federal authorities would likely be minimal because of the general permits that the Corps issues to reduce the regulatory requirements for these minor activities.

Benefits that accrue from this action include the value of the many ecosystem services provided by the small streams, wetlands, and other open waters protected by the many CWA provisions that would apply to them. These waters provide habitat and biodiversity, support recreational fishing and hunting, filter sediment and contaminants, reduce flooding, stabilize shorelines and prevent erosion, recharge ground water, and maintain biogeochemical cycling. Other benefits include government savings on enforcement expenses through reduced need for costly jurisdictional determinations where jurisdiction has been unclear under the current interpretation of the existing regulation. Business and government may also achieve savings from reduced uncertainty in where CWA jurisdiction applies.

Exhibit 16 displays a summary of costs and benefits. It includes costs and benefits derived from original analysis to support this proposed rule and costs and benefits derivative from previous economic assessments for other rules. Some values reflect a greater number of assumptions than others, as described in previous sections of this document. The values are not intended to be definitive, but merely illustrative. In addition, there are both costs and benefits that are not quantified in this analysis. The table includes costs and benefits that accrue to both private and public entities. For example, information presented in the table suggests that incremental costs to state governments in total would be approximately $1.1 million annually (CWA 401 and 402 Administration). Overall, a comparison indicates that the benefits justify the costs of this proposed action.

Exhibit 16. Estimated Incremental Annual Indirect Costs and Benefits (2010$ in millions)[1]

	COSTS		BENEFITS	
	low	*high*	*low*	*high*
CWA 404 Mitigation - Streams [2]	$8.7	$13.0		
CWA 404 Mitigation - Wetlands	$51.0	$100.5	$257.6	$345.1
CWA 404 Permit Application [3]	$19.7	$52.9		

	COSTS		BENEFITS	
	low	*high*	*low*	*high*
CWA 404 Administration	$7.4	$11.2		
CWA 401 Administration [(4)]	$0.7			
CWA 402 Construction Stormwater	$25.6	$31.9	$25.4	$32.3
CWA 402 Stormwater Administration	$0.2			
CWA 402 CAFO Implementation [(5)]	$5.5		$3.4	$5.9
CWA 402 CAFO Administration	$0.2			
CWA 402 Pesticide General Permit [(6)]	$2.9	$3.2		
CWA 311 Implementation	$11.7		$14.3	
Total	$133.7	$231.0	$300.7	$397.6

(1) Section 303 impacts are assumed to be cost-neutral; Section 402 impacts are components of costs and benefits previously identified for past actions, not new costs and benefits associated with this proposed rule.

(2) Benefits of stream mitigation are not quantified.

(3) Costs of potential delayed permit issuance and costs and benefits of avoidance/minimization are not quantified, nor are any benefits from reduced uncertainty.

(4) Costs to permittees and benefits of any additional requirements as a result of 401 certification are reflected in the mitigation estimates to the extent additional mitigation is the result, yet not calculated to the extent avoidance/minimization is the result.

(5) Benefits apply to large CAFOs only, which account for 85% of implementation costs and 66% of administrative costs.

(6) PGP benefits and government administrative costs are not available.

SECTION 11: ADDITIONAL CONSIDERATIONS FOR OTHER WATERS

"Other waters" is a regulatory term for wetlands and non-wetlands waters that do not fall into the category of waters susceptible to interstate commerce (e.g., a "traditional navigable waters" or TNWs), interstate waters, the territorial sea, tributaries, or waters adjacent to waters in one of the first four categories on this list. The Corps of Engineers ORM2 data base includes a category of aquatic resource type that represents "other waters" for purposes of determining the potential impacts of proposed new policies regarding assertion of CWA jurisdiction. All of the ORM2 FY2009-2010 "other waters" records are considered outside of assertion of CWA jurisdiction under current policies.

In the April 2011 draft guidance, EPA and the Corps (the agencies) suggested that “adjacent” wetlands and “proximate non-wetlands” are similarly situated and could be aggregated on a watershed scale for a significant nexus determination. An analysis of samples of “other waters” indicated that the agencies would assert jurisdiction for 17 percent of “other waters” under new policies proposed in the April 2011 draft guidance. Most of these (14 of the 17 percent) waters would be jurisdictional because they would be considered adjacent waters under the draft guidance. The sample review analysis indicated that an additional 3 percent were TNWs themselves, tributaries to TNWs, or proximate non-wetlands with a significant nexus. The sample review analysis indicated that the agencies would not assert jurisdiction under the April 2011 guidance policies for waters considered to be non-adjacent wetlands or non-proximate non-wetlands. These more remote or more isolated waters may include prairie potholes, vernal pools, playa lakes, and Carolina/Delmarva inland bays that have generally been considered “isolated, intrastate, non-navigable” and not under CWA jurisdiction since the 2001 SWANCC Supreme Court decision.

In the proposed rule, wetlands and non-wetlands that meet the definition of adjacent are considered jurisdictional per se because they have a significant nexus. Adjacent waters include those that are in a floodplain or riparian area, or have a surface or shallow sub-surface connection to jurisdictional waters. The proposed rule would have a result that is consistent with the sample review analysis that estimated the agencies would assert jurisdiction for 17 percent “other waters”. However, the April 2011 draft guidance policies differ from the policies in the proposed rule with respect to aggregation of the remaining “other waters” (i.e., non-adjacent wetlands and non-proximate non-wetlands) for a significant nexus evaluation. In the April 2011 draft guidance, the agencies stated that non-adjacent wetlands and non-proximate non-wetlands should only be aggregated if there is compelling science to do so. In the proposed rule, remaining other waters may be aggregated for a significant nexus determination if they perform similar functions and are located sufficiently close together to be evaluated as a single landscape unit in the same watershed. The policy articulated in the proposed rule could be more inclusive of waters in the ORM2 “other waters” group with respect to CWA coverage depending on how it is interpreted and applied.

It is not clear from examining the aforementioned sample review analysis results (that produced the 17 percent estimate) how the policy differences between the draft guidance and the proposed rule would affect the percent of non-adjacent "other waters" considered jurisdictional. The results of the sample review analysis were primarily driven by adjacency rather than the manner of aggregation within a watershed, and there is not sufficient information in the files that supported the analysis to consider watershed aggregation in a rigorous manner. It would take actual field experience to know the effect of the aggregation approach in the proposed rule with any precision.

In the proposed rule, aggregation of residual other waters (waters not meeting the definition of adjacent) can occur if 1) they perform similar functions and 2) they are located sufficiently close together (or close to a water of the U.S.) so that they can be evaluated as a single landscape unit with regard to their effect on the physical, chemical, or biological integrity of a TNW, interstate water, or territorial sea. In the preamble to the proposed rule, the agencies identify functions as including habitat, water storage, sediment retention, and pollution sequestration. They identify common soils, vegetation, and landforms as factors to be considered in understanding appropriate hydrologic and ecological bases for aggregation as well as the geographic distribution, distance between water bodies, and proximity to jurisdictional waters. Once aggregated, the group must then have a significant nexus to a traditional navigable water, interstate water, or territorial sea to be considered jurisdictional. Collectively, this is a multistep process that the agencies expect to be sufficiently documented. The intent of the policy is to focus on select areas where isolated waters are most concentrated and play an important role in watershed scale functions.

To ascertain the full potential impact of the proposed rule, an important question is what percent of the residual "other waters" (i.e., above and beyond the 17 percent which meet the definition of adjacent or are otherwise jurisdictional) would the agencies be likely to assert jurisdiction over. These residual "other waters" represent 83 percent of non-adjacent "other waters" in the sample review analysis. Thus, the total percent of "other waters" where the agencies would likely assert jurisdiction would be 100 percent of 17 percent (all "other waters" meeting the definition of adjacent or otherwise jurisdictional) plus "X" percent of 83 percent (a portion of the residual "other waters" that were not clearly adjacent in the sample review analysis). The following three-stage process can help identify "X":

1. Examine Information on Extent of Isolated Wetlands in a Watershed
2. Examine Models to Describe Probability of Aggregation and the Probability of Significant Nexus for Isolated Waters (these are two independent steps)
3. Select Model and Apply to Distribution of Extent of Isolated Wetlands

Step 1: Examine Information on Extent of Isolated Wetlands in a Watershed

The U.S. Fish and Wildlife Service published a study called *Geographically Isolated Wetlands: A Preliminary Assessment of Their Characteristics and Status in Selected Areas of the United States* on the extent and characteristics of isolated wetlands (Tiner et al., 2002).[14] This report focused on 72 study areas throughout the country. Although not statistically designed, it can offer some insight on the relative proportion of watersheds that have a significant amount of isolated wetlands. Each study area lies within a watershed boundary. The sites for this study represented two types of areas: 1) areas with an expected high concentration of isolated wetlands and 2) areas from major physiographic regions. The latter may or may not be typical of those regions, but in total there are representatives from each regions and the data set are inclusive of areas expected to contain a large amount of isolated wetlands. However, this group of study areas may be somewhat biased toward over-representation of areas with high concentrations of isolated wetlands. The isolated wetlands in these study areas could also lie within the floodplain or riparian area and thus be considered adjacent. Therefore, this information may also over-represent the residual "other waters" fraction the agencies seek to evaluate.

Tiner et al. (2002) present information on the number of study areas by the proportion of the total number of wetlands that are isolated in the study area (Exhibit 17) and the number of study areas by the proportion of the total wetlands acreage that are isolated in each study area (Exhibit 18). The isolated proportion of the total number of wetlands is often large because there tend to be a large number of small isolated wetlands and relatively smaller number of larger non-isolated wetlands in the study areas. A better indicator of the extent of isolated wetlands relevant to their relative importance in a watershed is the isolated proportion of total wetland acreage. The greater the proportion of isolated wetlands, the more likely there would be groups of isolated wetlands that are sufficiently close together to be evaluated as a single landscape unit for a case-specific significant nexus evaluation. The greater the proportion of isolated wetlands or groups of isolated wetlands in a watershed, the higher the likelihood of finding isolated wetlands, or groups of isolated wetlands, with a significant nexus.

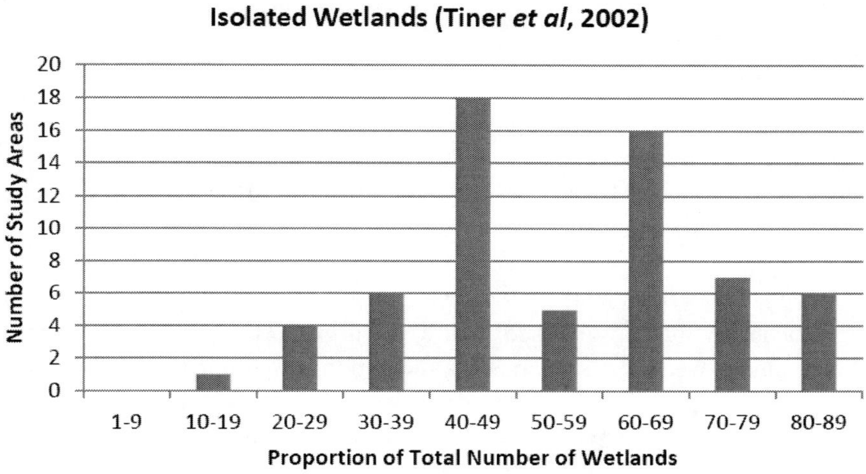

Exhibit 17. Isolated Wetlands in Proportion to Total Number of Wetlands in a Watershed.

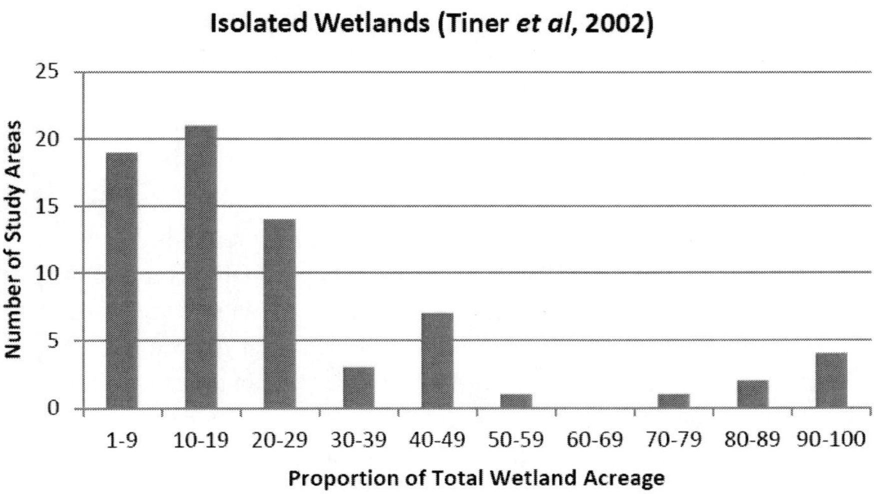

Exhibit 18. Isolated Wetlands in Proportion to Total Wetland Acreage in a Watershed.

Approximately 55 percent of the study areas have less than 20 percent of their wetland acreage as isolated wetlands, another approximate 35% percent of the study areas have between 20-50 percent of their wetlands as isolated wetlands. The remaining 10 percent of the study areas have a relatively high proportion (greater than 70 percent, with most greater than 90 percent) of their wetlands as isolated wetlands. These are study areas that would be most likely representative of watersheds with a large amount and a high density of isolated wetlands necessary to meet the aggregation requirements and then the significant nexus test in the proposed rule.

Step 2: Examine Models to Describe Probability of Aggregation and Significant Nexus

There are various mathematical relationships (models) that could describe the probability that a watershed with a given proportion of isolated wetlands will include wetlands that meet aggregation requirements and pass the significant nexus test. Each model should have the highest probability associated with the highest proportion of isolated wetlands, and the lowest probability with the lowest proportion of isolated wetlands. Exhibit 19 presents four such model relationships. The simplest model is where the probability increases at the same rate as the proportion isolated (LIN model). However, it is more likely that the probability increases at an increasing rate as the proportion isolated becomes larger (LOG model). It is also possible that the relationship starts in LOG model fashion, then hits a critical point where a critical mass of isolated wetlands (say 50 percent) makes aggregation/significant nexus more likely and the remaining incremental increases are small (SIG model).

A feature of these models is that they all key off a top level probability of aggregation and significant nexus (0.5 or 50 percent probability as shown in Exhibit 19). One may select alternative top level probabilities to see different outcomes once applied to the distribution of extent of isolated wetlands in step 3. In selecting the top level probability, it is important to recognize the bias toward watersheds with isolated wetlands in the distribution from step 1, the potential for adjacent wetlands to be included in the proportion isolated, and that application of a probability to a watershed implies that all isolated wetlands in the watershed would be jurisdictional. It is also important to recognize that aggregation and the significant nexus test are reliant on functional similarities (e.g., physical, chemical, and biological connections and processes) as well as location within the watershed. While proportion of total wetland acres is a good proxy for the likelihood of these similarities and connections, it is not the sole arbiter. For these reasons, the top level probability should be far less than 100 percent.

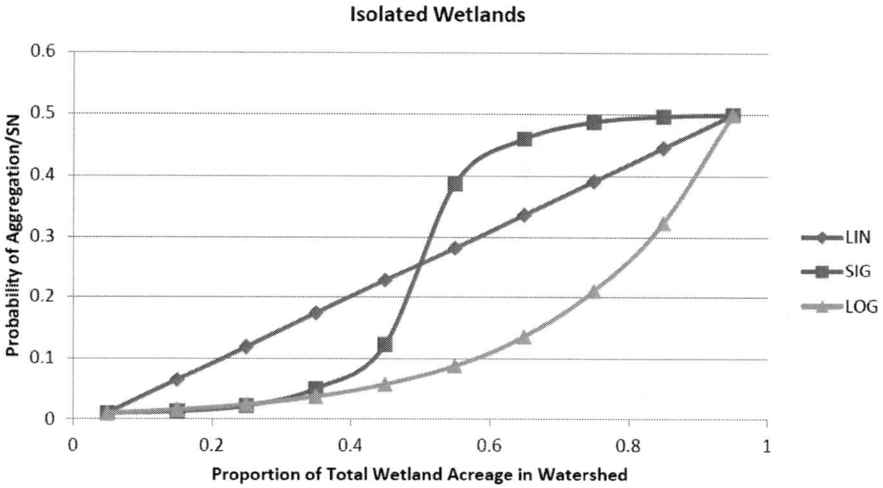

Exhibit 19. Probability Models for Isolated Wetlands Acreage.

Step 3: Select Model and Apply to Distribution of Extent of Isolated Wetlands

Applying a probability model (from step 2) to a distribution of extent of isolated wetlands (from step 1) yields an estimate of the percent of residual other waters where the agencies would assert jurisdiction. Exhibit 20 depicts this final step as a graph and Exhibit 21 shows the calculation for each category in the distribution for the sigmoidal (SIG model) and log (LOG model) relationships with a top level probability of 50 percent.

As described above, the top level probability can be changed. Exhibit 22 presented the results of each probability model for various top level probabilities. Not all these outcomes are considered likely, and not all outcomes are considered equally likely. The most likely estimates are for the LOG and SIG models with top level probabilities of aggregation/significant nexus between 0.4 and 0.6.

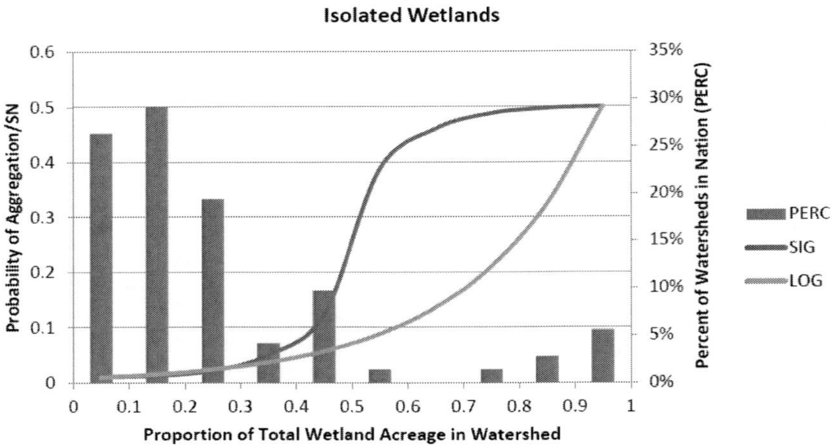

Exhibit 20. Application of Probability Model to Distribution of Extent of Isolated Waters.

Exhibit 21. Calculation of National Estimate of Percent of Jurisdictional Residual Other Waters Under Proposed Rule

Proportion of Isolated Wetlands	Number of Study Areas (Tiner et al., 2002)	Estimated Percent of National Watersheds[(1)]	Model Probability of Aggregation/Significant Nexus		
			LOG Model	SIG Model	LIN Model
90-100	4	6%	0.5	0.5	0.5
80-89	2	3%	0.323739	0.497198	0.445556
70-79	1	1%	0.209614	0.48812	0.391111
60-69	0	0%	0.135721	0.46026	0.336667
50-59	1	1%	0.087876	0.387231	0.282222
40-49	7	10%	0.056898	0.122769	0.227778
30-39	3	4%	0.03684	0.04974	0.173333
20-29	14	19%	0.023853	0.02188	0.118889
10-19	21	29%	0.015445	0.012802	0.064444
1-9	19	26%	0.01	0.01	0.01
TOTAL[2]	**72**	**100%**	**6%**	**8%**	**12%**
(1) Derived from the number of Tiner et al., 2002 study areas for each category of proportion of isolated wetlands.					
(2) Model probability totals are the sum of probability multiplied by the estimated percent of national watersheds for each category of proportion of isolated wetlands					

Exhibit 22. Various National Estimates of Percent of Jurisdictional Residual Other Waters Under Proposed Rule

Top Level Probability	Total Model Probability of Aggregation/Significant Nexus		
	LOG Model	SIG Model	LIN Model
0.1	2%	2%	3%
0.2	3%	4%	5%
0.3	4%	5%	8%
0.4	5%	6%	10%
0.5	6%	8%	12%
0.6	7%	9%	15%
0.7	8%	11%	17%
0.8	9%	12%	19%
0.9	9%	13%	22%
1.0	10%	15%	24%
gray shading represents unrealistic assumptions, orange shading represents best estimates			

Alternative Model for Estimating Additional Incremental Other Waters

The approach described above uses the proportion of total wetland acreage in a watershed that are isolated as the proxy for both aggregation and significant nexus. However, additional information in Tiner et al. (2002) allows consideration of a separate proxy for aggregation. Tiner et al. (2002) present total acreage for each study area. A measure of isolated wetland density can thus be calculated as the quotient of isolated wetland acreage divided by total watershed acreage. The greater this "density", the more likely isolated waters that perform similar functions would be sufficiently close to be evaluated as a single landscape unit. Exhibit 23 shows the distribution of isolated wetland density for the 72 study areas. Isolated wetland density ranges from less than a tenth of a percent to nearly 11 percent.

The same generalized probability models used above for proportion of total wetlands can be applied to these density categories for the aggregation step alone (see Exhibits 24 and 25). Without specific knowledge of a threshold density where aggregation would be more likely, a linear model may be most appropriate.

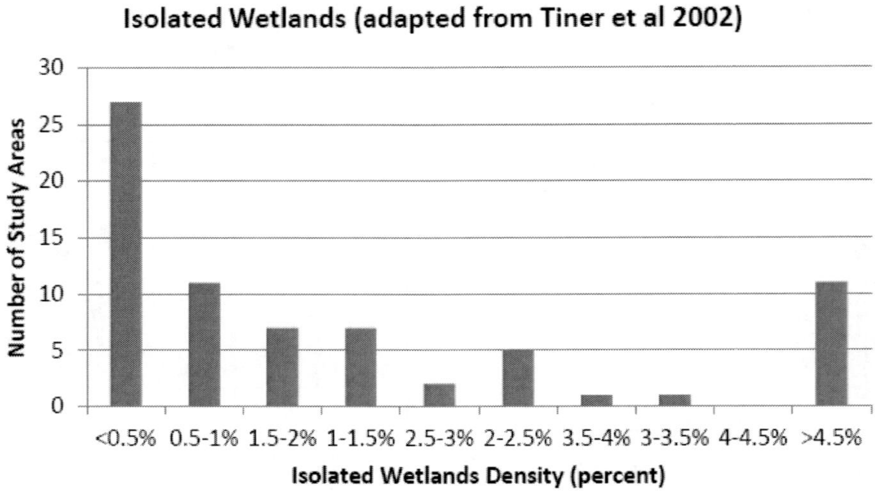

Exhibit 23. Distribution of Tiner et al. (2002) Study Areas by Isolated Wetland Density in Watershed.

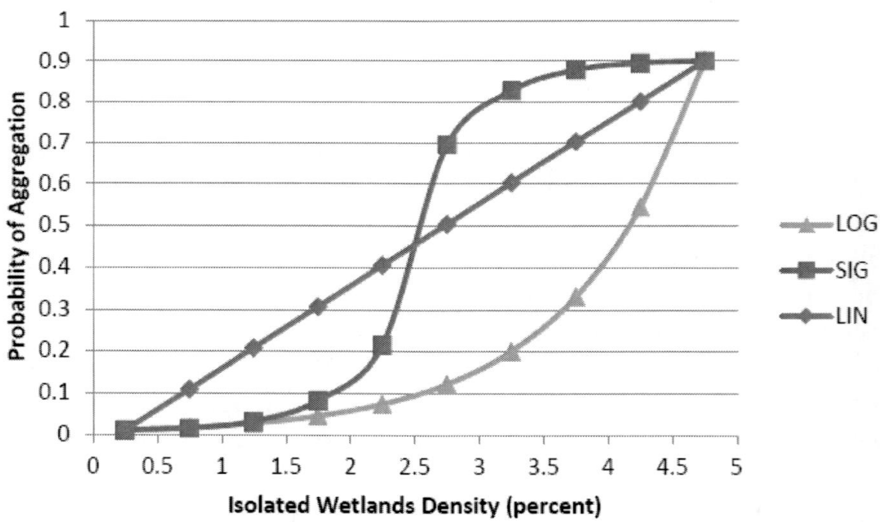

Exhibit 24. Probability Models for Isolated Wetlands Density.

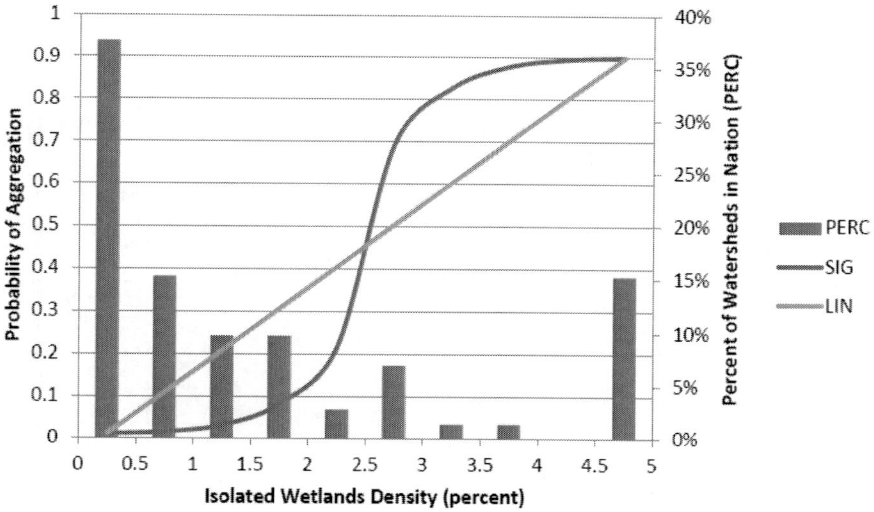

Exhibit 25. Application of Probability Model to Distribution of Isolated Waters Density.

Calculation of the overall estimate of the percent of residual other waters where the agencies would assert jurisdiction using this alternative model pairs the probability of aggregation using isolated wetlands density with the probability of significant nexus using proportion of total wetland acreage for each watershed. After normalizing for the fraction of all watersheds that each study area watershed represents (one out of 72, or approximately 1.4 percent), the products of each probability are summed for a national total. This approach is more complex because it requires selection of a probability model for density and for proportion of total wetland acreage and a selection of top level probability for each step. However, this added complexity offers the analyst greater flexibility and the ability to independently assess each step. The approach may better represent watersheds where density and proportion of total wetland acreage diverge, and can help further identify an appropriate range of percent of residual other waters for the impact analysis.

Exhibit 26 shows the results for various model combinations and for various top level probability combinations. The overall top level probability is the product of the two component top level probabilities, as each applies sequentially. To be most comparable to the previous estimates, the overall top level probability should align with the top level probability associated with the most likely estimates derived from the simpler approach presented in Exhibit 22 (i.e., approximately 0.4 to 0.6).

Exhibit 26. Various National Estimates of Percent of Jurisdictional Residual Other Waters Under Proposed Rule Using Alternative Approach

Top Level Probability		Total Model Probability of Aggregation and Significant Nexus (Model Used for Density/Proportion Isolated)								
Dens./ Prop.	Overall	LOG/ LOG	LOG/ SIG	SIG/ LOG	LIN/ LOG	SIG/ SIG	LIN/ SIG	LOG/ LIN	SIG/ LIN	LIN/ LIN
0.5/0.5	0.25	1.1%	1.3%	1.5%	1.6%	1.8%	2.0%	2.1%	2.6%	2.9%
0.7/0.5	0.35	1.5%	1.8%	2.1%	2.3%	2.5%	2.7%	2.8%	3.6%	4.0%
0.9/0.5	0.45	1.9%	2.3%	2.7%	2.9%	3.2%	3.5%	3.5%	4.6%	5.1%
0.7/0.7	0.49	2.0%	2.5%	2.9%	3.0%	3.5%	3.8%	3.9%	5.0%	5.5%
0.9/0.7	0.63	2.6%	3.1%	3.7%	3.8%	4.4%	4.8%	4.9%	6.4%	7.0%
0.9/0.9	0.81	3.2%	4.0%	4.6%	4.8%	5.6%	6.1%	6.3%	8.1%	9.0%
1.0/1.0	1.00	3.9%	4.8%	5.6%	5.8%	6.9%	7.5%	7.7%	10.0%	11.1%
gray shading represents unrealistic assumptions, orange shading represents best estimates										

This alternative approach tempers some of the previous estimates and indicates an upper bound estimate of 5 percent may be most likely. This analysis also further indicates that the agencies should not consider estimates beyond 10 percent. The agencies caution that the proxy values used in this analysis simply represent the best available information for this exercise, and should not be considered the means of determining aggregation or significant nexus in a case specific analysis.

Impacts of Additional Incremental Other Waters

The estimated impacts of asserting jurisdiction for 5 and 10 percent of residual other waters (non-adjacent waters) under the proposed rule are reflected in the scenarios described in Exhibit 27 below. Recall that residual other waters (non-adjacent waters) represent approximately 83 percent of other waters (the sample review exercise found 17 percent of other waters would be considered adjacent under the proposed policies).

The agencies also considered impacts from potential regulatory activity under the policies proposed that is not represented by ORM2 FY2009-2010 records. If a significant amount of waters are not included in the FY2009-2010 data because of presumed non-jurisdiction on the part of landowners and developers, then the overall percent increase in waters that become jurisdictional would be somewhat greater (other waters would represent more than 6 percent of the total records). To illustrate the effects of including waters not represented in ORM2 because potential applicants considered them non-jurisdictional and did not seek a jurisdictional determination, the agencies present the effect of doubling the number of other waters (effectively raising the share from 6 percent to 11 percent).

Exhibit 27 summarizes the various scenarios considered. Exhibits 28 and 29 present the results in terms of the effect on the range of total costs and benefits. The potential impact on all categories of costs and benefits are considered, not just the effect on mitigation, although those reflect the greatest degree of impact.

Exhibit 27. Scenarios for Consideration of Other Waters

Scenario	Description
Scenario A	5% of non-adjacent other waters are jurisdictional under the proposed rule
Scenario B	10% of non-adjacent other waters are jurisdictional under the proposed rule
Scenario C	There are double the number of other waters
Scenario D	There are double the number of other waters AND 5% of non-adjacent other waters are jurisdictional under the proposed rule
Scenario E	There are double the number of other waters AND 10% of non-adjacent other waters are jurisdictional under the proposed rule

Exhibit 28. Results of Scenarios for Other Waters on Costs and Benefits Estimates

Scenario	Percent of Other Waters Jurisdictional	Overall Percent Increment in Regulatory Actions	Low Range of Costs (2010$ millions)	High Range of Costs (2010$ millions)	Low Range of Benefits (2010$ millions)	High Range of Benefits (2010$ millions)
Base	17%	2.7%	$ 134	$ 231	$ 301	$ 398
Scenario A	21%	2.9%	$ 146	$ 251	$ 339	$ 449
Scenario B	26%	3.2%	$ 162	$ 278	$ 388	$ 514
Scenario C	17%	3.5%	$ 185	$ 328	$ 474	$ 629
Scenario D	21%	4.0%	$ 211	$ 372	$ 551	$ 733
Scenario E	26%	4.5%	$ 241	$ 422	$ 647	$ 861
This assumes for scenarios C, D, and E that the doubling of records includes both adjacent other waters and non-adjacent other waters in the same proportions as the original set of records.						

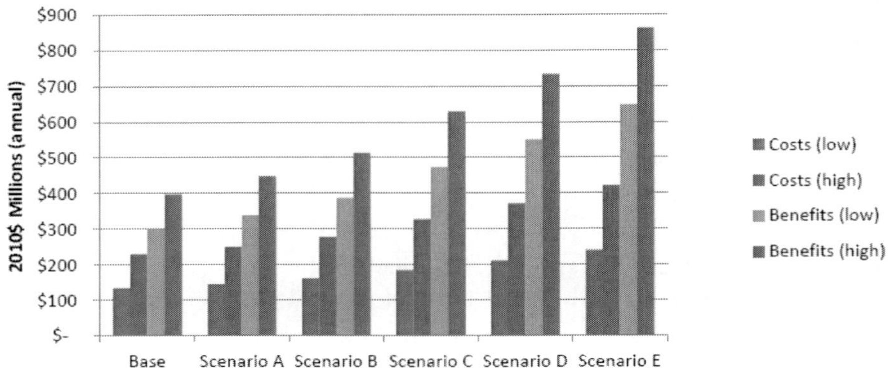

Exhibit 29. Results of Consideration of Other Waters on Costs and Benefits Estimates.

The difference in costs between scenario E and scenario C from Exhibit 28, the highest estimate of the effect of asserting jurisdiction over residual other waters, is between $56-94 million per year. As shown on Exhibit 28 and 29, because estimated benefits would also rise with more wetland protection, benefits would continue to justify costs.

An alternative way of calculating the impact on costs and benefits is to assume that the doubling of other water records (scenarios C, D, and E) do not include any additional "adjacent other waters" (assuming these types of waters are adequately represented in the Corps records), and that only the additional percentages for residual "non-adjacent other waters" apply to the doubling of other water records for scenarios D and E. In this way, scenario C simply becomes equal to the base because no residual non-adjacent other waters are assumed jurisdictional under this scenario. Exhibit 30 presents these results.

Exhibit 30. Alternative Results of Scenarios for Other Waters on Costs and Benefits Estimates

Scenario	Percent of Other Waters Jurisdictional	Overall Percent Increment in Regulatory Actions	Low Range of Costs (2010$ millions)	High Range of Costs (2010$ millions)	Low Range of Benefits (2010$ millions)	High Range of Benefits (2010$ millions)
Base	17%	2.7%	$ 134	$ 231	$ 301	$ 398
Scenario A	21%	2.9%	$ 146	$ 251	$ 339	$ 449
Scenario B	26%	3.2%	$ 162	$ 278	$ 388	$ 514
Scenario C	8.5%	2.7%	$ 134	$ 231	$ 301	$ 398

Scenario	Percent of Other Waters Jurisdictional	Overall Percent Increment in Regulatory Actions	Low Range of Costs (2010$ millions)	High Range of Costs (2010$ millions)	Low Range of Benefits (2010$ millions)	High Range of Benefits (2010$ millions)
Scenario D	13%	3.2%	$ 162	$ 278	$ 388	$ 514
Scenario E	18%	3.6%	$ 189	$ 325	$ 482	$ 640
This assumes for scenarios C, D, and E that the doubling of records includes only non-adjacent other waters, and that adjacent other waters are only represented in the original set of records.						

These alternative results may represent the more likely outcomes. Using 5 percent as a most likely upper bound on percent of non-adjacent other waters, scenario D from Exhibit 30 (orange shading) represents the agencies best estimate of the total costs and benefits that can be quantified. The difference in costs between scenario D and scenario C, the most likely estimate of the effect of asserting jurisdiction over non-adjacent other waters, is between $28-47 million per year.

APPENDIX A: SUPPLEMENTAL COST ANALYSIS INFORMATION

Exhibit 31. State-Level Unit Costs for Wetland and Stream Mitigation

State	Incremental Wetland Mitigation (Acres)	Unit Cost Per Acre of Wetland Mitigated		Incremental Stream Mitigation (Linear Feet)	Unit Cost Per Linear Foot of Stream Mitigated	
		Low	High		Low	High
AK	5	$500	$15,250	25.5	$170	$243
AL	8.2	$10,000	$15,000	580	$350	$619
AR	7.1	$2,000	$3,500	680.2	$170	$243
AZ	0	$9,000	$16,000	4.5	$170	$243
CA	102.8	$18,500	$159,250	6514.4	$170	$243
CO	93	$32,000	$66,000	307.4	$170	$243
CT	4.4	$124,000	$142,000	0	$170	$243
DE	3.9	$40,000	$40,000	0	$170	$243
FL	87.3	$35,000	$90,000	194.9	$170	$243

Exhibit 31. (Continued)

State	Incremental Wetland Mitigation (Acres)	Unit Cost Per Acre of Wetland Mitigated		Incremental Stream Mitigation (Linear Feet)	Unit Cost Per Linear Foot of Stream Mitigated	
		Low	High		Low	High
GA	43.3	$12,000	$67,000	1718.1	$106	$200
IA	14.6	$15,000	$15,000	470.4	$170	$243
ID	8.8	$40,000	$40,000	787.1	$170	$243
IL	64	$40,000	$120,000	294.6	$170	$243
IN	78	$40,000	$60,000	2680	$170	$243
KS	7.1	$50,000	$50,000	8746.1	$170	$243
KY	12.4	$30,000	$30,000	854.8	$170	$283
LA	38.5	$15,000	$32,500	912.2	$170	$243
MA	0.2	$124,000	$142,000	0	$170	$243
MD	92.2	$11,000	$34,500	25.1	$250	$442
ME	2.3	$125,000	$137,000	73.8	$170	$243
MI	4.9	$40,000	$60,000	16.6	$170	$243
MN	73.7	$4,000	$47,500	17.9	$170	$243
MO	18.3	$15,000	$20,000	825.2	$90	$145
MS	4.2	$3,000	$14,000	252.4	$170	$243
MT	9.5	$40,000	$40,000	150.4	$170	$243
NC	18.3	$23,000	$42,500	743.5	$256	$297
ND	279.3	$15,000	$15,000	123.7	$170	$243
NE	32.7	$15,000	$15,000	89.4	$170	$243
NH	2.3	$138,000	$168,000	5616.6	$170	$243
NJ	6.6	$80,000	$240,000	0	$170	$243
NM	2.7	$40,000	$50,000	196.4	$170	$243
NV	45.9	$55,000	$60,000	124.6	$170	$243
NY	134.7	$50,000	$60,000	852.6	$170	$243
OH	159.6	$15,000	$15,000	1526.6	$170	$243
OK	6.1	$12,000	$31,000	793.9	$170	$243
OR	11.7	$43,000	$84,000	23.1	$170	$243
PA	83	$12,000	$13,500	4151.3	$170	$243
RI	0.4	$124,000	$142,000	0	$170	$243
SC	107.9	$25,000	$62,500	52.7	$75	$138
SD	65.8	$15,000	$15,000	0	$170	$243
TN	10.6	$7,000	$13,500	878.7	$50	$125

State	Incremental Wetland Mitigation (Acres)	Unit Cost Per Acre of Wetland Mitigated		Incremental Stream Mitigation (Linear Feet)	Unit Cost Per Linear Foot of Stream Mitigated	
		Low	High		Low	High
TX	69.8	$15,000	$30,000	3491.5	$80	$142
UT	19.4	$55,000	$60,000	280.8	$170	$243
VA	22.2	$16,000	$78,000	1107.4	$300	$600
VT	4.6	$110,000	$121,000	0	$170	$243
WA	6	$100,000	$175,000	130.6	$170	$243
WI	81.9	$40,000	$40,000	0	$170	$243
WV	33.7	$30,000	$45,000	2759	$400	$600
WY	54	$15,000	$15,000	1	$170	$243
National	2,042	$24,989	$49,207	49,075	$177	$265

Exhibit 32. Labor Rates for Private Industry and Local, State, and Federal Government Positions

Position	Occupational Code[1]	Mean Hourly Wage[1]	Benefits Adjustment Factor[2]	Year Adjustment [3]	Total Hourly Adjusted Wage
Private Industry					
Environmental Scientist	19-2041	$35.32	1.292	1.0198	$46.54
Environmental Engineer	17-2081	$39.89			$52.56
Administrative Assistant	43-6011	$23.16			$30.52
Lawyer	23-1011	$65.65			$86.50
Economist	19-3011	$59.48			$78.37
Local Government					
Environmental Scientist	19-2041	$28.86	1.319	1.0258	$39.05
Environmental Engineer	17-2081	$35.89			$48.56
Administrative Assistant	43-6011	$22.03			$29.81
Lawyer	23-1011	$43.77			$59.22
Economist	19-3011	$34.27			$46.37

Exhibit 32. (Continued)

Position	Occupational Code[1]	Mean Hourly Wage[1]	Benefits Adjustment Factor[2]	Year Adjustment [3]	Total Hourly Adjusted Wage
State Government					
Environmental Scientist	19-2041	$27.15	1.319	1.0258	$36.73
Administrative Assistant	43-6011	$18.82			$25.46
Environmental Engineer	17-2081	$31.96			$43.24
Lawyer	23-1011	$39.78			$53.82
Economist	19-3011	$27.38			$37.05
Federal Government					
Environmental Scientist	19-2041	$45.05	1.3	1.0224	$59.88
Administrative Assistant	43-6011	$26.76			$35.57
Environmental Engineer	17-2081	$46.35			$61.60
Lawyer	23-1011	$61.32			$81.50
Economist	19-3011	$51.04			$67.84

1. Occupational codes and mean hourly wage from BLS (2009). Bureau of Labor Statistics (BLS), United States Department of Labor. 2009. Occupational Employment and Wages, December 2010. http://bls.gov/oes/2009/may/oes_nat.htm
2. Adjusted for benefits according to the Employment Cost for Employee Compensation Index for professional and related for private industry, local and state employees, and civilian workers.
3. Escalated to 2010 dollars using the Employment Cost Index for private industry (September 2010 = 113.3; June 2009 = 111.1), state and local employees (September 2010 = 115.3; June 2009 = 112.4) and civilian workers (September 2010 = 114.1; June 2009 = 111.6).

APPENDIX B: SUPPLEMENTAL BENEFIT ESTIMATE INFORMATION

Exhibit 33. Summary of Environmental Benefits by Wetland Types and Other Isolated Waterbodies Potentially Affected

Wetland Type	Distribution	Region	Environmental Benefits	Primary Threats
Rainwater Basin Wetlands	Southern Nebraska	Interior West	Very important habitat for waterfowl, Food chain support, Nutrient retention, Flood storage, Sediment trapping and shoreline anchoring	Agricultural activities such as drainage, clearing, and groundwater pumping
Sandhills Wetlands	North-Central and Northwestern Nebraska	Interior West	Habitat for migratory waterfowl and many threatened and endangered species	Ditching of wet meadows and cattle grazing
Prairie Potholes	North-Central U.S. (Iowa/South Dakota into Canada)	Midwest	Recharge and discharge areas for local groundwater flow and regional surface water flow; A great deal of storm water storage and flood protection; Concentric rings of vegetation zones create unique habitat areas; Waterfowl habitat (10% of breeding area; half of waterfowl); availability of large numbers of small wetlands allows dispersal	Agriculture, irrigation, and flood control projects

Exhibit 33. (Continued)

Wetland Type	Distribution	Region	Environmental Benefits	Primary Threats
Alvar Wetlands	Great Lakes region	Midwest	Provide habitat to rare species and a variety of hydrophytes	Quarrying, rural development, allterrain vehicles, and construction of cottages, vacation homes, and trailer parks
Woodland Vernal Pools	Northeastern U.S.	Northeast	Fluctuating water level prohibits establishment of fish populations, providing excellent breeding ground for amphibians and other species that spend most of their lives in the wooded areas around the pools	Often destroyed for development (since they are small and surrounded by upland), and are sometimes used as storm water detention basins. Drainage from agricultural fields or residential areas.
Delmarva Potholes	Delmarva Peninsula (Maryland, Delaware)	Northeast	Support populations of large quantities of amphibians and rare and endangered plants; Temporary storage of surface water and flood protection; Recharge regional groundwater supplies during dry periods	Drainage associated with agriculture or silviculture, and some development

Wetland Type	Distribution	Region	Environmental Benefits	Primary Threats
Kettle-hole Wetlands	New England and Midwest, north to Canada and Alaska	Northeast/ Midwest/ Alaska	Habitat for unique boreal plant species	Peat mining, drainage, and conversion to open waterbodies or commercial cranberry bogs; introduction of nutrients from lawn runoff
Wetlands of Washington' s Channeled Scablands	Eastern Washington (Cascade Mountains)	Pacific Coast	Habitat and staging grounds for migratory waterfowl; Habitat for resident waterfowl and some endangered plants	Impacts from livestock (cattle use as wallow) and overgrazing; some are drained and converted to hayfield or pasture.
Former Floodplain Wetlands	Alaska	Alaska	Important havens for waterfowl	
West Coast Vernal Pools	Southern Oregon to Northern Baja Mexico	Pacific Coast	Unpredictable flooding patterns promote endemism, creating unique flora and fauna, including many endangered species	Increasing urbanization and agricultural impacts
Pocosins	Atlantic-Gulf Coastal Plain, from Virginia to Florida	Southeast	Temporary storage of surface water to avoid quick runoff in estuaries (giving them time to assimilate freshwater); Habitat for many rare and endangered animal species	Ditching for drainage to increase timber production; agricultural conversion

Exhibit 33. (Continued)

Wetland Type	Distribution	Region	Environmental Benefits	Primary Threats
Cypress Domes	Florida and Southern Georgia	Southeast	Maintain regional biodiversity by providing important breeding grounds (especially for amphibians); Surface water storage, flood prevention, and groundwater recharge	Development, including conversion to residential subdivisions, commercial sites, and gold courses; drying out increases susceptibility to fire.
Sinkhole Wetlands	Karst landscapes (Southern U.S.)	Southeast	Productive amphibian breeding grounds, including for some endangered species; Unique habitat for cave-adapted animals	Water pollution from runoff or direct discharge, groundwater withdrawal, impoundment of local streams, timber harvest, fish stocking, and agricultural and residential development.
Carolina Bay Wetlands	Atlantic-Gulf Coastal Plain, from Virginia to Florida	Southeast	Habitat for abundant amphibian populations; Critical aquatic habitat for many species during droughts	Drainage for crop production
Coastal Zone Dune Swale and Deflation Plain Wetlands	U.S. Coastlines	Southeast/ Northeast/ Pacific Coast	Support a variety of hydrophytic plants (since they intersect groundwater tables); Food and habitat for migrating waterfowl; Habitat for a variety of species, including some unique	Residential housing, golf courses, and resort development

Wetland Type	Distribution	Region	Environmental Benefits	Primary Threats
Coastal Plain Ponds	Atlantic-Gulf Coastal Plain	Southeast/ Northeast	Fluctuating water levels and vegetation in concentric rings provide habitat supporting unique species	Coastal development, waste dumping, all-terrain vehicles, water withdrawal, and pollution from adjacent development.
Playas	Deserts, semi- arid prairies in Southwest (Texas and New Mexico)	Southwest	Characteristic fluctuating water levels promote nutrient cycling and biological productivity; Wintering grounds for waterfowl and shorebirds; Vital habitat for amphibians.	Poor water quality from adjacent crop land, discharge of water from oilfields, and effluent from livestock operations such as cattle feedlots; sedimentation from farmland, pit construction, and overgrazing
Salt Flat and Salt Lake Wetlands	Great Basin region -- Nevada and Utah	Southwest	Food and habitat for wildlife in an otherwise arid area	Road and utility construction; development pressures in urban areas
Desert Springs and their Wetlands	Southwest (California, Arizona, Nevada)	Southwest	Isolated populations of endemic species	Pumping of groundwater for agriculture and energy development lowers water levels

Source: USFWS (2002).

Exhibit 34. Types of Benefits Associated with Environmental Policies

Category	Examples	Valuation Methods
Human Health Improvements		
Mortality risk reductions	Reduced risk of fatality from cancer and acute health risks	Averting behavior, hedonics, stated preference
Morbidity risk reductions	Reduced risk of nonfatal illness	Averting behavior, hedonics, stated preference, cost of illness
Ecological Improvements		
Market products	Harvests or extraction of food, fuel, fiber, timber, fur, and leather	Production function
Recreation activities and aesthetics	Wildlife viewing, fishing, boating, swimming, hiking, scenic views	Production function, averting behaviors, hedonics, recreation demand, stated preference
Valued ecosystem functions	Climate moderation, flood moderation, groundwater recharge, sediment trapping, soil retention, nutrient cycling, pollination by wild species, biodiversity, water filtration, soil fertilization, pest control	Production function, averting behaviors, stated preference, hedonics
Nonuse values	Relevant species populations, communities, or ecosystems	Stated preference

Category	Examples	Valuation Methods
Other Benefits		
Aesthetic improvements	Visibility, taste, odor	Averting behaviors, hedonics, stated preference
Reduced materials damage	Reduced soiling and corrosion	Averting behaviors, production function, cost function, hedonics

Source: U.S. EPA (2010b; Table 7.1).

Summaries of Holistic Wetland Benefit Studies Used to Generate WTP Estimates

Azevedo et al. (2000) conducted a survey to understand how residents of Iowa value wetlands, specifically with regard to the following functions: wildlife viewing, fishing, biking, hiking, waterfowl and upland hunting. The 5-part survey collected information regarding wetland visitation patterns, perceived benefits and costs associated with wetlands, socioeconomic characteristics of respondents, and their WTP for preservation of existing wetlands and restoration of additional wetlands via two specific programs: the Prairie Pothole Joint Venture (PP) and the Iowa River Corridor Project (IRCP). The authors used contingent valuation to evaluate WTP for restoring additional wetlands through PP and ICRP. Results indicated that approximately 50% of Iowans would pay $25 in support of PP and less than $10 for ICRP (2000 dollars).

Mullarkey and Bishop (1999) conducted a study of WTP for a hypothetical rerouting of a highway expansion that would preserve 110 acres of wetlands in Wisconsin. The wetlands in question provide a range of services including flood control, water purification, bird/wildlife habitat, and for a portion of the affected wetlands, fish habitat. The study reported six estimates of WTP ranging from $13.68 to $57.83 (1999 dollars) depending upon whether respondents were informed that mitigation would be taking place if the wetland were destroyed and the degree of certainty respondents expressed in their answers.

Poor (1999) examined WTP to increase the area of wetlands in Nebraska's rainwater basin by an average of 41,000 acres across multiple survey versions. The basin is a large complex of 34,000 wetland acres, and a plan is already in place to create an additional 25,000 wetland acres. Wetland services in this study included flood control, water quality improvement, wildlife production and habitat, and bird watching/hiking. Median and mean household WTP were $4.17 and $21.05 (1995 dollars), respectively.

Blomquist and Whitehead (1998) conducted a contingent valuation study to estimate the value of four wetlands in Western Kentucky with differing characteristics. One was a freshwater marsh, one was a temporarily flooded bottomland hardwood forest, one was a seasonally flooded bottomland hardwood forest, and one was a bald cypress swamp. Wetland functions included flood control, water quality improvements, and wildlife production/habitat. WTP ranged from $1.69 (1990 dollars) for Flat Creek, a freshwater marsh, to $11.21 (1990 dollars) for Cypress Creek, a cypress swamp.

Roberts and Leitch (1997) conducted a contingent valuation study of the value of Mud Lake, a managed lacustrine wetland on the border of Minnesota and South Dakota. This study used a discrete choice survey to determine use, option/bequest, and existence values for Mud Lake. Use values, defined as WTP for management for water related recreation and fish/wildlife habitat ranged from $22,699 to more than $44,736 (1997 dollars) for all respondents in the sample. Option/bequest values ranged from $25,795 to more than $52,750 (1997 dollars) for all respondents in the sample. Existence values ranged from $18,508 to more than $40,451 (1997 dollars) for all respondents in the sample. Total overall median willingness to pay for the sample was estimated to be $102,000 (1997 dollars).

Dillman et al. (1993) estimated the WTP for preservation of 2,500 acres of wetlands in the Francis Biedler forest of South Carolina using dichotomous choice contingent valuation method. The study examined three types of wetland: frequently flooded bottomland (cypress-tupelo swamp), infrequently flooded bottomland hardwood forest, and nonbottomland pine plantation with hardwood runners.

These wetlands served the following functions: flood control, wildlife habitat, recreational activities, water supply, and aesthetic value. The mean WTP estimated was $16.74 (1993 dollars) per household (ranging from $6.82 for infrequently flooded bottomland hardwood forests to $19.57 for pine plantations with scattered hardwood runners).

Whitehead and Blomquist (1991) utilized contingent valuation to examine Kentucky residents' WTP for preservation of the Clear Creek wetland, a large natural wetland with hardwood trees, standing water, and nonwoody vegetation. The wetland provides a range of services including water quality maintenance, fish and wildlife habitat, flood and sediment control, groundwater recharge, biological productivity and outdoor recreation. The study used three different survey versions consisting of two WTP questions each, with the difference in each case reflecting a difference in information presented about the wetland quality that would result if Clear Creek is not preserved. WTP values ranged from $5.09 to $16.61 (1991 dollars) under the scenario discussing preservation and reclamation of Clear Creek itself, and from $3.75 to $8.13 (1991 dollars) under scenarios discussing preservation of other wetlands concurrent with reclamation of Clear Creek.

Johnson and Linder (1986) conducted a contingent valuation study to estimate the value of wetlands in South Dakota as a recreational resource for resident hunters. The study examined wetlands statewide, the majority of which are located in the eastern part of the state. Their results indicated that the total value for waterfowl, upland, big game, and predator hunting in South Dakota wetlands in 1986 dollars was $34 million, and that the average total per user value of wetlands was $289.90 for a single hunting season.

Loomis et al. (1991) studied California residents' willingness to pay additional taxes to preserve and restore wetlands in California's San Joaquin Valley. The study's focus was wetlands as a habitat for migratory birds. The study found that average annual household willingness to pay for a program to prevent further degradation of an existing 85,000 acres of wetlands was $174 in the San Joaquin Valley and $152 in the rest of the state, and willingness to pay for a program including both maintenance of existing acreage plus the restoration of an additional 40,000 acres was $286 in the San Joaquin Valley and $251 in the rest of the state (1990 dollars). The study also examined a program to reduce and prevent further pollution of wildlife habitat in the region, and to increase Chinook salmon populations.

Lant and Tobin (1989) studied willingness to pay higher state sales tax to improve water quality of riparian corridors in Iowa and Illinois. The study examined three river corridors utilizing face-to-face interviews: the Edwards River in Illinois, the South Skunk River in Iowa, and the Wapsipinicon River in Iowa. Value per person for improvement of quality in the Edwards River to that in the South Skunk was $8.85 per year, and value per person for improvement of quality in the South Skunk River to that in the Wapsipinicon was $20.37 per year. This study had a very small sample size.

Azevedo, C., J.A. Herriges, and C.L. Kling. 2000. Iowa Wetlands: Perceptions and Values. Center for Agricultural and Rural Development. Staff Report 00-SR 91.

Blomquist, G.C. and J.C. Whitehead. 1998. Resource Quality Information and Validity of Willingness to Pay in Contingent Valuation. Resource and Energy Economics 20: 179-196.

Dillman, B., L.J. Beran, and D.D. Hook. 1993. Nonmarket Valuation of Freshwater Wetlands: The Francis Beidler Forest. South Carolina Water Resources Research Institute, Clemson University.

Lant, C.L. and G.A. Tobin. 1989. "The Economic Value of Riparian Corridors in Cornbelt Floodplains: A Research Framework". Professional Geographer 41(3): 337-49.

Loomis, J., M. Hanemann, B. Kanninen and T. Wegge. 1991. "Willingness to Pay to Protect Wetlands and Reduce Wildlife Contamination from Agricultural Drainage." In A. Dinar and D. Zilberman (eds.), The

Economics and management of Water and Drainage in Agriculture. Boston, Massachusetts: Kluwer Academic Publishers, pp. 411-445.

Johnson, C.W. and R.L. Linder. 1986. An Economic Valuation of South Dakota Wetlands as a Recreation Resource for Resident Hunters. Landscape Journal 5(1): 33-38.

Mullarkey, D.J. and R.C. Bishop. 1999. Sensitivity to Scope: Evidence from a CVM Study of Wetlands. Presented at the Annual Meeting of the American Agricultural Economics Association, Nashville, TN, August 8-11, 1999.

Poor, P.J. 1999. The Value of Additional Central Flyway Wetlands: The Case of Nebraska's Rainwater Basin Wetlands. Journal of Agricultural and Resource Economics 24: 253-265.

Roberts, L.A. and J.A. Leitch. 1997. Economic Valuation of Some Wetland Outputs of Mud Lake, Minnesota-South Dakota. North Dakota Agricultural Experiment Station. Agricultural Economics Report No. 381.

Whitehead, J.C. and G.C. Blomquist. 1991. Measuring Contingent Values for Wetlands: Effects of Information about Related Environmental Goods. Water Resources Research 27: 2523-2531.

Exhibit 35. Studies of WTP for Preservation of Wetlands with Characteristics of Isolated Wetlands

Study	Publication Type	Year of Reported Dollar Values[2]	Location	Study Type	Survey Population	Response Rate
Azevedo et al. (2000)	Report	2000	IA	CVM, travel cost3	Random sample of Iowa residents statewide, additional random sample of a targeted group of hunters/anglers	58.1%[4]
Mullarkey and Bishop (1999)	Presentation	1999	WI	CVM	Random sample of Wisconsin residents statewide	43.5%
Poor (1999)	Journal article	1995	NE	CVM	Random statewide sample of Nebraska households	46%

Exhibit 35. (Continued)

Study	Publication Type	Year of Reported Dollar Values[2]	Location	Study Type	Survey Population	Response Rate
Blomquist and Whitehead (1998)	Journal article	1990	KY, IN, TN, IL, MO	CVM	Random dialing of households in Western Kentucky and nearby areas of Indiana, Tennessee, Illinois and Missouri from phone directories	66.7%
Roberts and Leitch (1997)	Report	1997	MN, SD	CVM	Minnesota and South Dakota households within a 30-mile radius of Mud Lake	62%
Dillman et al. (1993)	Report	1993	SC	CVM	Random sample of South Carolina households statewide	21%
Loomis et al. (1991)	Book chapter	1991	CA	CVM	Random telephone samples of California households statewide including random sample of targeted group, San Joaquin Valley residents	51%
Whitehead and Blomquist (1991)	Journal article	1991	KY	CVM	Random cluster sample of Western Kentucky households from phone directories	31%
Lant and Tobin (1989)	Journal article	1989	IA, IL	CVM	In person interviews with residents of towns near the three rivers surveyed	Not available
Johnson and Linder (1986)	Journal article	1986	SD	CVM	One percent random sample of a targeted group, South Dakota anglers and hunters statewide	61%
(1) Excludes studies of tidal wetlands or wetlands adjacent to navigable waters.						

(2) Where studies provided only the year a survey was conducted and did not specify dollar value years, we assumed publication year dollars rather than data year dollars, as this is the more conservative assumption.
(3) Non-CVM methodology estimates were excluded from meta-analysis.
58.1% represents average overall response rate for Azevedo et al. The response rate for the Prairie Pothole version of the survey was 58.9% and the response rate for the Iowa River Corridor version was 56.5%.

Exhibit 36. WTP for Preservation of Wetlands

Study	Wetland Type	Wetland Area (acres)	WTP [2,3]	WTP Description
Azevedo et al. (2000)	Depression/isolated, Riverine/floodplain	7,000 and 2,500 [4]	\$12.66 - \$31.66	Iowa residents' WTP to preserve and restore wetlands through the Prairie Pothole Joint Venture and Iowa River Corridor Project
Mullarkey and Bishop (1999)	Depression/isolated, Riverine/floodplain	110	\$247.10 - \$460.69	Individual WTP for a hypothetical rerouting of a highway expansion that would preserve 110 acres of wetlands in Wisconsin
Poor (1999)	Depression/isolated	41,000	\$415.86 - \$774.98	WTP to increase the area of wetlands in Nebraska's rainwater basin by an average of 41,000 acres
Blomquist and Whitehead (1998)	Emergent, Forested	500	\$38.92 - \$481.20	Household WTP for four wetlands with differing characteristics in western Kentucky
Roberts and Leitch (1997)	Emergent	5,000	\$124.59 – 232.29	Annual value to households of Mud Lake, a managed lacustrine wetland on the border of Minnesota and South Dakota
Dillman et al. (1993)	Forested	2,500	\$26.02	South Carolina households' one-time WTP for preservation of one of three 2,500 acre wetlands in the Francis Biedler forest of South Carolina
Loomis et al. (1991)	Riverine/ floodplain	85,000 and 125,000 [5]	\$243.35 - \$278.57 and \$401.85 – \$457.89	Annual California household WTP taxes to protect and restore San Joaquin Valley wetlands

Exhibit 36. (Continued)

Study	Wetland Type	Wetland Area (acres)	WTP [2,3]	WTP Description
Whitehead and Blomquist (1991)	Forested	5,000	\$112.46 - \$684.23	Kentucky households' WTP for preservation of the Clear Creek wetland, a large natural wetland with hardwood trees, standing water, and nonwoody vegetation
Lant and Tobin (1989)	Riverine/floodplain	1,406 and 1,663 [6]	\$23.05 - \$212.79	Individual WTP in Illinois and Iowa to improve water quality in the Edwards River to that in the South Skunk River, and to improve water quality in the South Skunk River to that in the Wapsipinicon River.
Johnson and Linder (1986)	Emergent	1,307,187	\$576.77	South Dakota hunters' individual WTP for wetlands statewide for hunting, the majority of which are located in the eastern part of the state

(1) Excludes studies of tidal wetlands or wetlands adjacent to navigable waters.
(2) For studies that provide only the year a survey was conducted and did not specify dollar value years, EPA assumed publication year dollars rather than data year dollars, as this is the more conservative assumption.
(3) If entity is not specified, EPA assumed WTP is on an individual basis. If frequency of payment is not specified, EPA assumed WTP is in terms of a one-time payment.
(4) Azevedo et al. present WTP values for two different study areas, sized 7,000 acres and 2,500 acres.
(5) Loomis et al. present WTP values to preserve existing wetlands of 85,000 acres and to preserve that acreage plus increase acreage by 40,000 to a total of 125,000.
(6) Lant and Tobin present WTP values for two different riparian corridors with different acreage.

End Notes

[1] The existing regulations represent one appropriate baseline for comparison, and because the proposed rule is narrower in jurisdictional scope then the existing (1986) regulations, there would be no additional costs in comparison to this baseline. A comparison to field practice following the 2008 guidance is also an appropriate baseline, and the agencies believe that baseline is the most useful for purposes of comparing the potential outcome of the proposed rule.

[2] The "other waters" group of ORM2 records represents a more inclusive set of waters than would be considered "other waters" as the term is used in the proposed rule. The "other waters" group of ORM2 records includes many wetlands and some non-wetlands waters that would meet the definition of "adjacent" under the proposed rule.

[3] U.S. Army Corps of Engineers. 2001. *Cost analysis for the 2000 issuance and modification of nationwide permits*. Institute for Water Resources. (August)

[4] D. Sunding and D. Zilberman. 2000. *Analysis of the Army Corps of Engineers' NWP 26 Replacement Permit Proposal*. Prepared for the National Association of Counties and the Foundation for Environmental and Economic Progress. (January).

[5] These details on the projects included in the survey sample are reported in: D. Sunding and D. Zilberman. 2002. "The economics of environmental regulation by licensing: An assessment of recent changes in the wetland permitting process." *Natural Resources Journal*. V. 42, Winter.

[6] The range of NWP application costs in the survey was between $2,000 and $140,076; the median cost was $11,800, and the mean cost was $28,915. The range of IP application costs in the survey was between $7,000 and $1,530,000; the median cost was $155,000 and the mean cost was $271,596. (All estimates are presumed to reflect 1999$)

[7] The sample analysis of "other waters" indicated that none of the 145 waters examined in the state of California would become jurisdictional. While the analysis suggested no change in jurisdictional status of "other waters" in the state of California, the agencies applied a 5 percent change in jurisdiction to be conservative.

[8] The value of a bundle of services is generally not the same as the sum of values for individual services that comprise the bundle estimated separately. The independent valuation and then aggregation of multiple service values can introduce systemic bias in total value estimates because independent valuation does not account for the potential interdependence (e.g., complementarily) among services. Use of CV to estimate total values for all services collectively avoids this problem by estimating values for resource changes while considering the potential interdependence among individual resource services.

[9] Moeltner, K. and R. Woodward. 2007. Meta-Functional Benefit Transfer for Wetland Valuation: Making Most of Small Samples. UNR Joint Economics Working Paper 07-012. Paper presented at the W1133 Annual Meetings, Richmond, VA, March 28-30, 2007.

[10] Heimlich, R.E., R. Claassen, K.D. Wiebe, D. Gadsby, and R.M. House. 1998. Wetlands and Agriculture: Private Interests and Public Benefits. AER-765, U.S. Dept. Agr. Econ. Res. Serv., Aug.

[11] Brown, T. C., Measuring nonuse value: A comparison of recent contingent valuation studies, W-133 Sixth Interim Rep., Dep. of Agric. and Appl. Econ., Univ. of Ga., Athens, 1993.

[12] Carson, R.T., Mitchell, R.C., 1993. The value of clean water: the public's willingness to pay for boatable, fishable, and swimmable quality water. Water Resources Research 29 (7), 2445–2454

[13] EPA focused this estimate on state implementation and did not attempt to quantify potential impacts on tribes.

[14] Tiner, R.W., H.C. Bergquist, G.P. DeAlessio, and M.J. Starr. 2002. Geographically Isolated Wetlands: A Preliminary Assessment of their Characteristics and Status in Selected Areas of the United States. U.S. Department of the Interior, Fish and Wildlife Service, Northeast Region, Hadley, MA.

In: U.S. Waters Protected …
Editor: Caroline M. Ednie

ISBN: 978-1-63321-275-6

Chapter 3

THE WETLANDS COVERAGE OF THE CLEAN WATER ACT (CWA): *RAPANOS* AND BEYOND*

Robert Meltz and Claudia Copeland

SUMMARY

In 1985 and 2001, the Supreme Court grappled with issues as to the geographic scope of the wetlands permitting program in the federal Clean Water Act (CWA). In 2006, the Supreme Court rendered a third decision, *Rapanos v. United States*, on appeal from two Sixth Circuit rulings. The Sixth Circuit rulings offered the Court a chance to clarify the reach of CWA jurisdiction over wetlands adjacent only to *non*navigable tributaries of traditional navigable waters—including tributaries such as drainage ditches and canals that may flow intermittently. (Jurisdiction over wetlands adjacent to traditional navigable waters was established in the 1985 decision.)

The Court's decision provided little clarification, however, splitting 4-1-4. The four-Justice plurality decision, by Justice Scalia, said that the CWA covers only wetlands connected to relatively permanent bodies of water (streams, rivers, lakes) by a continuous surface connection. Justice Kennedy, writing alone, demanded a substantial nexus between the wetland and a traditional navigable water, using an ambiguous ecological

* This is an edited, reformatted and augmented version of Congressional Research Service Publication, No. RL33263, dated November 6, 2013.

test. Justice Stevens, for the four dissenters, would have upheld the existing broad reach of Corps of Engineers/EPA regulations.

Because no rationale commanded the support of a majority of the Justices, lower courts are extracting different rules of decision from *Rapanos* for resolving future cases. Corps/EPA guidance issued in December 2008 says that a wetland generally is jurisdictional if it satisfies either the plurality or Kennedy tests. In April 2011, the agencies proposed revised guidance intended to clarify whether waters are protected by the CWA, but this proposal was controversial. The ambiguity of the *Rapanos* decision and questions about the agencies' guidance have increased pressure on EPA and the Corps to initiate a rulemaking to promulgate new regulations. In September 2013, EPA and the Corps withdrew the controversial proposed guidance and submitted a draft rule to the Office of Management and Budget for review. The substance of the draft rule, and when it might be proposed, are unknown for now. There also has been pressure on Congress to provide legislative clarification. In the 111th Congress, legislation intended to do so was approved by a Senate committee, but no further legislative action occurred. Similar legislation was not introduced in the 112th Congress or so far in the 113th Congress. Instead, proposals to bar issuance of the Corps/EPA revised guidance and to narrow the regulatory scope of the CWA have been introduced.

The legal and policy questions associated with *Rapanos*—regarding the outer geographic limit of CWA jurisdiction and the consequences of restricting that scope—have challenged regulators, landowners and developers, and policymakers for 40 years. The answer may determine the reach of CWA regulatory authority not only for the wetlands permitting program but also for other CWA programs, since the CWA uses but one jurisdiction-defining phrase ("navigable waters") throughout the statute.

While regulators and the regulated community debate the legal dimensions of federal jurisdiction under the CWA, scientists contend that there are no discrete, scientifically supportable boundaries or criteria along the continuum of wetlands to separate them into meaningful ecological or hydrological compartments. Wetland scientists believe that all such waters are critical for protecting the integrity of waters, habitat, and wildlife downstream. Changes in the limits of federal jurisdiction highlight the role of states in protecting waters not addressed by federal law. From the states' perspective, federal programs provide a baseline for consistent, minimum standards to regulate wetlands and other waters. Most states are either reluctant or unable to take steps to protect non-jurisdictional waters through legislative or administrative action.

INTRODUCTION

In 2006, the Supreme Court decided *Rapanos v. United States,*[1] the most recent and well-known of three Supreme Court decisions wrestling with the question of which wetlands are covered by the wetlands permitting program in the Clean Water Act (CWA).[2] Since then, numerous decisions from the lower federal courts have sought to divine what criteria to draw from the fractured opinions in *Rapanos* as to which wetlands are "jurisdictional" (within the CWA's reach), and which are not. At the same time, the agencies charged with administering the wetlands permitting program, the U.S. Army Corps of Engineers and Environmental Protection Agency (EPA), have issued several guidance documents seeking to explain their view of their jurisdiction post-*Rapanos*.

This report provides background including the pre-*Rapanos* Supreme Court opinions, then moves on to *Rapanos* itself and the Corps/EPA guidance documents.

BACKGROUND

From the earliest days, Congress has grappled with where to set the line between federal and state authority over the nation's waterways. Typically, this debate occurred in the context of federal legislation restricting uses of waterways that impaired navigation and commerce. The phrase Congress often used to specify waterways over which the federal government had authority was "navigable waters of the United States."[3] This "navigable waters" concept proved an elastic one: in Supreme Court decisions from the early to mid-20th century, "navigability" underwent a substantial expansion "from waters in actual use to those which used to be navigable to those which by reasonable improvements could be made navigable to nonnavigable tributaries affecting navigable streams."[4]

Notwithstanding the Court's enlargement of "navigability," the Congress considering the legislation that became the CWA of 1972[5] felt that the term was too constricted to define the reach of a law whose purpose was not maintaining navigability, as in the past, but rather preventing pollution. Accordingly, Congress in the CWA retained the traditional term "navigable waters," but defined it to mean "waters of the United States"[6]—seemingly minimizing the constraint of navigability. The conference report said that the new phrase was intended to be given "the broadest possible constitutional interpretation."[7]

Among the provisions in the 1972 clean water legislation was Section 404,[8] which together with Section 301(a) requires persons wishing to discharge dredged or fill material into "navigable waters," as newly defined, to obtain a permit from the U.S. Army Corps of Engineers.[9] The Corps' initial response to Section 404 was to apply it solely to waters traditionally deemed navigable (which included few wetland areas), despite the broadening "waters of the United States" definition and conference report language. Under a 1975 court order,[10] however, the Corps issued new regulations that swept in a range of wetlands.[11] This broadening ushered in a debate, continuing today, as to *which* wetlands Congress meant to reach in the Section 404 permit program. At one time or another, the debate has occupied all three branches of the federal government.

Wetlands, with a variety of physical characteristics, are found throughout the country. They are known in different regions as swamps, marshes, fens, potholes, playa lakes, or bogs. Although these places can differ greatly, they all have distinctive vegetative assemblages because of the wetness of the soil. Some wetland areas may be continuously inundated by water, while other areas may not be flooded at all. In coastal areas, flooding may occur on a daily basis as tides rise and fall.

Riverside Bayview Homes

The Supreme Court's first foray into the Section 404 jurisdictional quagmire came in 1985, in *Riverside Bayview Homes, Inc. v. United States.*[12] There, the Court unanimously upheld as reasonable the Corps' extension of its Section 404 jurisdiction to "adjacent wetlands"—as one component of the agency's definition of "waters of the United States."[13] Under the Corps regulations, adjacent wetlands are wetlands adjacent to any non-wetland waterbody that constitutes a water of the United States—such as navigable bodies of water or interstate waters, or their tributaries. The Court reasoned that the water-quality objectives of the CWA were broad and sensitive to the fact that water moves in hydrologic cycles. Due to the frequent difficulties in defining where water ends and land begins, the Court could not say that the Corps' conclusion that adjacent wetlands are inseparably bound up with "waters of the United States" was unreasonable, particularly given the deference owed by courts to the Corps' and EPA's ecological expertise. Also persuasive was the fact that in considering the 1977 amendments to the CWA, Congress vigorously debated but ultimately rejected amendments that would have narrowed the Corps' asserted jurisdiction under Section 404.

SWANCC

In 2001, the Court returned to the geographic reach of Section 404. The decision in *Solid Waste Agency of Northern Cook County v. U.S. Army Corps of Engineers* (*SWANCC*)[14] directly involved the "isolated waters" component of the Corps' definition of "waters of the United States,"[15] rather than the "adjacent wetlands" component at issue in *Riverside Bayview Homes*. "Isolated waters," in CWA parlance (the regulations don't actually use the phrase), are waters that are not traditional navigable waters, are not interstate, are not tributaries of the foregoing, and are not hydrologically connected to navigable or interstate waters or their tributaries—but whose "use, degradation, or destruction [nonetheless] could affect interstate commerce."[16] Illustrative examples listed in the regulations include "intrastate lakes, rivers, streams (including intermittent streams), mudflats, sandflats, *wetlands*, sloughs, [or] prairie potholes"[17] with an interstate commerce nexus, or connection. The issue before the Court was whether "waters of the United States" is broad enough to embrace the Corps' assertion of jurisdiction over such "isolated waters" purely on the ground that they are or might be used by migratory birds that cross state lines—known as the Migratory Bird Rule.

In a 5-4 ruling, the Court held that the Migratory Bird Rule was not authorized by the CWA. The decision's rationale was much broader, however, appearing to preclude federal assertion of 404 jurisdiction over isolated, nonnavigable, intrastate waters on *any* basis—indeed, over wetlands not adjacent to "open water."[18] This disparity between the Court's holding and its rationale occasioned considerable litigation in the lower courts, the majority of which opted for a narrow reading of *SWANCC*, hence a broad reading of remaining Corps jurisdiction under Section 404. Such uncertainties as to the Corps' isolated waters jurisdiction after *SWANCC* focused attention on the alternative bases in Corps regulations for asserting 404 jurisdiction—such as the existence of "adjacent wetlands." Neither the Corps of Engineers nor EPA, however, has modified its Section 404 regulations since *SWANCC*.[19]

The new spotlight on the concept of "adjacent wetlands" became the backdrop for the Supreme Court's *Rapanos* decision, the Court's second encounter with this phrase after *Riverside Bayview Homes.*

RAPANOS

Rapanos was actually a consolidation of two cases, Rapanos and Carabell, on appeal from the Sixth Circuit. Though both cases involved issues as to what constitutes "adjacent wetlands," the issues in each are different.

The Sixth Circuit Decisions

Rapanos in the Sixth Circuit involved the Corps' assertion of 404 jurisdiction over a wetland adjacent to a tributary (man-made ditch) that ultimately flowed, miles later, into a traditional navigable water. As in Riverside Bayview, the issue was the Corps' jurisdiction under the "adjacent wetlands" component of its regulations defining "waters of the United States." In particular, plaintiffs argued that SWANCC did more than throw out the Migratory Bird Rule; it also barred Section 404 regulation of wetlands that do not physically abut a traditional navigable water.

In ruling that Section 404 reached the Rapanos's wetlands, the Sixth Circuit held that immediate adjacency of the wetland to a traditional navigable water is not required. Rather, what is needed is a "significant nexus"—a ubiquitous phrase in Section 404 court decisions lifted from SWANCC's explanation of Riverside Bayview[20]—between the wetlands and traditional navigable waters. "Significant nexus," in turn, can be satisfied by the presence of a "hydrological connection." Thus, the fact that the Rapanos's wetlands had surface water connections to nearby tributaries of traditional navigable waters was sufficient for Section 404 jurisdiction. Nor did it seem to matter to the court that the hydrological connection to traditional navigable waters was, for at least one of the Rapanos wetlands, distant—surface waters from this wetland flow into a man-made drain immediately north of the site, which empties into a creek, which flows into a navigable river. According to the record, this wetland is between 11 and 20 miles from the nearest navigable-in-fact water. In ruling that a surface water connection to a tributary of a navigable water was enough, the circuit aligned itself with the large majority of appellate courts to rule on this issue since SWANCC.

In its petition for certiorari to the Supreme Court, the Rapanoses asked whether the CWA's reach extends to nonnavigable wetlands "that do not even abut a navigable water."

Carabell in the Sixth Circuit involved the Corps' assertion of jurisdiction over a wetland adjacent to a tributary (man-made ditch) that ultimately flowed into traditional navigable waters—but the wetland was separated from the tributary by a manmade berm.

The Sixth Circuit held that "adjacent wetlands" jurisdiction existed under the Corps regulations, even though the wetland was separated from a tributary of "waters of the United States" by a four-foot-wide manmade berm that blocked immediate drainage of surface water from the parcel to the tributary.[21] The existence of the berm meant, critically, that unlike the wetlands in Rapanos, the wetlands here lacked any hydrological connection to navigable waters at all. Parenthetically, the fact that the "tributary" was merely a man-made ditch (which emptied into a creek, which flowed into a navigable lake) did not appear to be an issue in the case, as it was in Rapanos. Finally, the court endorsed the view of the majority of courts addressing the question that SWANCC spoke only to the Corps' "isolated waters" jurisdiction; it did not narrow the agency's "adjacent wetlands" authority involved here and broadly construed in Riverside Bayview.

In its petition for certiorari, the Carabells asked whether Section 404 extends to "wetlands that are hydrologically isolated from any of the 'waters of the United States.'"

The Supreme Court Decision

For many who had waited so long to have "waters of the United States" clarified, the *Rapanos* decision (addressing the Sixth Circuit decisions in both *Rapanos* and *Carabell*) was a disappointment. In three major opinions, the Court split 4-1-4 as to whether the Corps' assertions of 404 jurisdiction in the two cases before it comported with the CWA—that is, involved "waters of the United States." Justice Scalia wrote a four-Justice plurality opinion, ruling that the Corps had overreached and thus the Sixth Circuit decisions must be vacated and remanded for further proceedings applying the plurality's rule. Justice Kennedy, in a lone concurrence, also disagreed with the Corps' interpretation of the CWA, but would have applied a different approach than the plurality. He supplied the fifth vote supporting the vacation and remand, making that the judgment of the Court. (Five votes is a majority on the

Supreme Court.) Finally, Justice Stevens wrote a four-Justice dissent upholding the Corps' reading of its jurisdiction. Accordingly, he would have affirmed the decisions below.[22]

The problem is that no single rationale in these three opinions commands the support of a majority of the Justices. Thus, lower courts addressing challenges to Corps 404 jurisdiction since *Rapanos* have struggled with what rule of decision to extract from the decision. Does the Scalia plurality decision control? Or does the Kennedy concurrence provide the test? Or is satisfying either of these adequate to support jurisdiction?

Justice Scalia's plurality opinion asserts what is probably the narrowest view of 404 jurisdiction in the three major opinions, at least in most circumstances. His opening paragraphs set the tone by describing the substantial costs of applying for 404 permits, and the "immense expansion of federal regulation of land use that has occurred under the Clean Water Act."[23] This critical tone continues with the opinion's description of how the lower courts, "[e]ven after *SWANCC*," have continued to uphold the "sweeping" assertions of jurisdiction by the Corps over tributaries and adjacent wetlands.[24]

Justice Scalia goes on to construe "waters" in "waters of the United States" to mean only *relatively permanent, standing or flowing bodies of water*, such as streams, rivers, lakes, and other bodies of water "forming geographic features."[25] This definition leads him to exclude "channels containing merely intermittent or ephemeral flow."[26] Wetlands, our topic here, are included as "waters of the United States"—that is, are "adjacent" in the Corps' language—only when they have a *"continuous surface connection"* to bodies that are "waters of the United States" in their own right. By contrast, wetlands with only an intermittent, physically remote hydrological connection to "waters of the United States" are not covered by Section 404, according to the Scalia opinion.

Importantly, the plurality sought to calm concerns that a narrow reading of Section 404 would eviscerate other sections of the CWA, particularly the point-source permitting program under Section 402 that is the heart of the act. That section, the plurality explained, does not require that the point source discharge *directly* into a jurisdictional water. It is enough that the discharged pollutant is likely to ultimately be carried downstream to such a jurisdictional water. Thus, unlike with Section 404, discharges into non-covered waters could still be regulated.

Justice Kennedy's concurring opinion, in contrast to the absolute rules proposed by the plurality, offers a case-by-case test. He picks up on the "significant nexus" test used by the Sixth Circuit and many other courts—but while the lower courts defined significant nexus as having a *hydrological connection* with traditional navigable waters,[27] Justice Kennedy used an ambiguous *ecological* test.[28] A wetland, he declared, has the requisite significant nexus if, alone or in combination with similarly situated lands in the region, it significantly affects the chemical, physical, and biological integrity of traditional navigable waters.[29] These ecological functions include flood retention, pollutant trapping, and filtration. Under Kennedy's opinion, the waters that perform these functions may be intermittent or ephemeral, and they need not have a surface hydrological connection to other waters. When, in contrast, their effects on water quality are speculative or insubstantial, the wetland is beyond Section 404's reach.[30]

This formulation, Justice Kennedy explained, allows that when the Corps seeks to regulate wetlands adjacent to *navigable-in-fact* waters, adjacency is enough for jurisdiction. In contrast, for wetlands sought to be regulated based on adjacency to *non-navigable tributaries*, a significant nexus must be shown on a case-by-case basis. Importantly, however, the Justice did allow that the Corps might adopt regulations at some point declaring certain categories of wetlands to have a significant nexus per se, obviating the case-by-case approach for those wetlands.

Each of the foregoing views, the plurality's and Justice Kennedy's, rejects the hitherto prevailing view that any hydrological connection to a traditionally navigable water, no matter how distant, is sufficient for coverage. This "any hydrological connection" test had been a key element of the United States' assertions of "adjacent wetlands" jurisdiction.

The four dissenters found the Corps' assertion of jurisdiction reasonable in both cases. The Court's earlier decision in *Riverside Bayview*, the dissenters argue, was not confined to wetlands having continuous surface flow with traditional navigable waters or their tributaries. Rather it had endorsed jurisdiction over non-isolated wetlands generally, without case-by-case analysis. The plurality's concerns about the costs of applying for a permit, they continued, are more properly addressed to Congress, not to a court.

LEGAL ANALYSIS OF *RAPANOS*

The jurisdictional questions raised by Rapanos and Carabell presented the Supreme Court with a "perfect storm" of hot-button issues. First, there is the federalism matter: Where do CWA Section 404 and the Constitution's Commerce Clause draw the line between federal and state authority over wetlands? Second, there are property rights concerns. Some 75% of jurisdictional wetlands in the lower 48 states are on private property, with the result that protests from property owners denied Section 404 permits (or subjected to unacceptable conditions on same) are often heard— sometimes in the courts through Fifth Amendment takings suits. Third, Rapanos and Carabell have pervasive significance within the CWA itself, since "waters of the United States" governs not only the Section 404 wetlands permitting program, but also multiple other provisions and requirements of that law (see discussion below under "Policy Implications"). In addition, the Corps' broad reading of its jurisdiction created novel semantics (such as viewing dry arroyos as "waters," and manmade ditches as "tributaries") that Justices inclined to more literal readings of statutory language would have a hard time accepting.

It was not surprising in light of the above themes that the Justices split as they did: the four more "conservative" Justices rejecting the Corps' expansive view of its adjacent wetland jurisdiction, the four "liberal/moderates" upholding it, and Justice Kennedy coming down in between (as he often does) with a case-by-case test, at least until the Corps adopts new rules. The question, as noted earlier, is what rule of decision the lower courts will discern in Rapanos, with its absence of a majority rationale, for use in future cases. In practice, courts often look for common approaches supported by a majority of the Justices, looking both to the views of plurality Justices (supporting the judgment of the court in the case) and those of the dissenters (who do not support the judgment).

Thus far, lower courts applying Rapanos have drawn different tests from the decision, as was predicted based on its fractured nature. Nine of the thirteen federal circuits have ruled so far, an indication of the frequency with which CWA jurisdictional questions arise.[31] Two federal circuits held that the Kennedy "significant nexus" test alone controls;[32] two applied the Kennedy test but reserve for another day the question whether the plurality test as well is valid;[33] three accepted Justice Stevens's suggestion that a wetland satisfying either the Kennedy or plurality tests is jurisdictional;[34] and two avoided the issue altogether by finding that the Kennedy test and plurality test were both satisfied by the particular wetland in the case.[35] (See Figure A-1 in the Appendix to this report.) No circuit decision has opted for the plurality test alone. As the footnotes below show, the Supreme Court has declined to review every one of these circuit decisions where a petition for certiorari has been filed. The likely reason for these consistent denials is that with no change in the Justices since Rapanos that is likely to make a difference in their voting pattern, the Court may see little point to taking another case in the area.

District court decisions, at least the reported ones, seem to all follow either the Kennedy test alone or the Kennedy-or-plurality test view.[36] As with the appellate decisions, there appears to be no reported district-court decision squarely holding that the plurality test alone governs.[37]

To a considerable extent, the court decisions turn on how the courts read Supreme Court guidance on what rule of law may be inferred from decisions of the Court in which no rationale commands the support of five or more Justices. The United States, for its part, has consistently taken the Kennedy-or-plurality position in litigation, as it did in congressional testimony soon after the Rapanos decision[38] and in the Corps/EPA guidance on interpreting Rapanos (discussed below).

In the wake of Rapanos, several factors arguably put pressure on the Corps and EPA to do a rulemaking on the scope of "adjacent wetlands" permitting jurisdiction under the CWA (assuming Congress does not act). One is the fact that no fewer than three of the opinions in Rapanos urged the agencies to do so.[39] A second factor is the labor-intensive nature (and vagueness) of the Kennedy case-by-case approach, requiring empirical study of each wetland near a non-navigable tributary. The third factor is the divergence of the lower courts as to the rule to be applied after Rapanos. One can be confident, however, that anything the Corps and EPA promulgate will find its way into the courts. The agencies stated in guidance issued in 2008 that "further consideration of jurisdictional issues, including clarification and definition of key terminology, may be appropriate in the future, either through issuance of additional guidance or through rulemaking."[40]

All of the Rapanos opinions that mention SWANCC seem to accept, without discussion, that SWANCC eliminates jurisdictional coverage of all isolated, intrastate, nonnavigable waters—not just those isolated, intrastate, nonnavigable waters where the sole basis for asserting jurisdiction was the Migratory Bird Rule. Most lower court decisions to broach this issue had adopted the latter narrower reading of SWANCC. Thus, although only adjacent wetlands were directly involved in Rapanos, there may be impacts on the Corps' authority over isolated, intrastate, nonnavigable waters also.

Finally, although both petitions for certiorari in Rapanos raised the Commerce Clause issue, the decision in Rapanos, as expected, was on purely statutory grounds. The plurality, however, did assert that the Corps view of its adjacent wetlands jurisdiction "stretches the outer limits of Congress' commerce power,"[41] using this as one of several reasons for adopting a narrow reading of that jurisdiction. This plurality view is plainly relevant to congressional bills seeking to overturn SWANCC and Rapanos by amending the CWA to explicitly assert jurisdiction over waters to the fullest extent consistent with the Constitution (see "Legislative Consideration").

THE EPA/CORPS GUIDANCE ON *RAPANOS*

On December 2, 2008, EPA and the Corps of Engineers issued guidance to their field offices on how *Rapanos* should be interpreted in jurisdictional determinations, agency enforcement actions, and other agency actions. The guidance does not impose legally binding requirements on EPA or the Corps, and may not apply in a particular circumstance.

The Corps and EPA had previously issued other guidance, attempting to clarify the Court's rulings on the jurisdictional issues discussed here. Following the *Rapanos* ruling, the agencies first issued informal guidance in 2006; it was replaced by formal guidance in June 2007. The December 2008 guidance made limited changes to the 2007 guidance and supersedes it.[42] The 2008 revisions were made after review of public comments on the 2007 guidance and evaluation of the agencies' own implementation of the guidance. However, they noted in 2008, "The agencies will continue to monitor implementation of the Rapanos Guidance and, as we gain experience, consider appropriate opportunities to provide additional guidance or to initiate rulemaking."[43] This statement encouraged those who argue that revised regulations are needed to resolve lingering interpretive questions. Others contend that a legislative remedy is required. The potential for litigation to challenge the guidance itself is unclear.

The 2008 guidance adopts the Kennedy-test-or-plurality-test view, with the addition of agency interpretation of vague phrases in the Kennedy and plurality opinions. It has three parts, addressing waters that are (1) categorically within the scope of "waters of the United States"; (2) within "waters of the United States" or not, on a case-by-case basis; or (3) categorically outside the scope of "waters of the United States."

1) Waters categorically labeled "waters of the United States"—that is, without a case-by-case inquiry into whether there is a "significant nexus" with a traditional navigable water—are first, traditional navigable waters[44] and their adjacent wetlands. Under this test, the existence of a continuous surface connection, as demanded by the

plurality, but not Kennedy or the dissenters, is required to establish adjacency. Categorical "waters of the United States" also include non-navigable tributaries of traditional navigable waters, where such tributaries are "relatively permanent waters" (i.e., typically flowing year-round or at least seasonally) and adjacent wetlands with a continuous surface connection to such tributaries (not separated by uplands, berms, etc.). The 2008 guidance clarifies that a wetland is adjacent if it has an unbroken hydrologic connection to jurisdictional waters, or is separated from those waters by a berm or similar feature, or if it is in reasonably close proximity to a jurisdictional water.

2) Waterbodies that are "waters of the United States" on a case-by-case basis are those dependent on a finding of a "significant nexus" with a traditional navigable water, per the Kennedy concurrence. They include non-navigable tributaries that are not relatively permanent (such as intermittent and ephemeral streams) and their adjacent wetlands, and wetlands adjacent to but that do not directly abut a relatively permanent non-navigable tributary. The 2008 guidance states that, in making the site- and fact-specific analysis to determine "significant nexus," the agencies will evaluate hydrology (e.g., proximity to traditional navigable waters), ecologic factors (e.g., ability of wetlands to trap and filter pollutants or store flood waters), and flow characteristics (flow and functions of the tributary and adjacent wetlands). The purpose of these tests is to demonstrate a connection and the role of a tributary and any adjacent wetlands in protecting the chemical, physical, and biological integrity of downstream traditional navigable waters.
3) Waterbodies not generally considered "waters of the United States" are swales or erosional features (e.g., gullies) and ditches (including roadside ditches) excavated wholly in and draining only uplands, and that do not carry a relatively permanent flow of water. The agencies generally will not assert jurisdiction over these waterbodies.

To provide greater transparency of decisionmaking, the 2007 guidance required the Corps and EPA to be more thorough in documenting their jurisdictional determinations than in the past. To meet this requirement, which continues under the 2008 guidance, the Corps uses a standardized documentation form and posts results on District websites.[45] These steps respond to criticism, such as detailed in a GAO report, that Corps district offices have used differing practices in making jurisdictional determinations and that few districts made their documentation public.[46]

Overall, stakeholder groups, including industry, environmental advocates, and states, expressed disappointment or frustration with the 2007 guidance and the 2008 revision—some believing that it goes too far in narrowing protection of wetlands and U.S. waters, others believing that it does not go far enough. Generally, most agree that implementing the "significant nexus" test is especially difficult, because the guidance is complicated and vague. Industry groups said that because there are no clear guideposts on this key point, the guidance fails to provide the certainty desired by the regulated community. Environmentalists said that the "significant nexus" test in the guidance is more limited than the standard described by Justice Kennedy, because although his opinion recognizes the impact of losing wetlands or other small tributaries on large waters,[47] the guidance does not account for cumulative effects. In evaluating "significant nexus," the guidance focuses only on a tributary and wetlands adjacent to that tributary. The 2008 revised guidance did not modify the 2007 guidance with respect to evaluating "significant nexus." Overall, industry groups reportedly believe that the 2008 revisions provide modest improvement over the earlier guidance and could make some jurisdictional determinations easier, but environmental advocates assert that the guidance substantially limits the waters that will be protected by the Clean Water Act.[48]

One issue that has caused considerable confusion following the *Rapanos* ruling concerns CWA jurisdiction over wetlands not immediately adjacent to traditional navigable waters—including how jurisdiction will be applied in states within the Fourth, Seventh, Ninth, and Eleventh Circuits, where appellate courts have subsequently said that the Kennedy test alone is controlling. As noted, the 2008 guidance adds some clarification about determining adjacency, but continuing questions about this and other interpretive issues are possible.

Since the initial 2007 guidance was issued, the CWA permitting process has become more complex and is slower, according to many participants and observers. A revealing EPA memorandum in March 2008 reports that since July 2006 (shortly after *Rapanos* was decided), the *Rapanos* ruling or the 2007 guidance negatively affected approximately 500 enforcement cases, a "significant portion" of the CWA enforcement docket.[49] The breakdown identified in the EPA memo is 304 instances in which EPA regions decided not to pursue formal enforcement because of jurisdictional uncertainty, 147 instances where the enforcement priority of a case was lowered due to jurisdictional concerns, and 61 cases where lack of CWA jurisdiction has been asserted as an affirmative defense in an enforcement case. The memorandum goes on to say the greatest burden on the government results from "the implied presumption of non-jurisdiction [in the plurality test] for the most common types of waters in our country, intermittent and ephemeral tributaries to traditionally navigable waters and headwater wetlands. This presumptive exclusion can only be overcome by a resource-intensive 'significant nexus analysis' [the Kennedy test] described in the Guidance." The memorandum recommended "a few targeted revisions" to the guidance that OECA believes would address these issues, while remaining consistent with the *Rapanos* decision. For example, it recommended revising the guidance to incorporate Justice Kennedy's suggestions that, when evaluating jurisdiction, it is appropriate to consider wetlands either alone or in combination with other similarly situated lands in the region. The 2008 revised guidance did not address this recommendation.

Echoing the EPA memorandum, a Corps official stated at a May 2008 conference that making jurisdictional determinations is 8 to 10 times more resource-intensive for Corps staff who must consider a multitude of factors to determine what constitutes a "significant nexus." Representatives of developers and environmental advocates concurred that the joint guidance exacerbates permitting delays.[50] Concern about this reported impact on CWA enforcement drew the attention of two House committee chairmen in 2008. Their staffs reviewed a large number of EPA and Corps documents and concluded that there had been a significant decline in CWA inspections, investigations, and enforcement actions since the *Rapanos* ruling and the 2007 guidance.[51]

2011 Proposed Revised Guidance

At the end of 2010, the Obama Administration weighed into the CWA jurisdiction debate as EPA and the Corps drafted new joint agency guidance to clarify regulatory jurisdiction over U.S. waters and wetlands and to replace the agencies' 2008 guidance.

The document underwent several months of interagency review before release in April 2011 in the form of proposed revised guidance, subject to public comment until July 1, 2011. In releasing the proposal, the agencies said that once finalized, the revised guidance would supersede the 2008 guidance; until then, the existing guidance remains in effect. Also, the agencies said that after issuance of final guidance, they expected to propose revisions to regulations to further clarify which waters are subject to CWA jurisdiction, consistent with the Supreme Court's rulings.[52] As noted previously, three of the *Rapanos* opinions had argued for such a rulemaking.[53]

Status of the 2011 Proposed Guidance

As described below (see "Policy Implications"), in September 2013, the 2011 proposed guidance was withdrawn, prior to issuance in final form, and EPA and the Corps drafted a rule to clarify regulatory jurisdiction of the CWA. The draft rule is undergoing interagency review at the Office of Management and Budget (OMB). The following portion of this report discusses the proposed guidance. Although it has now been withdrawn, interest in the 2011 proposal remains high, particularly as an indication of policy that may be contained in the draft rule.

Like the 2008 guidance, the 2011 revisions proposed to adopt the Kennedy-test-or-plurality-test view of *Rapanos*. However, the agencies believed that a wider evaluation of jurisdiction is possible than the 2008 guidance suggests, stating, "after careful review of these opinions, the agencies concluded that previous guidance did not make full use of the authority provided by the CWA to include waters within the scope of the Act, as interpreted by the Court."[54] EPA and the Corps acknowledged that, compared with the existing guidance, the proposed revisions were likely to increase the number of waters identified as protected by the CWA.

> The agencies expect, based on relevant science and recent field experience, that under the understandings stated in this draft guidance, the extent of waters over which the agencies assert jurisdiction under the CWA will increase compared to the extent of waters over which jurisdiction has been asserted under existing guidance, though certainly not to the full extent that it was typically asserted prior to the Supreme Court decisions in *SWANCC* and *Rapanos*.[55]

EPA and Corps officials believed that the likely increase in jurisdictional waters would occur because, in their view, the existing guidance under-protects waters and has created uncertainty about many gray areas of jurisdiction, which the revised guidance was intended to clarify. Officials believed that additional acreage likely to be jurisdictional would not be large, but they did not estimate how much expansion would occur. Certain types of aquatic resources were likely to benefit, because they generally are non-jurisdictional under the existing guidance (for example, some prairie potholes). Although there still would be need for case-by-case determination of "significant nexus" waters (i.e., to demonstrate potential hydrologic or ecological connections to jurisdictional waters), the proposed revisions were intended to make such evaluations clearer.

The proposed revisions were built on the existing guidance with modifications that the agencies believed were consistent with the CWA, the Court's rulings, and science. According to EPA and the Corps, the guidance was focused on protection of smaller waters that feed into larger ones, to keep downstream water safe from upstream pollutants. The focus was also on reaffirming protection for wetlands that filter pollution and store water in order to help keep communities safe from floods. Two key changes in the proposed revisions, discussed below, were (1) inclusion of all interstate waters in those that are categorically labeled "waters of the United States," and (2) an expanded characterization of "adjacency" for waters and wetlands that must demonstrate a significant nexus to a jurisdictional water.

Like the existing guidance, the 2011 proposed revisions interpreted phrases in the plurality and Kennedy opinions in order to clarify waters that (1) are categorically within the scope of "waters of the United States;" (2) are "waters of the United States" if they meet a case-by-case test of "significant nexus" to a jurisdictional water; or (3) are generally outside the scope of "waters of the United States."

(1) Waters categorically labeled "waters of the United States" were those that are traditional navigable waters, wetlands adjacent to traditionally navigable waters or interstate waters, non-navigable tributaries of traditional navigable waters or interstate waters that are relatively permanent (i.e., they meet the plurality standard), and wetlands that directly abut relatively permanent waters. Existing regulations define "adjacent" to mean bordering, contiguous, or neighboring. Regarding categorically protected waters, the proposed guidance made two changes compared to the existing guidance: (a) all interstate waters were considered categorically jurisdictional, whereas under the existing guidance, interstate waters are not mentioned and their treatment is unclear, and (b) the standard for non-navigable tributaries that are "relatively permanent" was modified. Under the 2008 guidance, "relatively permanent" means a water that typically flows year-round or has continuous flow at least seasonally (meaning, e.g., typically for three months). Under the proposed revisions, seasonal flow making a water relatively permanent meant that the water typically flows during the wet season of the region in which the water is located.

(2) Waters over which the agencies generally would assert jurisdiction were those that are not categorically jurisdictional but have "significant nexus" to a jurisdictional water. Under the Kennedy standard in *Rapanos*, waters have a "significant nexus" if, either alone or in combination with similarly situated waters in the region, they significantly affect the chemical, physical, or biological integrity of traditional navigable waters. The existing guidance says that the agencies will assert jurisdiction over non-navigable tributaries that are not relatively permanent and their adjacent wetlands, and over wetlands adjacent to but not directly abutting a relatively permanent tributary based on a fact-specific evaluation of significant nexus.

The 2008 guidance defines tributaries for the purpose of the "significant nexus" determination as a single stream reach of the same order.[56] It then limits "similarly situated" waters (described in the Kennedy standard) to a single stream reach or to wetlands that are adjacent to the same single stream reach. Aggregation of streams or stream reaches is not allowed under the 2008 guidance, and jurisdiction for tributaries under the "significant nexus" test is considered in isolation, that is, not together with other waters in the area.

The 2011 proposed guidance was broader and would allow watershed-wide aggregation for similarly situated wetlands and tributaries. Under the proposed guidance, a tributary would be jurisdictional if it is a tributary to a navigable-in-fact water or an interstate water and, alone or in combination with other tributaries in the watershed, has a significant nexus to such water. It essentially defined tributaries as those features that flow into another jurisdictional water and have a bed (the bottom of the channel) and bank, which is generally indicated by an ordinary high water mark.

Under the 2008 guidance, in evaluating significant nexus, EPA and the Corps can consider the flow characteristics (volume, duration, and frequency of flow) and ecological factors such as potential of the tributary to carry pollutants downstream to a traditional navigable water, or the potential of wetlands to trap and filter pollutants. The 2011 proposed guidance would allow consideration of other factors such as maintenance of habitat that provides spawning areas for species in downstream waters. It stated that all wetlands within a wetland mosaic (a landscape of wetlands and non-wetlands) should ordinarily be considered collectively when determining adjacency. As a result, wetlands likely to be considered jurisdictional under the revised guidance would be those that are adjacent to a newly identified traditional navigable water, or those that are adjacent to other jurisdictional non-wetland waters based on a more expansive "significant nexus" determination of adjacency.

Under the proposed revisions, so-called "other waters"[57] would require case-by-case evaluation and would be divided into two categories. First, physically proximate (see above) "other waters" that would satisfy the regulatory definition of "adjacent" if they were wetlands would be evaluated in the same manner as adjacent wetlands to determine significant nexus. Second, non-physically proximate "other waters" that do not meet the definition of "adjacent" in the proposed guidance (e.g., there is no demonstrable ecological interconnection to a jurisdictional waterbody) cannot be easily evaluated for significant nexus to jurisdictional waters. Thus the revised guidance proposed to continue the current practice of referring such waters to agency Headquarters for evaluation.

(3) Regarding waters that generally are not waters of the United States and over which the agencies will not assert jurisdiction, the existing guidance and 2011 proposed revisions were similar. Both would exclude geographic features such as swales, gullies, and ditches that are not tributaries or wetlands. The revised guidance also specifically identified a number of other examples of non-jurisdictional waters (e.g., waters that are excluded from coverage by statute or existing regulation; artificial lakes or ponds that are created by excavating and/or diking dry land and are used exclusively for purposes such as stock watering or irrigation; and artificially irrigated areas that would revert to upland should irrigation cease).

Release of the proposed revisions was accompanied by a preliminary economic analysis document prepared by EPA. It examined a range of indirect costs and benefits resulting from implementing guidance to clarify the scope of CWA jurisdiction. The analysis indicated that the majority of costs would result from incremental permitting costs and mitigation expenses incurred by entities seeking CWA Section 404 permits. Economic benefits also would result from water quality improvements such as protecting additional small streams and wetlands. EPA's analysis estimated that the benefits of implementing the proposed guidance would range from $162 million to $328 million annually, while the incremental costs would be between $87 million and $171 million. EPA acknowledged that valuing the benefits of the new guidance to wetlands and other waters poses many challenges, and the precision and accuracy of results were highly uncertain; nevertheless, EPA concluded that the analysis suggested that benefits were likely to justify costs.[58] Preparing an economic analysis to accompany the proposed guidance was a somewhat unusual step for EPA, likely reflecting anticipated significant interest in the new guidance. Economic analyses are typically developed to support formal regulatory proposals, rather than non-binding agency guidance.

Critical reaction to the proposed revisions began even before release of the document in April 2011. While the guidance was being developed and reviewed internally, press reports suggested that it would substantially increase waters subject to CWA regulation, raising concern among industry and some other groups that was confirmed when the proposed guidance was released.[59] Industry criticism focused on two issues: (1) the revised guidance would broaden the number and kinds of waters subject to regulation, in their view beyond what the CWA and the Supreme Court's rulings permit; and (2) government was attempting to effect policy change through nonbinding guidance that generally is not reviewable by courts. EPA and Corps officials responded that the guidance would not extend federal protection to any waters not historically protected under the Clean Water Act and would be fully consistent with the law, including decisions of the Supreme Court. Most state and local officials were supportive of clarifying the scope of CWAregulated waters, but some were concerned that expanding the CWA's scope could impose costs on states and localities as their own actions (e.g., transportation projects) become subject to new requirements. Environmental advocacy groups welcomed the new guidance, which would more clearly define U.S. waters that are subject to CWA protections but would not, they said, expand the reach of the law.

The proposed guidance drew congressional attention, as well, both before and after its release. Some Members wrote letters supporting issuance of new guidance to address the confusion resulting from the Supreme Court's rulings.[60] Others criticized the revised guidance as going beyond clarification and thus amounting to a *de facto* rule, instead of advisory guidelines.[61]

Legislative provisions to prohibit the agencies from funding activities related to revising the guidance were included in several appropriations bills in the 112th Congress, but none of these provisions was enacted. Similar provisions in 113th Congress appropriations bills also have not been enacted. Interest in legislation concerning the guidance also is evident with bills in the 113th Congress to prevent the agencies from finalizing the 2011 draft guidance (S. 861, S. 1006, S. 1514, and H.R. 1829). Other legislation would amend the CWA with a narrow definition of waters that are subject to the act's jurisdiction (S. 890 and H.R. 3377).

POLICY IMPLICATIONS

As with the legal questions, the policy questions associated with the Supreme Court cases—what *should be* the outer limit of CWA regulatory jurisdiction and what are the consequences of restricting that jurisdiction—also have challenged regulators, landowners and developers, and policymakers since passage of the act in 1972. The act prohibits the discharge of dredged or fill material into navigable waters without a permit, and it also prohibits discharges of pollutants from any point source to navigable waters without a permit. Disputes have centered on whether wetlands and other waters are "navigable waters," a legal term of art. The answer to this question is important, because it may determine the extent of federal CWA regulatory authority not only for the Section 404 program, but also for purposes of implementing other CWA programs. Critics of the Section 404 regulatory program, such as land developers and agriculture interests, argue that the Corps' wetlands program has gradually and illegally expanded its asserted jurisdiction since 1972. They want the Corps and EPA to give up jurisdiction over most non-navigable tributaries and allow other federal and state programs to fill whatever gap is created. Waters that are jurisdictional are subject to the multiple regulatory requirements of the CWA: standards, discharge limitations, permits, and enforcement. Non-jurisdictional waters, in contrast, do not have the federal legal protection of those requirements. The act has one definition of "navigable waters" that applies to the entire law. The definition applies to federal prohibition on discharges of pollutants (§301), requirements to obtain a permit prior to discharge (§§402 and 404), water quality standards and measures to attain them (§303), oil spill liability and oil spill prevention and control measures (§311), certification that federally permitted activities comply with state water quality standards (§401), and enforcement (§309). It impacts the Oil Pollution Act and other environmental laws, as well. For example, the reach of the Endangered Species Act (ESA) is affected, because that act's requirement for consultation by federal agencies over impacts on threatened or endangered species is triggered through the issuance of federal permits.[62] Thus, by removing the need for a CWA permit, a non-jurisdictional determination would eliminate ESA consultation, as well. As discussed above, the Scalia opinion in *Rapanos* concluded that a narrow interpretation of the Corps' 404 jurisdiction would not impact these other provisions, but many observers contend that the question is not fully resolved. EPA said that it might issue additional guidance concerning the effect of *Rapanos* on other CWA programs that use the common "waters of the United States" definition, but it has not done so. In March 2008, EPA officials reportedly asked states to assist in developing guidance to govern CWA jurisdiction decisions under Section 402, because of continuing uncertainty on the law's scope, especially in western states that have a preponderance of intermittent and ephemeral streams.[63] *SWANCC* found invalid the assertion of CWA jurisdiction over isolated, non-navigable intrastate waters solely on the basis of their use (or potential use) as habitat by migratory birds. Most of the post-*SWANCC* cases have instead addressed tributaries and adjacent wetlands, asking which of these have the "significant nexus" to navigable waters that *SWANCC* was interpreted to say is necessary to establish federal jurisdiction.

Wetlands are an important part of the total aquatic ecosystem, with many recognized functions and values, including water storage (mitigating the effects of floods and droughts), water purification and filtering, recreation, habitat for plants and animals, food production, and open space and aesthetic values. Functional values, both ecological and economic, at each wetland depend on its location, size, and relationship to adjacent land and water areas. To the layman, many of these values are more obvious for wetlands adjacent to large rivers and streams than they are for wetlands and small streams that are isolated in the landscape from other waters. Many of the functions and values of wetlands have been recognized only recently. Historically, many federal programs encouraged wetlands to be drained or altered because they were seen as having little value. Even today, while more federal laws either encourage wetland protection or regulate their modification, pressure exists to modify, drain, or develop wetlands for uses that some see as more economically beneficial.

While regulators and the regulated community debate the legal dimensions of federal jurisdiction, scientists contend that there are no discrete, scientifically supportable boundaries or criteria along the continuum of waters/wetlands to separate them into meaningful ecological or hydrological compartments. Numerous scientific studies define and describe the importance of the functions and values of wetlands, in support of their significant nexus to navigable waters.[64] In all but some very narrow instances, scientists say, terms such as "isolated waters" and "adjacent wetlands" are artificial legal or regulatory constructs, not valid scientific classifications. From this perspective, even waters and wetlands that lack a direct surface connection to navigable waters or that only flow intermittently are connected to the larger aquatic ecosystem via subsurface or overflow hydrologic connections. Wetland scientists believe that all such waters/wetlands are critical for protecting the integrity of waters, habitat, and wildlife downstream.

In *SWANCC*, the Supreme Court did not draw a bright line for purposes of determining the limits of federal jurisdiction (many wetland scientists do not believe that a bright line is possible, in any case). While the ruling reduced federal jurisdiction over some previously regulated wetlands, even more than a decade later it remains difficult to determine the precise effect of that decision. Many affected interests (states and the regulated community) contend that the 2003 guidance from the Corps and EPA did not adequately define the scope of regulated areas and wetlands affected by *SWANCC* and subsequent court rulings.[65] The Rapanoses and the Carabells had hoped that the Supreme Court would clarify the jurisdiction issue and that the Court would further narrow the program's geographic reach. Other interest groups disagreed with the petitioners' views on the issues, but also had hoped for clarity. Most say that the 4-1-4 ruling, in which the three main opinions did not agree on what constitutes "waters of the United States," did not bring the desired clarity of meaning in legal and policy terms. Estimates of the types of wetlands and amounts of acreage affected by *SWANCC, Rapanos*, and subsequent lower court rulings depend on interpretation of the cases and on assumptions about defining key terms such as "adjacent," "tributary," and "significant nexus." Because in its regulations before *SWANCC* the Corps had broadly defined "waters of the United States," including those encompassed by the Migratory Bird Rule, nearly all U.S. wetlands and waters were subject to CWA jurisdiction, since practically all are used to a greater or lesser extent by migratory birds.[66] Depending on how key terms are defined, reduced federal jurisdiction could affect very small or very large categories of waters and wetlands. Reflecting the uncertainties about how broadly or narrowly *SWANCC* would be interpreted, one estimate made after that decision found that the possible changes in jurisdiction could range from 20% to 80% of the nation's total estimated 100 million acres of wetlands.[67] Following the *Rapanos* decision, concern was expressed particularly about that ruling's impacts in arid and semi-arid western states to exclude intermittent or ephemeral streams and adjacent wetlands and riparian areas from CWA jurisdiction. A reduction in CWA jurisdiction affects implementation of the 404 and possibly other CWA programs. Early in 2006, EPA estimated conservatively that the extent of non-navigable tributaries and adjacent wetlands that could be affected by the narrow reading of the Clean Water Act that was advocated by the *Rapanos* and *Carabell* petitioners was up to 59% of the total length of streams in the United States, excluding Alaska. EPA also estimated that 34% of industrial and municipal dischargers that are subject to CWA Section 402 permits are located on these stream segments and that public drinking water systems which use intakes on these segments provide drinking water to over 110 million people.[68] Because there is no national database of non-navigable tributaries, EPA analyzed surrogate data on the linear extent of intermittent/ephemeral streams and stream segments that lie at the head of tributary systems and have no other streams flowing into them. Some estimate that the smallest, or headwater, first- and second-order streams represent more than 75% of the nation's stream network. These streams, if left unprotected by expansive interpretation of the Court's rulings, are at risk from a variety of polluting activities due to urbanization, construction, and channelization for flood control purposes.[69] As noted, the uncertainties resulting from the *Rapanos* decision led to widespread anticipation that the Corps and EPA would take administrative action to clarify how they interpret the ruling and its impact on waters that are protected by the Clean Water Act. Corps and EPA officials testified before a Senate subcommittee in August 2006 that the agencies were working on substantive interpretive guidance to clarify CWA jurisdiction in light of the decision[70]—the guidance that was eventually released in June 2007 and was revised in December 2008. While many observers acknowledged that guidance is useful, some argued that the Corps must initiate a rulemaking to revise its regulations—especially since three Justices in some fashion suggested one. This view is, in fact, widely held by many diverse stakeholders—environmental groups, industry, and states—who disagree on the substance of the guidance proposed by EPA and the Corps in April 2011. The Administration's schedule for either final guidance or new regulations was uncertain until recently. Final guidance was submitted to the White House Office of Management and Budget (OMB) for review in February 2012, but it was not released. In September 2013, EPA and the Corps announced that the guidance document had been withdrawn (a listing for the guidance was removed from OMB's list at http://www.reginfo.gov of all regulations under active review), and at the same time, the agencies submitted a draft regulation to OMB for review. The substance of this proposal, and when it might be proposed, are unknown for now. New regulations may clarify many current questions, but they are unlikely to please all of the competing interests, as one environmental advocate observed.

> However, a rulemaking would only benefit wetlands if it did not reduce the jurisdiction offered by current regulations and if the Administration remained faithful to sound science. If politics were to trump science in the rulemaking process, the likelihood of such a protective rule would not be promising. Also, rules are subject to legal

challenge and can be tied up in court for years before they are implemented.[71]

Also in September, EPA released a draft report that reviews and synthesizes the peer-reviewed scientific literature on the connectivity or isolation of streams and wetlands relative to large water bodies such as rivers, lakes, estuaries, and oceans. The purpose of the review, according to EPA, is to summarize current understanding about these connections, the factors that influence them, and mechanisms by which connected waters affect the function or condition of downstream waters.[72] The focus of the report is on small or temporary non-tidal streams, wetlands, and open waters. Based on the reviewed literature, it makes certain findings.

- All tributary streams, including perennial, intermittent, and ephemeral streams, are physically, chemically, and biologically connected to downstream rivers.
- Wetlands and open waters in riparian areas and floodplains also are physically, chemically, and biologically connected with rivers and serve an important role in the integrity of downstream waters. In these types of wetlands, water-borne materials can be transported from the wetland to the river network and vice versa (e.g., water from a stream flows into and affects the wetland).
- Wetlands and open waters where water only flows from the wetland to a river network, such as many prairie potholes, vernal pools, and playa lakes, occur on a gradient of connectivity, making it difficult to generalize about their effects on downstream waters from the currently available literature.

EPA has asked its Science Advisory Board (SAB) to review the draft report and to comment on whether its conclusions and findings are supported by the available science. The SAB review, which includes public meetings in mid-December, will presumably influence a final report at some future time. Earlier versions of the science report, in 2011, received interagency and external peer review, but were not released for public or SAB comment. The draft report is not intended as a policy document—it does not reference either the Scalia plurality or Kennedy tests in *Rapanos*, nor does it address legal standards for CWA jurisdiction. Nevertheless, EPA and the Corps say that the draft rule now at OMB takes into consideration the latest peer-reviewed science reflected in the draft science report. The report, when finalized, will provide a scientific basis needed to clarify CWA jurisdiction, according to EPA.[73] Some stakeholders have expressed concern that the scientific study could allow the agencies to assert jurisdiction in a blanket fashion over ephemeral and intermittent streams, rather than subjecting them to case-by-case determination of a "significant nexus" to downstream navigable waters.[74]

Filling the Gaps

Whatever gaps in wetland regulation result from reduced federal jurisdiction arguably could be filled, at least in part, by other federal or state and local programs and actions. For example, some assert that wetland restoration and creation programs, such as the Wetlands Reserve Program and the Coastal Wetlands Restoration Program, or private conservation efforts can provide protection, even if the wetland is no longer jurisdictional under federal law.[75] However, others respond that such programs are likely to be incomplete in filling gaps, since they apply primarily to rural areas and do not apply to the one-third of the nation's lands in federal ownership. Moreover, they were never intended to be a seamless group that would fill all possible gaps.

SWANCC, Rapanos, and the subsequent lower court decisions also highlight the role of states in protecting waters not addressed by federal law. From the states' perspective, the federal Section 404 program provides the basis for a consistent national approach to wetlands protection. But if a larger portion of wetlands are no longer jurisdictional, they say, it can be argued that the Section 404 program no longer provides a baseline for consistent, minimum standards to regulate wetlands. None of these court rulings prevents states from protecting non-jurisdictional waters through legislative or administrative action, but few states have done so. Prior to *SWANCC*, 15 states had programs that regulate isolated freshwater wetlands to some degree, but state officials acknowledge that these programs vary substantially from some that are comprehensive in scope to others that are limited by wetland size or have exemptions for agriculture and other activities.[76] Since 2001, a few states have passed new legislation or updated water quality regulations; the issue remains under consideration in several states, where competing proposals that are viewed by some as strengthening and by others as weakening wetland protection have been debated.[77]

Although some states have authorities to regulate waters of their state, their ability to regulate effectively may be compromised, because state rules often are tied to federal definitions. The gap produced by reduced federal jurisdiction is most evident in the 32 states that have no independent wetlands programs and that typically have relied on CWA Section 401 water quality certification procedures to protect wetlands. Pursuant to Section 401, applicants for a federal permit must obtain a state certification that the project will comply with state water quality standards. Consequently, by conditioning certification, states have the ability to affect the federal permit and to exercise some regulatory control over wetlands without the expense of establishing independent state programs. However, as described previously, diminished CWA jurisdiction which affects the Section 404 program also limits the reach of other CWA programs, including Section 401.

Analysts familiar with the political and fiscal environments of states believe that most states are either reluctant or unable "to step boldly into the breach in federal wetlands protection.... The Corps and the U.S. Environmental Protection Agency, not to mention Congress, have little cause to rely on the notion that states will effectively backstop federal protection for isolated wetlands."[78] Many states are barred from enacting laws more stringent than federal rules, or are reluctant to take action, due to budgetary and resource concerns, as well as apprehension that regulation will be judged to involve "taking" of private property and require compensation.

Legislative Consideration

Some argue that what is needed—regardless of interpretive guidance or rulemaking by the Corps and EPA—is legislative action to affirm Congress's intention regarding CWA jurisdiction. Others contend that, although the *Rapanos* decision did not resolve the issues, it also did not substantially affect Congress's willingness or interest in acting on issues that have been pending for several years without congressional action. Related to this is the view that, because the current questions are highly technical in nature, a simple fix may not address the problem, or may create others, such as impacting rights that the CWA reserves to states. In the 109th Congress, bills were introduced to address the CWA jurisdictional issues in different ways, but Congress took no action. One proposal (the Clean Water Authority Restoration Act of 2005) would have provided a broad statutory definition of "waters of the United States"; would have clarified that the CWA is intended to protect U.S. waters from pollution, not just maintain their navigability; and would have included a set of findings to assert constitutional authority over waters and wetlands. Other legislation intended to restrict regulatory jurisdiction also was introduced (the

Federal Wetlands Jurisdiction Act of 2005). It would have narrowed the statutory definition of "navigable waters" and defined certain isolated wetlands that are not adjacent to navigable waters, or non-navigable tributaries and other areas (such as waters connected to jurisdictional waters by ephemeral waters, ditches or pipelines), as not being subject to federal regulatory jurisdiction.

Legislation similar to the Clean Water Authority Restoration Act of 2005 was introduced in the 110th Congress (H.R. 2421 and S. 1870, a slightly different bill). The House Transportation and Infrastructure Committee held hearings on H.R. 2421 and related jurisdictional issues in July 2007, and a third hearing in April 2008. The Senate Environment and Public Works Committee held a non-legislative hearing on issues related to the *Rapanos* and *SWANCC* rulings in December 2007, and a legislative hearing on S. 1870 in April 2008.

Proponents of legislation contend that Congress must clarify the important issues left unsettled by the Supreme Court's 2001 and 2006 rulings and by the Corps/EPA guidance. Bill sponsors argued that the legislation would "reaffirm" what Congress intended when the CWA was enacted in 1972 and what EPA and the Corps had subsequently been practicing until recently, in terms of CWA jurisdiction. However, critics asserted that by making *activities* that affect waters of the United States (in addition to discharges) subject to the CWA's jurisdiction, the legislation would expand federal authority, and thus would have consequences that are likely to increase confusion, rather than settle it. Critics questioned the constitutionality of the bill, arguing that, by including all non-navigable waters in the jurisdiction of the CWA, it would exceed the limits of Congress's authority under the Commerce Clause. Supporters contended that the legislation is properly grounded in Congress's commerce power. The Bush Administration did not take a position on any legislation to clarify the scope of "waters of the United States" protected under the CWA. Congressional attention resumed in the 111th Congress, especially after statements by Obama Administration officials supporting the need for legislative clarification of these issues. In May 2009, the heads of EPA, the Corps, the Department of Agriculture, the Department of the Interior, and the Council on Environmental Quality jointly wrote to congressional leaders to identify certain principles that might help guide legislative and other actions: Broadly protect the nation's waters; make the definition of covered waters predictable and manageable; promote consistency between CWA and agricultural wetlands programs; and recognize long-standing practices, such as exemptions now in effect only through regulations or guidance.[79] A modified version of legislation from the previous Congress was introduced in the Senate (S. 787, the Clean Water Restoration Act), and in June 2009, the Senate Environment and Public Works approved it with an amendment in the nature of a full substitute to the bill as introduced. As approved by the committee, S. 787 would have deleted "navigable waters" from the CWA and use "waters of the United States" directly to define jurisdiction. It defined "waters of the United States" by a rewritten version of the regulatory definition in use by EPA and the Corps—

> The term "waters of the United States" means all waters subject to the ebb and flow of the tide, the territorial seas, and all interstate and intrastate waters including lakes, rivers, streams (including intermittent streams), mudflats, sandflats, wetlands, sloughs, prairie potholes, wet meadows, playa lakes, and natural ponds, all tributaries of any of the above waters, and all impoundments of the foregoing.

In response to prior criticism, the definition did not encompass *activities* that affect waters of the United States (see above). The bill as reported also instructed that "waters of the United States" be construed consistently with (1) how EPA and the Corps interpreted and applied "waters of the United States prior to January 9, 2001, the day before *SWANCC* was decided, and (2) Congress's constitutional authority. The bill would have excluded, as in current EPA-Corps regulations, prior converted cropland and waste treatment systems. It also included a savings section that referenced without paraphrasing eight provisions in CWA §§402(l) and 404(f) which exempt certain types of discharges from CWA permits, such as discharges from normal farming activities, and discharges from maintenance of drainage ditches. The full Senate did not take up the bill.[80] Legislation similar to the bills in the 111th Congress was not re-introduced in the 112th Congress or so far in the 113th Congress, while, as described above, bills have been introduced to block EPA and the Corps from issuing revised "waters of the United States" guidance, as well as other bills to narrow the statutory definition of waters that are subject to CWA jurisdiction. In light of the widely differing views of proponents and opponents, future prospects for legislation on the geographic scope of CWA jurisdiction are highly uncertain. One difficulty of legislating changes to the CWA in order to specify which waters and wetlands are subject to the act's jurisdiction results from the fact that the complex scientific questions about such areas are not easily amenable to precise resolution in law. Debates over whether and how to revise the act highlight the challenges of trying to use the law to do so.

APPENDIX. WHICH *RAPANOS* TEST GOVERNS?

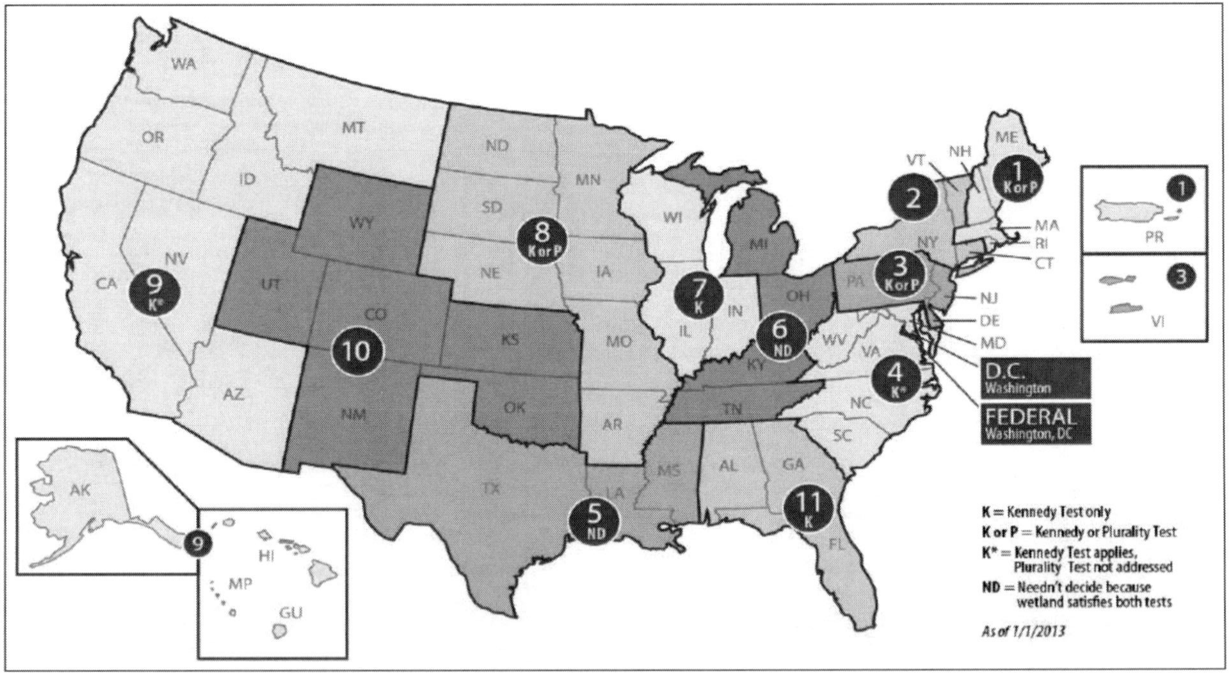

Source: Compiled by CRS.

Notes: The 13 Federal Judicial Circuits (See 28 U.S.C.A. §28).

Figure A-1.Which *Rapanos* Test Governs? Rulings of Federal Circuit Courts of Appeal Only.

End Notes

[1] 547 U.S. 715 (2006).
[2] 33 U.S.C. §§1251-1387.
[3] See in particular two precursors of the CWA: Rivers and Harbors Act of 1899 §§10 (33 U.S.C. §403), and 13 (33 U.S.C. §407). Section 13 covers tributaries of navigable waters as well.
[4] William H. Rodgers, Jr., Handbook on Environmental Law 401 (1977) (footnotes omitted).
[5] P.L. 92-500. To be precise, the 1972 enactment was titled the Federal Water Pollution Control Act Amendments of 1972. It was only after the 1977 amendments thereto that the act as a whole became known as the Clean Water Act.
[6] CWA §502(7), 33 U.S.C. §1362(7).
[7] Conference report S.Rept. 92-1236 at 144, *reprinted in* 1972 U.S. Code Cong. & Admin. News 3776, 3822.
[8] 33 U.S.C. §1344.
[9] Section 301(a), 33 U.S.C. §1311(a), prohibits the discharge of any pollutant into navigable waters, except in compliance with various CWA sections, including Section 404.
[10] NRDC v. Callaway, 392 F. Supp. 685 (D.D.C. 1975).
[11] 40 Fed. Reg. 31320 (July 25, 1975), amending 33 C.F.R. part 209.
[12] 474 U.S. 121 (1985).
[13] 33 C.F.R. §328.3(a)(7). An identical EPA definition is at 40 C.F.R. §230.3(s)(7).
[14] 531 U.S. 159 (2001).
[15] 33 C.F.R. §328.3(a)(3). An identical EPA definition is at 40 C.F.R. §230.3(s)(3).
[16] 33 C.F.R. §328.3(a)(3).
[17] *Id.* (emphasis added).
[18] In *SWANCC* dictum, the Court stated: "In order to rule for the [Corps of Engineers], we would have to hold that the jurisdiction of the Corps extends to ponds that are *not* adjacent to open water. But we conclude that the text of the statute will not allow this." 531 U.S. at 168 (emphasis in original).
[19] The agencies did consider initiating a rulemaking to consider "issues associated with the scope of waters that are subject to the Clean Water Act" in light of *SWANCC*, 68 *Fed. Reg.* 1991 (2003), but the effort was abandoned in December 2003.
[20] *SWANCC*, 531 U.S. at 167.
[21] Corps of Engineers regulations define the word "adjacent" in "adjacent wetlands" to mean "bordering, contiguous, or neighboring. Wetlands separated from other waters of the United States by man-made dikes or barriers ... are 'adjacent wetlands.'" 33 C.F.R. §328.3(c).
[22] In addition to these three major opinions, Chief Justice Roberts wrote a brief opinion concurring with the plurality, and Justice Breyer wrote a brief opinion concurring with the dissenters.
[23] 547 U.S. at 722.
[24] *Id.* at 726.
[25] *Id.* at 732-733.
[26] *Id.* at 733-734.
[27] Hydrological connection is the test that the Corps has used to demonstrate significant nexus.
[28] Soon after *Rapanos* was decided, a federal district court commented that Justice Kennedy's opinion "advanced an ambiguous test—whether a 'significant nexus' exists to waters that are/were/might be navigable.... This test leaves no guidance on how to implement its vague, subjective centerpiece." United States v. Chevron Pipe Line Co., 437 F. Supp. 2d 605 (N.D. Tex. 2006).

[29] 547 U.S. at 780.

[30] *Id.*

[31] Going back to the CWA's enactment in 1972, several of the federal circuits have addressed issues as the scope of CWA jurisdiction—that is, the scope of "waters of the United States"—on ten or more occasions. See Marjorie A. Shields, *What Are "Navigable Waters Subject to Federal Water Pollution Control Act*," 160 A.L.R. Fed. 585 (updated weekly).

[32] United States v. Robison, 505 F.3d 1208 (11th Cir. 2007), *cert. denied*, 129 S. Ct. 627 (2008); United States v. Gerke Excavating, Inc., 464 F.3d 723 (7th Cir. 2006), *cert. denied*, 552 U.S. 810 (2007);

[33] Northern California River Watch v. Wilcox, 2011 Westlaw 238292, *1 (9th Cir. Jan. 26, 2011), *clarifying* Northern California River Watch v. City of Healdsburg, 496 F.3d 993 (9th Cir. 2007), *cert. denied*, 552 U.S. 1180 (2008); Precon Development Corp. v. U.S. Army Corps of Engineers, 2011 Westlaw 213052 (4th Cir. Jan. 25, 2011).

[34] United States v. Donovan, 661 F.3d 174 (3d Cir. 2011), *cert. denied*, 132 S. Ct. 2409 (2012); United States v. Bailey, 571 F.3d 791 (8th Cir. 2009); United States v. Johnson, 467 F.3d 56 (1st Cir. 2006), *cert. denied*, 552 U.S. 948 (2007).

[35] United States v. Cundiff, 555 F.3d 200 (6th Cir.), *cert. denied*, 130 S. Ct. 74 (2009); United States v. Lucas, 516 F.3d 316 (5th Cir.), *cert. denied*, 129 S. Ct. 116 (2008).

[36] See, e.g., United States v. Evans, 2006 Westlaw 2221629 (M.D. Fla. 2006) (Kennedy test or plurality test); Environmental Protection Information Center v. Pacific Lumber Co., 469 F. Supp. 2d 803 (S.D. Cal. 2007) (bound by *City of Healdsburg* to apply Kennedy test only); Simsbury-Avon Preservation Soc'y, LLC v. Metacon Gun Club, Inc., 472 F. Supp. 2d 219 (D. Conn. 2007) (Kennedy test or plurality test).

[37] One reported decision took its cue from the Scalia plurality view, though principally relying on circuit precedent. United States v. Chevron Pipe Line Co., 437 F. Supp. 2d 605 (N.D. Tex. 2006). This decision actually involved the amendments to the CWA made by the Oil Pollution Act, which uses the same definition of "waters of the United States" as CWA Section 404. A second decision holds that the significant nexus test is inapplicable outside the isolated wetlands context (with the implication that the plurality test alone applies). Sierra Club v. City and County of Honolulu, 2008 Westlaw 3850495, *7 (D. Hawaii August 18, 2008).

[38] Cruden, John C., Deputy Assistant Attorney General, Environment and Natural Resources Division, U.S. Department of Justice, "Statement Concerning Recent Supreme Court Decisions Dealing with the Clean Water Act," before the Subcommittee on Fisheries, Wildlife and Water, U.S. Senate Committee on Environment and Public Works, August 1, 2006, p. 16.

[39] See opinions of Justice Kennedy, Justice Breyer, and Chief Justice Roberts.

[40] U.S. Environmental Protection Agency, U.S. Army Corps of Engineers, "Clean Water Act Jurisdiction Following the U.S. Supreme Court's Decision in *Rapanos v. United States & Carabell v. United States*," December 2, 2008, p. 3.

[41] 547 U.S. at 738.

[42] "Clean Water Jurisdiction Following the Supreme Court's Decision in Rapanos v. United States and Carabell v. United States," Dec. 2, 2008, see http://water.epa.gov/lawsregs /guidance/wetlands/CWAwaters.cfm, under "Previous EPA Statements on Waters of the US." This webpage contains the 2008 guidance and the 2007 guidance, now superseded. It also includes a legal memorandum issued in January 2003 that continues to govern the agencies' interpretation of jurisdiction over the "isolated waters" addressed in the Supreme Court's 2001 *SWANCC* ruling.

[43] "Questions and Answers Regarding the Revised *Rapanos & Carabell* Guidance, December 2, 2008," p. 3, http://water.epa.gov/lawsregs/guidance/wetlands/upload/2008_12_5_wetlands_Rapanos_-20Guidance_QA20120208.pdf.

[44] These include all waters described in 33 C.F.R. §328.3(a)(1) (Corps of Engineers) and 40 C.F.R. §230.3(s)(1) (EPA). The 2008 guidance provides clarification of the scope of traditional navigable waters and guidance to field staff on making such a determination.

[45] The Corps has eight U.S. Divisions (which generally follow watershed boundaries), further subdivided into 38 Districts.

[46] U.S. General Accounting Office (now Government Accountability Office), "Waters and Wetlands, Corps of Engineers Needs to Evaluate Its District Office Practices in Determining Jurisdiction," February 2004, GAO-04-297.

[47] 547 U.S. at 775 (2006).

[48] American Rivers, "Bush Administration's So-called Revised Guidance on Clean Water is Just More of the Same," press release, December 3, 2008.

[49] Memorandum from Granta Nakayama, EPA Ass't Administrator for Enforcement and Compliance Assurance, to Benjamin Grumbles, EPA Ass't Administrator for Water, "OECA's Comments on the June 6, 2007 Memo, *Clean Water Act Jurisdiction Following the U.S. Supreme Court's Decision in Rapanos v. United States and Carabell v. United States*," dated March 4, 2008, on file with authors. EPA informs us that the "June 6, 2007 Memo" is the same as the June 2007 guidance referred to in footnote 42.

[50] Jeff Kinney, "Clean Water Act Jurisdictional Decisions Slower, More Complex, Amy Corps Says," *Daily Environment Report*, May 20, 2008, p. A-3.

[51] "Decline of Clean Water Act Enforcement Program," Majority Staff Memorandum to Representative Henry Waxman, Chairman, House Committee on Oversight and Government Reform, and Representative James L. Oberstar, Chairman, House Committee on Transportation and Infrastructure, December 16, 2008, 21 p., on file with authors.

[52] Environmental Protection Agency and Department of Defense, "EPA and Army Corps of Engineers Guidance Regarding Identification of Waters Protected by the Clean Water Act," 76 *Federal Register* 24479, May 2, 2011.

[53] See note 39 and accompanying text.

[54] Environmental Protection Agency and Army Corps of Engineers, "Draft Guidance on Identifying Waters Protected by the Clean Water Act," April 27, 2011, p. 2, on file with authors.

[55] *Id.* at 3.

[56] Stream order is a measure of the relative size of streams and is a method for stream classification based on relative position within a river network. Stream sizes range from the smallest, first-order, to the largest, the twelfth-order (e.g., the Amazon River). Headwater streams (first- and second-order) are the most abundant stream type in most river networks, and they supply most of the water in rivers. See http://www.cotf.edu/ete/modules wqphysmethods.html.

[57] "Other waters" are waters that are geographically separated in that they do not have a hydrological connection to jurisdictional waters. Jurisdiction previously was asserted under Corps regulations (33 CFR §328.3(a)(3)) which provide for CWA jurisdiction over "[a]ll other waters ... the use, degradation or destruction of which could affect interstate or foreign commerce...." Geographically isolated, non-navigable intrastate waters were at issue in *SWANCC*.

[58] U.S. Environmental Protection Agency, "Potential Indirect Economic Impacts and Benefits Associated with Guidance Clarifying the Scope of Clean Water Act Jurisdiction," April 27, 2011, on file with authors.

[59] Inside E.P.A., "EPA's Draft Guidance Seeks To 'Increase Significantly' Water Act's Scope," February 17, 2011.

[60] Letter from Honorable Benjamin L. Cardin et al. to President Barack Obama, March 31, 2011, on file with authors.

[61] Letter from Honorable Bob Gibbs et al. to Lisa P. Jackson, EPA Administrator, and Jo-Ellen Darcy, Assistant Secretary of the Army for Civil Works, April 14, 2011; and Letter from Honorable John Barrasso et al. to Lisa P. Jackson, EPA Administrator, May 27, 2011, on file with authors.

[62] 16 U.S.C. §1536.

[63] "EPA Eyes Guide to Clarify Water Act's Scope for Discharge Permits," *Inside EPA*, Vol. 29, no. 10, March 7, 2008.

[64] Scott G. Leibowitz, "Isolated Wetlands and Their Functions: An Ecological Perspective," *Wetlands*, vol. 23, no. 3, September 2003, pp. 517-531.

[65] See, e.g., U.S. Congress, House of Representatives, Committee on Transportation and Infrastructure, Subcommittee on Water Resources and Environment, "Inconsistent Regulation of Wetlands and Other Waters," Hearing, 108th Congress, 2d Session, March 30, 2004 (H.Hrg. 108-58), 200 p.

[66] Jon Kusler, The Association of State Wetland Managers, "'Waters of the U.S.' After SWANCC," August 12, 2005 (draft), p. 6.

[67] Jon Kusler, The Association of State Wetland Managers, "The SWANCC Decision: State Regulation of Wetlands to Fill the Gap," March 2004, pp. 6-8. Hereafter, Kusler.

[68] Benjamin H. Grumbles, Assistant Administrator for Water, EPA, letter to Ms. Jeanne Christie, Association of State Wetland Managers, January 9, 2005 (sic), p. 3. The letter was written in January 2006, not 2005.

[69] American Rivers and Sierra Club, "Where Rivers Are Born: The Scientific Imperative for Defending Small Streams and Wetlands," February 2007, p. 7.

[70] Benjamin H. Grumbles, Assistant Administrator for Water, EPA, and John Paul Woodley, Assistant Secretary of the Army for Civil Works, Department of the Army, Statement before the Subcommittee on Fisheries, Wildlife, and Water of the U.S. Senate Committee on Environment and Public Works, August 1, 2006, 109th Congress, 2d session.

[71] James Murphy, "*Rapanos v. United States*: Wading Through Murky Waters," *National Wetlands Newsletter*, vol. 28, no. 5, September-October 2006, p. 19.

[72] U.S. Environmental Protection Agency, Office of Research and Development, *Connectivity of Streams and Wetlands to Downstream Waters: A Review and Synthesis of the Scientific Evidence*, External Review Draft, EPA/600/R-11- 098B, September 2013, http://yosemite.epa.gov/sab/sabproduct.nsf/0/7724357376745F48852579E60043E88C/$File / WOUS_ERD2_Sep2013.pdf.

[73] See U.S. Environmental Protection Agency, "Clean Water Act Definition of 'Waters of the United States,'" http://water

[74] Amena H. Saiyid, "EPA Study Could Be Used to Expand Reach of Law Over Waters, Wetlands," *Daily Environment Report*, September 27, 2013, pp. BB-1.

[75] U.S. Environmental Protection Agency, "Advance Notice of Proposed Rulemaking on the Clean Water Act Regulatory Definition of 'Waters of the United States,'" 68 *Federal Register* 1994-95, January 15, 2003.

[76] Kusler, p. 15.

[77] Jan Goldman-Carter, "Isolated Wetland Legislation: Running the Rapids at the State Capitol," *National Wetlands Newsletter*, May-June 2005, pp. 27-29.

[78] Turner Odell, "On Soggy Ground—State Protection for Isolated Wetlands," *National Wetlands Newsletter,* September-October 2003, p. 10.

[79] See http://epw.senate.gov/public/index.cfm?FuseAction=Majority.PressReleases&ContentRecord_id=64739ae3- 802a-23ad-4c30-36fc58cc1014&Region_id=&Issue_id=.

[80] The committee report on the bill, S.Rept. 111-361, was filed in December 2010, 18 months after the committee's action to approve the amended legislation. Companion legislation was introduced in the House in the 111th Congress (H.R. 5088), but no further action occurred.

INDEX

D

E

F

G

H

I

J

K

L

M

Q

R

S

T

U

V

W